UNIVERSI
LIBRAF

Burn Trauma
Management and Nursing Care

CORNWALL COLLEGE
LIBRARY

SWNHS

C20100804

Burn Trauma

Management and Nursing Care

Second Edition

Edited By

Chrissie Bosworth Bousfield

MSc, BSc (Hons), PGDip Ad Ed, RGN
Health Lecturer, School of Nursing, Faculty of Medicine
and Health Sciences,
University of Nottingham and
Clinical Nurse Specialist, Burns and Tissue Viability
The Harley Street Clinic, London

W
WHURR PUBLISHERS
LONDON AND PHILADELPHIA

© 2002 Whurr Publishers

First published 2002 by
Whurr Publishers Ltd
19b Compton Terrace, London N1 2UN, England
325 Chestnut Street, Philadelphia PA19106, USA

All rights reserved. No part of this publication may be reproduced, stored in a retrieval system, or transmitted in any form or by any means, electronic, mechanical, photcopying, recording or otherwise, without the prior permission of Whurr Publishers Limited.

This publication is sold subject to the conditions that it shall not, by way of trade or otherwise, be lent, resold, hired out, or otherwise circulated without the Publisher's prior consent, in any form of binding or cover other than that in which it is published, and without a similar condition including this condition being imposed upon any subsequent purchaser.

British Library Cataloguing in Publication Data

A catalogue record for this book is available from the British Library.

ISBN 1 86156 240 3

Printed and bound in the UK by Athenaeum Press Limited, Gateshead, Tyne & Wear.

Contents

Contributors

David Anderton, BSc, SRD, Senior Dietitian, City Hospital NHS Trust, Nottingham.

Fiona Bailie, MB, BCh, BAO, FRCS (Ed), formerly Consultant in Burns and Plastic Surgery, Department of Plastic, Reconstructive and Burns Surgery, City Hospital NHS Trust, Nottingham.

Deborah Beeby, BSc (Hons), Dip Health Studies, RGN, RSCN, Staff Nurse, Childrens Unit, Ipswich Hospital, Ipswich.

Jill Blunt, BSc (Hons), RGN, Sister, Pain Services, formerly Clinical Leader, Burns Unit, City Hospital NHS Trust, Nottingham.

Chrissie Bousfield, MSc, BSc (Hons), PGDipAdEd, RGN, Health Lecturer, School of Nursing, Faculty of Medicine and Health Sciences, University of Nottingham, and Clinical Nurse Specialist Burns and Tissue Viability, Harley Street Clinic, London.

Deborah Cook, MSc, BSc (Hons), RNT, RGN, Emergency Nurse Practitioner, Acute Medicine, City Hospital NHS Trust, Nottingham.

Nicole Glassey, MCSP, Senior Physiotherapist, Department of Plastic, Reconstructive and Burns Surgery, City Hospital NHS Trust, Nottingham.

Rosemary Gollop, DipCot, SROT, Senior Occupational Therapist, Department of Plastic, Reconstructive and Burns Surgery, City Hospital NHS Trust, Nottingham.

Lynn Hubbard, BSc, SRD, Senior Dietitian, Selly Oak Hospital, Birmingham.

Owen Jones, RNMH, RGN, DipNursing (Child), Unit Manager, Burns Unit, City Hospital NHS Trust, Nottingham.

David Knights, BMedSci, BM, BS, FRCS, Consultant Burns Anaesthetist, City Hospital NHS Trust, Nottingham.

Sarah Pankhurst, BSc (Hons), RGN, Clinical Nurse Specialist – Tissue Viability, Wollaton Vale Health Centre, Nottingham.

Tinaz Pochkhanawala, RGN, Clinical Leader, Burns Unit, City Hospital NHS Trust, Nottingham.

Stephen Regel, MA, PGCE, Cert Behav Psych, RN, Senior Lecturer in Trauma Studies, Nottingham Trent University, Nottingham.

David Wilson, MB, BS, FRCS (Plast), Consultant in Burns and Plastic Surgery, Department of Plastic, Reconstructive and Burns Surgery, City Hospital NHS Trust, Nottingham.

Preface

Burn injuries, a unique form of trauma, are in many respects the worst injuries an individual can experience (Wachtel et al., 1983). The management of care for an individual following burn trauma is a specialized area that requires a wealth of knowledge and a wide range of clinical skills from the members of a large multidisciplinary team.

The burn patient, during the course of the resulting injury, undergoes a variety of physical and psychological changes, and in order for members of the multidisciplinary team effectively to treat the patient and support the family, it is essential to have a clear understanding of the pathophysiological effects and the management required at each stage of recovery.

This book has been written as a resource for all grades of staff within the multidisciplinary team caring for patients of all ages with different types of burn injury, in a variety of clinical environments. Its aim is to increase the reader's understanding of the effects of burn trauma on the individual, and it outlines the management of care that will be required during the course of hospitalization. It should also prove to be an additional resource for those nurses undertaking diploma- or degree-level nurse education programmes and/or continuing professional development relating to the speciality of burn care.

Selected members of the multidisciplinary team with expertise in their clinical fields have contributed chapters providing a wide range of information using a research-based evidence approach and up-to-date references to ensure that patients receive the high standards of care they deserve. I would like to acknowledge and thank all of the contributing authors who have shared their knowledge and clinical expertise.

Finally, I dedicate this book to all the nurses who care for individuals who have sustained a burn injury, and especially to the burn patients themselves, facing the challenge of recovery from what must be a devastating experience in their lives.

Chrissie Bousfield

Reference

Wachtel TL, Kahn V, Frank HA (1983) Rehabilitation of the burn injured patient. Current Topics in Burn Care. Rockville, MD: Aspen Systems Corporation. pp 217–20.

Acknowledgements

Grateful thanks are extended to the Photographic Department and to John Houghton, Clinical Leader, Burns Unit, at the City Hospital NHS Trust, Nottingham, for their assistance in producing the illustrations in Chapters 9, 11 and 13.

Introduction

CHRISSIE BOUSFIELD

History of Burn Care

Ever since our ancestors discovered fire, man has knowingly risked his life to reap its benefits. This has inevitably led to accidental burn injuries, and many have paid the price of discovery with suffering, scarring and death (Kemble and Lamb, 1987).

In the writings of ancient Egypt and Greece (1600 BC), there are records of treating burns with oil-soaked cloths made from animal fat (Bryan, 1930). This may be considered as the ancient counterpart of the modern paraffin gauze dressing, which is still often used today. The Roman Empire (1st century AD) emphasized the use of herbs for wound therapy and even then practised surgical excision of contracted burn scars (Schumann, 1991).

There have been other major historical developments in the care of burns. In 1607, Hilanus described the three degrees of a burn, and in the 1800s Guillaume Dupuytren described six depths of burn injury. In 1897, the first saline solution infusions were given by Tommasoli in Sicily for fluid replacement in major burns, and in 1905, Wiedenfeld and Zumbush performed early wound excision within the first three days of a burn injury occurring (Haynes, 1987).

Underhill and associates in 1921 conducted a research study which demonstrated that burns shock was primarily a result of fluid loss during the initial burn period. Much of their research laid the foundation for modern fluid and electrolyte therapy, and served as a basis for further study into the pathophysiology of burns (Underhill et al., 1923).

The advent of skin grafting started with the techniques of the Swiss surgeon Reverdin, who performed the first epithelial graft in 1869 (Haynes, 1987), laying the foundation for modern split-thickness skin grafting (Schumann, 1991). However, the dermatome was not introduced until 1939 (Archambeault-Jones and Feller, 1981), and then prompted a move towards early wound closure and reduced mortality.

In 1954, Leidberg, Reis and Artz discovered that septicaemia was a common cause of death in individuals following burn trauma (Leidberg et al., 1954) and this led to vigorous research on topical antimicrobial agents, which still continues today. Since then, advances in burn therapy have escalated dramatically. Half a century ago, an individual who had sustained burn trauma was one of the most neglected in surgery. Now, in specialized Burns Units, the patient is the object of keen competitive multidisciplinary care (Marvin, 1991).

The history of burn care would not be complete without mentioning Boston's Cocoanut Grove fire disaster of 1942, in which 492 lives were lost and hundreds of individuals were treated for burn injuries. This created a public movement for changes in building codes, building designs and standards of fire protection and prevention efforts, which are still prevalent today.

Burn Prevention/Health Promotion

Burn prevention efforts have traditionally been directed at public education, and, despite numerous campaigns at international, national and local level, burn injuries continue to be a considerable health hazard for many people worldwide (Linares and Linares, 1990).

Many burn prevention campaigns are aimed at public education and increased awareness of burn safety, with behaviour modification as the ultimate goal. Some worldwide education programmes undoubtedly have been successful in lowering burn injury rates and have been reported by Waller (1985), Herd et al. (1986) and Keswani (1986).

However, these few successes notwithstanding, it is evident that after years of public education efforts, education alone has seldom resulted in a marked decrease in burn injuries. One important concept to consider is the attenuation effect that occurs normally from the implementation of an educational programme on prevention (McLoughlin et al., 1982).

Many research findings have documented the striking limitations of health education alone in motivating people to change their behaviour, and acknowledge that an increase in knowledge and awareness does not necessarily lead to a change in behaviour or lifestyle. Why then does health education have such little impact? The Health Belief Model formulated by Rosenstock (1974) and later modified by Becker et al. (1974) helps to explain why some people follow recommended prevention measures while others do not. The Health Belief Model assumes that individuals are likely to take a health preventative action if, first, they believe they are susceptible to the injury, or that the injury could have serious effects on their life, second, they are aware of actions that can be taken and believe these actions may reduce the likelihood or severity of the injury, and, third, they believe that the threat to them of taking such action(s) is not as great as the injury itself.

An individual's subjective perception of contracting or encountering a specific health problem has been shown to be a strong indicator of taking preventative health actions (Janz and Becker, 1984). Thus, in the long term, increasing a person's perceived susceptibility to a burn injury may potentially lead to a change in behaviour, and when planning educational programmes directed at burn prevention, one may need to take motivational variables into account.

Motivation to change behaviour or to take a health action may be prompted by increasing an individual's perceived threat of a burn injury. For example, people may know it is dangerous to store flammable liquids in the garage, but if they do not perceive themselves or their family to be at risk or do not believe that a fire or explosion may result, they will, out of habit or a sense of 'it will not happen to me', continue with the practice. Therefore, it is important to modify an individual's perceived susceptibility to the injury (Linares and Linares, 1990).

We can no longer afford to implement educational programmes that simply have as their major goal an increase in knowledge and awareness. A more successful approach to reducing the occurrence of burn injuries is likely to be one that combines education and legislation to achieve behaviour change, environmental control and product modification. Burn prevention campaigns should aim to increase motivation to change behaviour by raising perceived susceptibility to burn injury, to produce more pressure from the public for manufacturers to develop safer products, and to press for legislation for more effective environmental controls (Linares and Linares, 1990).

The approach to burn prevention must be based on a solid knowledge of the aetiology of burn injuries, taking into account geographic variations and socio-economic backgrounds. Prevention methods must also be accepted in response to current and changing causation factors.

Legislation, standards and regulations already exist which are pertinent to burn prevention together with organizations concerned with fire safety. British Standards are subject to regular scrutiny and revision. Leaflets and booklets on legal aspects of safety are obtainable from the Department of Trade and Industry and the Consumer Safety Act of 1987 makes it a criminal offence to supply unsafe consumer goods in the United Kingdom. Burn prevention is an educational matter (Linares and Linares, 1990): however, it is uncertain how and by whom education is best implemented. The Royal Society for Prevention of Accidents and the Child Accident Prevention Trust encompass the extensive field of accident prevention and produce regular reports and statistics. Media publicity is often used to support prevention campaigns but this is difficult to organize and is costly (Lawrence, 1996).

Modification of products or environmental control can successfully reduce the incidence of certain burn injuries; for example, the Child and Young Persons Act (1914) makes it an offence if a child suffers a burn when there is no fireguard present. The Heating Appliances Act (1945/1971) and the Fireguards Act (1952) makes it an offence to offer for sale new gas or electric fires not fitted with a fireguard to safety standard of BSI specification BS1945 (1971). The Night-dresses for Children Act (1962) makes it illegal to offer for sale children's night-dresses that are not flame resistant to BSI specifications BS3121 (1967) and BS5722 (1979) (Leveridge, 1991). However, there is still no legislation relating to children's pyjamas.

Product modification is also evident in the introduction of coiled kettle flexes designed to reduce the incidence of scald injuries caused by children pulling trailing electric flexes attached to kettles.

Modification of the environment, such as decreasing the hot water temperature to 130°F (54.4°C) or below, effectively lowers the risk of scald injuries, as it increases the exposure time for a full thickness burn to occur (Feldman et al., 1978). Environmental control through the installation of smoke detectors should also effectively decrease housefire-related deaths.

Implementation of preventative measures need not rely purely on legislation: the publicity relating to firework hazards associated with annual November 5th activities, together with the voluntary code of practice agreed with firework manufacturers has resulted in a decline of such accidents. Organized public displays and the increased cost of fireworks are other contributory factors (Lawrence, 1996).

Passive manoeuvres that protect the public through product modification, environmental redesign or control and legislation are generally more effective in preventing injuries than are active measures that depend on persistent long-term behavioural or lifestyle change. However, future efforts aimed at public education and promotion of legislation should continue, with the support of responsible authorities who understand the problems and authorize adequate funds to support them (Linares and Linares, 1990).

Health promotion appears to lend itself well to the domains of burn care, and in essence the burn is just the beginning. Health promotion is a positive team approach, and nurses and other members of the multidisciplinary team are in a unique position that allows them to assist individuals in promoting, protecting and maintaining their health care status during the course of recovery and rehabilitation.

The Burns Team

The management of care for an individual following burn trauma has changed dramatically over the past twenty years, leading to decreased morbidity and improved survival, function and cosmetic results in the long term (Marvin, 1991). These changes have been accomplished by the dedication of a wide range of professionals working together as a multidisciplinary Burns team.

Teamwork is an essential part of the management of the burn patient (Leveridge, 1991), and has proved to be effective in dealing with even the most complex patient scenario. Although each member of the team – nurse, surgeon, anaesthetist, physiotherapist, occupational therapist, dietitian and psychologist – has a specific role, many of the roles overlap and require a coordination of activities to promote high-quality care and successful patient outcomes.

The nurse provides critical care, wound care and rehabilitation, promoting the return to activities of daily living. The role also involves giving emotional support to both the patient and the family, together with coordinating multidisciplinary team activities. The surgeon provides comprehensive medical/surgical care that promotes wound healing, while the anaesthetist directs anaesthesia for operative and major wound care procedures and coordinates the management of patients with inhalation burn injuries. The roles of the physiotherapist and occupational therapist are to assist patients in regaining optimal physical function, and the dietitian is responsible for providing nutritional advice and support. The psychologist aims to improve patients' psychological and psycho-social well-being, as well as providing emotional support for the family and, additionally, members of the multidisciplinary team.

It is therefore evident that the management of care for an individual following a burn injury requires a unique body of knowledge and skills from a range of multidisciplinary team members, and encompasses a wide variety of roles and responsibilities.

To this end, the following chapters seek to provide a comprehensive text for a variety of professionals in different clinical settings, whether it is the Accident and Emergency department, the Intensive Care Unit or the Burns Unit itself. The contents aim to outline burn trauma, methods of treatment and the overall management of care provided by members of the multidisciplinary team, while reflecting the philosophical foundation 'to provide and maintain high standards of care in an individual and family-centred environment'.

References

Archambeault-Jones CA, Feller I (1981) Burn care. Cited in Kinney MR et al. (1981) ACCN's Clinical Reference for Critical Care Nursing. New York: McGraw-Hill. pp 741–42.

Becker MH, Drachman RH, Kirscht JP (1974) A new approach to explaining sick role behaviour in low income populations. American Journal of Public Health 6: 205.

Bryan CP (1930) Ancient Egyptian Medicine. The Papyrus. Ares, London: Ebers.

Feldman KW, Schaller TS, Feldman JA et al. (1978) Tap water scald burns in children. Paediatrics 62: 1.

Haynes BW (1987) The history of burn care. Cited in Beswick JA, The Art and Science of Burn Care. Rockville, MD: Aspen. pp 3–7.

Herd AN, Widdowson P, Tanner NSB (1986) Scalds in the very young – prevention or cure? Burns Journal 12: 246.

Janz NK, Becker MH (1984) The health belief model – a decade later. Health Education 11: 1.

Kemble JVH, Lamb BE (1987) Practical Burns Management. London: Hodder and Stoughton.

Keswani MH (1986) The prevention of burn injury. Burns Journal 12: 533.

Lawrence JC (1996) Burns and scalds: aetiology and prevention. Cited in Settle JAD, (Ed) Principles and Practice of Burns Management. Edinburgh: Churchill Livingstone.

Leidberg NC, Reiss E, Artz CP (1954) Infection in burns, III. Septicaemia, a common cause of death. Surgery, Gynaecology and Obstetrics 99: 151.

Leveridge A (1991) Therapy for the Burns Patient. London: Chapman and Hall.

Linares AZ, Linares HA (1990) Burn prevention – the need for a comprehensive approach. Burns Journal 16: 281–85.

McLoughlin E, Vince C, Lee AM et al. (1982) Project burn prevention: outcome and implications. American Journal of Public Health 72: 241.

Marvin J (1991) Cited in Trofino RB, Care of the Burn Injured Patient. Philadelphia: FA Davis.

Rosenstock IM (1974) Historical origins of the health belief model. Health Education Monograph 2: 328.

Schumann L (1991) History of burn care. Cited in Trofino RB, Care of the Burn Injured Patient. Philadelphia: FA Davis. pp 3–7.

Underhill EP et al. (1923) Blood concentration changes in extensive superficial burns and their significance for systemic treatment. Archives of International Medicine 32: 31.

Waller JA (1985) Injury Control – a Guide to the Causes and Prevention of Burn Trauma. Lexington, MA: Lexington Books. pp 318–19.

CHAPTER 1

Pathophysiology of Burns

DEBORAH COOK

Burn trauma represents a major injury in terms of the physical and psychological damage to the individual. For the members of the multidisciplinary team to effectively treat the patient and support the family, an understanding of the pathophysiology of burn trauma is essential.

This chapter discusses the normal anatomy of the skin and the physiological responses that occur as a result of a burn injury.

Normal Anatomy of Skin

Structurally the skin consists of two principal parts: the outer, thinner epithelium called the epidermis and the inner, thicker connective tissue part called the dermis. Beneath the dermis is a subcutaneous layer which consists of areolar and adipose tissue (Figure 1.1).

The epidermis is organized into four or five cell layers, depending on its location in the body. Where exposure to friction is greatest, such as the palms and soles, the epidermis has five layers. In all other parts it has four layers. The basement layer of cells divides and gradually sheds towards the surface. The cells lose their nuclei to become the dead horny keratin surface layer. A cell migrates from the basement membrane to the keratin layer in about 19 days. Passing through the epidermis are the hairs, secretions from the sebaceous glands and the ducts of the sweat glands.

The dermis is composed of connective tissue containing collagenous and elastic fibres. The dermis is very thick in the palms and soles and very thin in the eyelids, penis and scrotum. It also tends to be thicker on the dorsal aspects of the body than the ventral, and thicker on the lateral aspects of extremities than medial aspects. Numerous blood vessels, lymphatics, nerves, glands and hair follicles are embedded in the dermis.

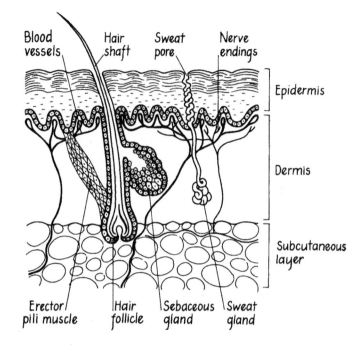

Figure 1.1 Anatomy of the skin.

The sweat glands, sebaceous glands and hair follicles are derived from the epidermis, growing down into it during embryonic development.

The combination of collagenous and elastic fibres in the dermis provides the skin with strength, extendibility and elasticity. The ability of the skin to stretch can readily been seen in pregnancy, obesity and oedema. The dermis is attached to underlying organs, such as bone and muscles, by the subcutaneous layer. Beneath the dermis is a plexus of capillaries and the subdermal layer of fat.

Functions of Skin

For the average adult, the skin occupies a surface area of approximately 1.8m². The skin is quite complex in structure and serves several functions essential for survival.

Maintenance of Body Temperature

The body temperature is normally maintained at an average of 36.8°C. If the temperature is raised, metabolism increases and if it is lowered, metabolism decreases. The skin helps to ensure a fine balance is maintained between heat produced by the body and heat lost to the environment, 97% of heat lost from the body being via the skin.

The amount of heat lost from the skin depends to a great extent on the amount of blood in the vessels in the dermis. As the amount of heat produced by the body increases the arterioles become dilated and more blood pours into the capillary network in the skin. In addition to increasing the amount of sweat produced, the temperature of the skin rises. When this happens heat is lost through the following processes:

Radiation – exposed parts of the body allow heat to radiate away into the environment (provided the air temperature is below surface body temperature).

Conduction – the clothes in contact with the body carry heat away.

Convection – the air passing over the exposed parts of the body and clothing carries heat away with the rising current.

Evaporation – sweat is discharged onto the skin surface and evaporates.

Protection

The skin protects the deeper and more delicate organs and acts as the main barrier against the invasion of micro-organisms and other harmful agents.

The sebaceous glands pour their secretion, sebum, into the hair follicles and onto the skin. Sebum provides some waterproofing, keeps the skin soft and pliable, acts as a bactericidal agent preventing the successive invasion of micro-organisms, and prevents drying, especially on exposure to heat and sunshine.

Also, melanocytes in the basement layer of skin react to ultraviolet radiation by the production of melanin pigment, which absorbs ultraviolet rays.

Perception of Stimuli

The skin contains numerous nerve endings and receptors that detect stimuli related to temperature, touch, pressure and pain. The presence of the sensory nerve endings enables the body to react by reflex action to unpleasant or painful stimuli, thus protecting itself from further injury.

Fluid and Electrolyte Balance

Intact keratin is nearly waterproof, whereas dermis denuded of epidermis is permeable. Except via glandular secretion, little or no fluid, protein or electrolytes pass through intact skin. However, copious sweating will cause loss of sodium and chloride ions as well as of water.

Synthesis of Vitamin D

Ultraviolet light from sunlight converts 7-dehydrocholesterol in the skin into vitamin D. It is used with calcium and phosphorus in the formation and maintenance of bone. Excess of requirements is stored in the liver.

Local Pathology

Burn injury to the skin deranges these functions and causes the following pathophysiological changes:

- When damage is small, such as light sunburn, capillaries in the dermis become widely dilated, resulting in redness. Some fluid loss from the capillaries into the tissues may cause a rise in interstitial tissue pressure, stimulation of nerve endings and pain.
- In a more severe burn, the fluid loss from the capillaries accumulates as blisters, either within the dermis or at the junction of dermis with epidermis. The overlying epidermal cells die and must be regenerated from adjacent epithelium.
- When a burn destroys the upper part of the dermis in addition to the epidermis, regeneration has to take place from epithelial elements in the glands and hair follicles. This can take 10 to 14 days.
- A more severe injury will destroy the dermis leaving a few epithelial remnants in glands and hair follicles only in the subdermal fat layer. Deep dermal burns will only re-epithelialize slowly, resulting in poor, thin skin.
- Destruction of all skin elements may also burn underlying muscle, bone or tendon. Such a burn will not heal without surgical intervention.

Circumferential burns may compromise blood supply to the limbs or breathing if the neck or chest are involved (see Chapter 4).

Systemic Pathophysiology

Burn injury can destroy the proteins in the exposed cells and cause cell injury or death. The injury to tissues directly or indirectly in contact with the damaging agent, such as the skin, or the linings of the respiratory and digestive tracts, is the local effect of the burn.

Generally, however, the systemic effects of a burn are a greater threat to life than the local effects. Among the systemic effects of a burn are the following:

Cardiovascular Effects

Reduction in the volume of blood in active circulation is a common denominator in shock, and the central role of hypovolaemia in burns shock was emphasized by Blacock in 1931. However, it was not until the 1940s that the magnitude of the fluid shift in burns began to be elucidated (Cope and Moore, 1947). Prior to this, it was thought that the only loss of plasma from the circulation was that which could be seen leaving the surface of the wound.

Within minutes of a burn being sustained, oedema begins to gather beneath the damaged areas, as a result of changes in capillary permeability in tissues affected, but not devitalized by heat. The development of this oedema appears to be obligatory: as yet no treatment has been found which will stop the plasma leak from the affected vessels. The amount of oedema that occurs depends partly upon the circumstances of the burn, i.e. the temperature and the time of exposure, and partly upon the elasticity and tissue tension of the part affected. Thus, in the face, where the tissues are relatively lax and easily distensible, the swelling will be great and obvious, while in places with a high tissue elasticity, such as limbs, much less swelling will occur (Muir et al., 1987).

The composition of the burn oedema is essentially that of plasma but with rather less protein. This is due to the dilutional effect of fluid drawn from the uninvolved interstitial compartment. The oedema continues to accumulate until a new balance is struck between the intravascular and extravascular compartments (Arturson, 1979).

This leakage is maximal in the first 8 hours after the burn and then gradually decreases until after 48 or 72 hours when the patient creates more fluid in their circulatory system, has a diuresis and becomes more stable (Pitt et al., 1987; Pruitt and Mason, 1971). This timing varies at either end of the age scale, being quicker to settle in younger patients, and is slower in deeper, larger burns.

In a burn of up to 30% body surface area, the leakage is around the injured area, but when it is over 30% the leakage becomes generalized. The loss of plasma from the capillaries leads to haemoconcentration, i.e. an increase in the ratio of red cells to plasma in the blood. The blood becomes more viscous, and circulation in the capillaries may be slowed or stopped. Because of poor tissue perfusion, the depth of the burn will be increased because of lack of oxygen supply to the tissues.

Without treatment the haematocrit will progressively rise; by the time one half of the plasma volume has been lost into the burn, the haematocrit will be between 60 and 70%. One third of the total blood volume will then have been lost, the signs and symptoms of severe shock will be present, and the patient's life will be in danger. Without treatment, the patient with an extensive burn (over 50% body surface area) reaches this stage within 3 to 4 hours of the accident.

The loss of this protein-rich fluid from the plasma at the site of the burn is the factor of overriding importance in the causation of the clinical condition of shock in burned patients.

Signs and symptoms of shock

The signs and symptoms of shock vary with the severity of the condition but among the characteristic signs are the following:

- Hypotension, in which the systolic blood pressure is lower than 90mmHg, due to generalized vasodilatation and decreased cardiac output.
- Cool, clammy, pale skin, due to vasoconstriction of peripheral circulation, and sweating due to sympathetic stimulation and increased levels of adrenaline.
- Reduced urine output, inadequate for effective clearance of waste products normally dealt with by the kidney, due to hypotension and increased levels of aldosterone and ADH.
- Altered mental status due to cerebral ischaemia: initially the patient may be alert and apprehensive, but as shock progresses, they become disturbed, disorientated and restless to an extreme degree; consciousness may only be lost as a pre-terminal event.
- Weak, thready pulse due to generalized vasodilatation and reduced cardiac output, with little evidence of capillary filling; tachycardia due to sympathetic stimulation and increased levels of adrenaline.
- Thirst, due to loss of extra-cellular fluid; administration of fluids by mouth usually produces vomiting.
- Breathing which at first is rapid and shallow, but later becomes gasping and is described as air hunger; the build up of lactic acid leads to acidosis.

It is essential to realize that all of these features are the result of inadequate perfusion of the body tissues. They are evidence of compensatory mechanisms, both reflex and hormonal, which serve to maintain blood flow to the cerebral and coronary vessels until the last possible moment. There is no treatment for them other than restoration of the circulation (Figure 1.2).

Following major burn injury, cardiac output falls within half an hour or so to a third of normal. This initial fall is obligatory and is unaffected

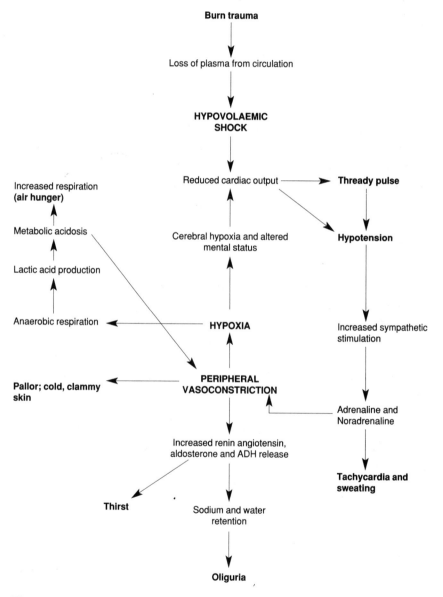

Figure 1.2 Pathophysiology of shock.

by rapid transfusion (Horton et al., 1989). However, transfusion to replace circulating fluid volume can prevent or reduce a later fall in cardiac output from 6 to 8 hours post-injury. The initial fall is thought to be due to factors released into the plasma (Raffa and Trunkey, 1978). As fluid therapy is administered, cardiac output progressively returns to normal or above by 24 to 36 hours.

Red blood cells undergo changes after a burn injury. There is an immediate haemolysis in the region of the burn, and if the quantity destroyed is sufficient this will become manifest as obvious haemoglobinaemia and haemoglobinuria. Additionally, however, red cells have a reduced lifespan, becoming abnormally fragile and removed by the reticuloendothelial system, so that the haemoglobin level may fall markedly within a few days of injury (Muir et al., 1987).

Transfused blood will undergo the same haemolysis as the patient's own cells and may increase the already elevated blood viscosity, leading to further impairment of the microvascular flow. White cell count is usually raised following burn injury, but function is poor, reducing resistance to infection.

Renal Fluid and Electrolytes

Renal blood flow and urine output diminish after a severe burn, under the action of angiotensin, catecholamines and the antidiuretic hormones of the posterior pituitary (Le Quesne, 1957). Acute tubular necrosis may follow inadequate fluid replacement. In deep burns affecting muscle or bone – typically, high voltage electrical burns – myoglobinuria or haemoglobinuria may be present due to the destruction of erythrocytes or muscle, blocking tubules and giving a pigmented urine. Unless treated this can lead to rapid renal failure.

Glycosuria occurs in patients with large burns and who are stressed. This is due to depletion of pancreatic insulin. This pseudo-diabetes usually lasts for up to 48 hours, is unaccompanied by symptoms, and is differentiated from true diabetes by the absence of ketones in the urine and by a glucose tolerance test (Bailey, 1966).

The large volumes of fluid which move from one compartment to another in burns shock are associated with corresponding shifts of electrolytes. Damaged collagen in the burned area absorbs sodium selectively, and the membranes of damaged cells allow sodium to leak into the cells and potassium to leak out. Hypokalaemia may be severe enough to warrant replacement therapy.

Pulmonary Changes

The incidence of pulmonary complications associated with burn injury is approximately 22% but the mortality of this group is of the order of 80% (Achauer et al., 1973). Lung damage initially may occur from the inhalation of hot gases, from irritants such as smoke, or from anoxia.

The upper airway, nasal passages, mouth, pharynx and trachea respond by the formation of oedema, which may continue for up to 48 hours, leading to obstruction of the airway. The bronchioles and alveoli also become oedematous and perfusion becomes inadequate. Acidosis may ensue as carbon dioxide is not cleared.

As airway oedema subsides, over the 3 to 4 days after the injury, increased mucus production along with reduction in cilial activity combine to increase the risk of infection. Debris becomes detached from the small airways, which then become obstructed, thus adding to the increased shunt fraction seen following major burns.

Adult respiratory distress syndrome (ARDS) is well described in association with major burn injury, possibly due to mediators released from the burn or resulting from inhalation injury damaging the pulmonary capillary-endothelial membrane.

Ventilation may also be hampered by encircling eschar around the chest or neck, by the outpouring of transudate into the alveolar spaces, and by elevation of the diaphragm by intestinal ileus.

Metabolic Effects

Large quantities of heat may be lost from the burned patient due to:

• loss of the thermoregulatory function of damaged skin
• increased evaporation of fluid from the weeping burn

Under the abnormal conditions of additional water loss in a burned patient, heat loss may exceed body heat production, unless additional energy is supplied in the form of a high ambient room temperature (up to 28°C or more), and additional calories from nutrition.

In the healthy body, protein synthesis and breakdown are in equilibrium. In the burned patient, synthesis is usually normal but breakdown is greatly accelerated. This is shown by an increase in urine urea and creatinine.

Gastrointestinal Tract Effects

Early vomiting, often experienced when giving oral fluids to the recently burned patient, is the result of gastric dilatation and intestinal ileus due to splanchnic vasoconstriction, and may occur several days after burn injury. It may be associated with electrolyte imbalance, and is also a sign of sepsis.

Unexplained hypotension, haematemesis or melaena may result from ulceration of the gastro-intestinal tract, usually from multiple points. Gastric perforation is more likely with larger burns and can occur some 10 to 14 days after injury. This is the ulcer that was described by Curling in 1842, and is usually known by his name.

Endocrine Effects

Burn injury is associated with a marked endocrine response (Dolecek, 1989). Catecholamines and cortisol are raised and impaired glucose tolerance is a common feature.

Immune function is suppressed more in burned than other trauma patients, rendering them highly susceptible to infection. Various immunosuppressive factors have been isolated from burn serum; they may originate from burn tissue or be released by an intense local inflammatory response following a severe burn injury (Hansborough et al., 1990).

Endotoxin, released from macrophages, elicits the production of tumour necrosis factor (TNF), which causes coagulopathy, shock, fluid and electrolyte sequestration, and widespread organ damage, and is in itself a pyrogen. The resetting of the hypothalamic thermostat will make the patient pyrexial, usually at 38–39°C (Marano et al., 1990).

Pathophysiology of Electrical Burns

The pathophysiology of electrical burn injury may appear mild when viewed as only local pathology: the severity of the damage, however, may be much worse systemically. Electrical current enters the body at the point of contact, travels along planes and structures of low resistance, and exits through the earth contact.

Only the contact points initially produce visible skin injury. Factors which influence the amount of tissue damage include the following:

Voltage

High-tension voltages ionize the air particles and may arc across several metres (making physical contact with the electrified victim unnecessary for the sustaining of injury). Voltages as small as 45 volts have been fatal.

Amperage

Current determines the heat generated. Ventricular fibrillation has been induced by 100 amps on the heart, and the effect of amperage is related to the length of time it is applied.

Resistance

In ascending order of resistance, blood vessels, nerve, muscle, skin, tendon, fat and bone provide a pathway for passage of the current. Thrombosis of blood vessels may result in ischaemic or venous gangrene of tissue supplied by those vessels, at some distance from the burn injury. Skin immersed in water has a reduced resistance to dry skin.

Damage is produced by:

- heat from the passage of the current through tissues
- damage to vessels producing ischaemic necrosis
- interference with electrical conductivity of organs such as the heart and nerves
- tetanic contraction of muscle
- thermal injury from ignition of clothing
- forceful propulsion of the body, producing spinal or limb fractures, intraperitoneal and intrathoracic injury

Unexplained hypokalaemia may occur within a few hours of injury and persist for several weeks. This may be explained by alteration of the cell membrane potential caused by the electrical injury affecting electrolyte exchange across the cell wall.

Burning by contact with electrical current which passes through the body has effects upon the heart, brain, abdominal cavity, muscles, or blood vessels and nerves. In addition, it destroys the skin which comes into contact with the electrical source. For this reason, the estimation of the extent of the burn by measuring the percentage body surface area of the burn is valueless. Considerably greater quantities of tissue may be destroyed beneath intact skin than is superficially apparent.

References

Achauer BM, Allyn PA, Furnas DW et al. (1973) Pulmonary complications of burns; the major threat to the burn patient. Annals of Surgery 177: 311–19.

Arturson G (1979) Microvascular permeability to macromolecules in thermal injury. Acta Physiologica Scandinavica 463(suppl): 111.

Bailey BN (1966) Hyperglycaemia in burns. British Medical Journal 2: 1783.

Blacock A (1931) Experimental shock VIII: the importance of the local loss of fluid in the production of the low blood pressure after burn. Archives of Surgery 22: 610.

Cope O, Moore FD (1947) The redistribution of body water and the fluid therapy of the burned patient. Annals of Surgery 126: 1010.

Dolecek R (1989) Endocrine changes after burn trauma – a review. Keio Journal of Medicine 38: 262–76.

Hansborough JF, Zapata-Sirvent R, Hoyt D (1990) Postburn immunosuppression: an inflammatory response to the burn wound? Journal of Trauma 30: 671–75.

Horton JW, Baxter CR, White DJ (1989) Differences in cardiac responses to resuscitation from burn shock. Surgery, Gynecology and Obstetrics 168: 201.

Le Quesne LP (1957) Fluid Balance in Surgical Practice. 2nd edn. London: Lloyd-Luke.

Marano MA, Fong Y, Moldawer LL et al. (1990) Serum cachectin/tumour necrosis factor in critically ill patients with burns correlates with infection and mortality. Surgery, Gynecology and Obstetrics 170: 32–38.

Muir IFK, Barclay TL, Settle JAD (1987) Burns and their Treatment. 3rd edn. London: Butterworths.

Pitt RM, Parker JC, Jurkovich GJ et al. (1987) Analysis of altered capillary pressure and permeability after thermal injury. Journal of Surgical Research 42: 693.

Pruitt BA, Mason AD (1971) Haemodynamic studies of burned patients during resuscitation. In Research in Burns: Transactions of the Third International Congress on Research in Burns. Bern, Switzerland: Hans Huber. pp 42–48.

Raffa J, Trunkey DD (1978) Myocardial depression in acute thermal injury. Journal of Trauma 18: 90–93.

CHAPTER 2

Classification of Burn Trauma

DEBORAH COOK

Rarely a week goes by without reports of the death of one or more people involved in a house fire. Although serious burns are less common than minor ones, they are an important cause of mortality and morbidity. In England and Wales during 1988, 900 people died from the effects of fire and 15 000 required admission to hospital (Wardrope and Smith, 1992). A much larger number of patients are managed in Accident and Emergency departments – approximately 150 000 new patients will attend Accident and Emergency departments each year with a burn injury; many of these represent the smaller and usually superficial burns (Westaby, 1989). This chapter looks at the causes of burn trauma, and the methods of classifying injuries according to their depth and body surface area. Severity of injury and related mortality is also discussed.

Although burns are often unpredictable, particular patterns to burn accidents can be identified in specific age groups. Under the age of 3, scalds predominate, most happening in or near the kitchen or bathroom. Some 70% of superficial burns occur in children under 5 years, with a peak incidence at 1 to 2 years, when children have attained both mobility and curiosity without having achieved caution. From ages 3 to 14, most injuries are due to clothes catching fire or are the result of conflagration. From 15 to 60, industrial accidents predominate, while after the age of 60 the general effects of ageing result in an increased risk of thermal injury (Dyer and Roberts, 1990). Abuse of cigarettes, drugs and alcohol are frequently responsible for the more serious complications of burns in the adult population. In almost all age groups, there are proportionally more burn injuries to males than females. Boys are frequently burned whilst experimenting with chemicals, fireworks, or by grabbing onto high-tension cables when climbing. Young girls are often burned whilst helping in the kitchen.

The type of injury varies according to such factors as the rural or industrial nature of the environment, the predominant type of heating in the homes, and so on. The majority of fire casualties occur in houses; and scald injuries to children occur almost exclusively in homes. Only 18% of non-fatal and 10% of fatal fire injuries occur in buildings such as factories, hotels, schools and restaurants. Cooking appliances left on or unattended are responsible for starting 35% of all home fires, and account for 27% of non-fatal and 6% of fatal casualties. More devastating still are cigarettes, cigars, pipe ash and matches, which are responsible for 28% of non-fatal and 39% of fatal casualties. Heating appliances such as electric and gas fires and heaters lead to 13% of non-fatal and 19% of fatal casualties (Kemble and Lamb, 1987).

Types of Burn

There are several types of burn injury:

- **Scalds** – injury from hot fluids such as tea, coffee, bath water, saucepans. Although most scalds will result in superficial skin loss, boiling water from a domestic kettle will cause full thickness skin loss in a few seconds. Steam will cause greater damage, owing to the release of the latent heat of vaporization. Boiling fat is at a higher temperature and deeper damage results.
- **Flame** – ignition of clothing from unguarded gas and electric fires, matches, open coal fires, explosion of paraffin- and petrol-ignited bonfires or barbecues. In the elderly, a cigarette dropped into the armchair or bedclothes is all too often fatal. Burns from clothing that has caught fire are almost always serious. Flash burns occur when skin is momentarily exposed to high temperatures, e.g. lightning.
- **Chemical** – napalm and phosphorus, used in military combat; bleaches, domestic cleaners, industrial acids and alkalis, agricultural lime, cement. Cytotoxic drugs injected extravenously by accident can produce extensive tissue necrosis. The severity of the burn will depend on the type of chemical, its concentration, and the contact time.
- **Electrical** – high-tension overhead or underground power cables carry 32 000 volts or more. Contact with the cable may be accompanied by violent propulsion of the patient in the explosion, causing fractures or intraperitoneal bleeding. High voltage supply will cause severe

and extensive burns with massive tissue destruction. Domestic burns (240 volts AC) occur when a live terminal or wire is touched, while the patient is earthed.

- **Radiation** – the commonest burns of this nature are those caused by exposure to sunlight or sunbeds, and are usually superficial. Other causes are inadvertent escape of nuclear fuels, accidents during radiotherapy, or deliberate use of destructive weapons. These wounds are slow to heal because of the induced thrombo-angitis, and the resulting scar tissue is prone to further ulceration.
- **Contact** – with hot metals, domestic appliances such as irons or ovens, bitumen. Also, contact with extreme cold temperatures as in frostbite. Friction burns may result from road traffic or other accidents resulting in shearing of the skin against another surface.
- **Inhalation** – of hot gases or smoke, usually when the incident occurs within a confined space. Inhalation injury greatly increases the risk of mortality.

Abuse

Abuse is the cause of many thermal burns in children (Purdue et al., 1988). A careful social history may reveal abuse in other family members or previously unexplained injuries on the victim. Risk is increased for male children, less than 3 years of age, who are left alone with a babysitter or boyfriend, although women also may abuse children. A delay in seeking medical attention for the child more than 30 minutes after the injury should raise the question of abuse (Hobbs, 1986). Specific patterns of injury have been identified. Circular burns from cigarettes, and scald injuries with sharply defined margins, especially in a stocking or glove distribution, must be suspect. Perineal burns in children who are not yet toilet trained should always be reported as possible abuse (Purdue et al., 1988).

Degree of Injury

The depth of burn will depend on:

the **intensity/concentration** of the burning agent
the **time** the agent is in contact with the skin (Dyer, 1988)

When patients are first seen, an attempt should be made to assess the depth of the burn injury. Describing the injury as a first-, second- or third-degree burn can be misleading, as these terms do not have a uniform meaning. It is less likely to cause misunderstanding if descriptive terms are used.

The most important aspect of the depth of the burn is whether or not the skin has been destroyed in its entire thickness and it is this distinction which should be attempted during early assessment (see Table 2.1). When the burned areas are mapped out on a body outline chart, some simple form of shading should indicate which parts are thought to be full thickness skin destruction and which parts only partial thickness skin damage.

Table 2.1 Characteristics of burns (Reproduced from Kemble and Lamb, 1987, with permission)

	Partial thickness	Full thickness
Length of contact with burning agent	Momentary	More than a few seconds
Temperature of burning agent	40–55°C	Boiling water, hot metal
Electrical injury	Unlikely	Probable
'Flash' burn without contact	Probable	Possible
Soles of feet and back of trunk	Probable	Possible
Amount of pain in burn	Painful	Painless
Appreciation of sharpness to pinprick test	'Sharp'	Appreciates touch or anaesthesia
Pressure on burn with forceps	Blanches	No change
Removal of forceps	Circulation returns	No change
Circulation in subcutaneous veins	Present	Absent, thrombosed
Appearance	Pink, blistering	White or charred

Unfortunately, there is no simple test which will enable this distinction to be made with certainty on all occasions. However, it is usually well worthwhile testing the burned areas for sensation to pinprick. If the patient feels pain when the skin is pricked firmly with a sterile needle, viable cells must be present and the burn is of partial thickness (Jackson, 1953). The majority of flash burns and scalds are of this type. Burns from blazing clothing – particularly when saturated with paraffin or petrol – which are dark brown, leathery hard, and show evidence of thrombosed veins, are obviously full thickness skin destruction and are analgesic to needles and scalpels.

Some burns and scalds have a mottled red and white appearance, with a moist surface from which the most superficial layers of the skin have been lost or removed. These burns are quite often analgesic to pin prick and yet are capable of re-epithelialization from epithelial elements surviving in the deepest parts of the sweat glands and hair follicles. It can be seen then that sensation to pinprick is significant when present but less so when absent (Muir et al., 1987). (See Table 2.2.)

Table 2.2 Clinical depth of burn (Reproduced from Kemble and Lamb, 1987, with permission)

	History	Appearance	Blisters	Sensation	Result
Superficial	Momentary exposure or sunburn	Red, bloated	Absent	Painful	Heals in approximately 7 days
Partial Thickness	Scalds of limited duration	Red or pink, with capillary return	Present, or surface wet or waxy	Painful	Heals in approximately 14 days
Full Thickness	Contact with high temperature or chemicals, or electrical injury	Charred, brown or white, dry thrombosed vessels	Absent	Painless	Granulates

A superficial burn involves only the surface epithelium. It is characterised by mild pain, erythema (redness), dry skin, slight oedema, and no blisters. Skin functions remain intact. Generally it will heal within 2 to 3 days and may be accompanied by flaking or peeling. A typical sunburn is an example of this (see Figure 2.1).

A partial thickness burn involves the deeper layers of the epidermis or the upper levels of the dermis and skin functions are lost. In a superficial partial thickness burn, the deeper layers of the epidermis are injured and

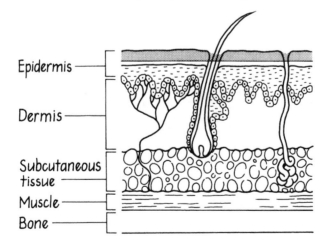

Figure 2.1 Superficial burn.

there is characteristic erythema, blister formation, marked oedema, and pain, although the hair follicles, sebaceous glands and sweat glands are spared. Such an injury usually heals within 7 to 10 days with mild or no scarring (see Figure 2.2). In a deep partial thickness burn, there is destruction of the epidermis as well as the upper levels of the dermis and only the deeper parts of the hair follicles or the sweat glands survive. If there is no infection, these burns may heal without grafting in about 3 to 4 weeks, although scarring may occur (see Figure 2.3).

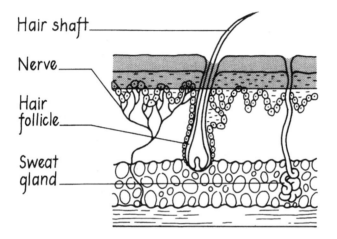

Figure 2.2 Partial thickness burn.

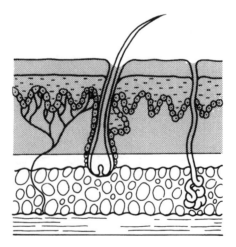

Figure 2.3 Deep partial thickness burn.

A full thickness burn involves destruction of the epidermis, dermis, and the epidermal derivatives and skin functions are lost. Such burns vary in appearance from marble-white to mahogany coloured, to charred, dry wounds. Thrombosed vessels may be visible beneath the injured skin. There is marked oedema and such a burn is not usually painful to the touch due to destruction of the nerve endings. Regeneration is slow and much granulation tissue forms before being covered by epithelium (see Figure 2.4). Even if skin grafting is commenced early, full thickness burns may quickly contract and produce scarring.

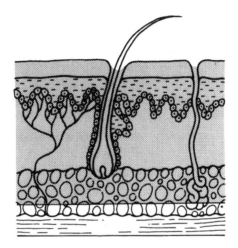

Figure 2.4 Full thickness burn.

Extent of Injury

When a patient with a thermal injury is first seen, estimation of the area burned is important. For adults the extent of the injury can be estimated by using the rule of nines (Wallace, 1951), which indicates, in an easily remembered form, the percentage of total body surface area accounted for by various parts of the body: 9% each for arms and head; 18% each for the legs, front of trunk and back of trunk (see Figure 2.5).

In children these percentages change, since the head and trunk represent a larger proportion of the total body surface area. The Lund-Browder chart more accurately determines the extent of the burn (Lund and Browder, 1944: see Figure 2.6). In addition a series of body charts have been designed that are more representative of changing body proportion with increasing age. Being easier to use, it was found that these charts led to a better estimate by the Accident and Emergency doctor of the body

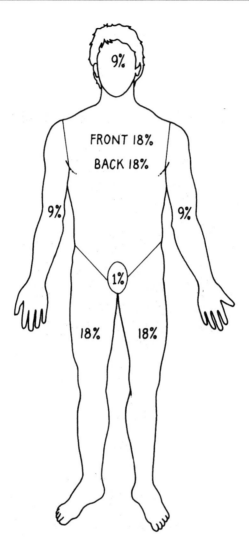

Figure 2.5 Rule of Nines.

surface area that had been burned (Wilson et al., 1987: see Figures 2.7a–h). For parts of the body that have only small areas of burn it is useful to remember that the palmar surface of the patient's hand constitutes about 1% of the body surface area. Areas of erythema should not be included as burned tissue.

A major burn is defined as any burn involving greater than 15% total body surface area in an adult, or 10% in a child, and these burns should be transferred to a Burns Unit as soon as possible. Similarly, burns in critical areas including the hands, face, feet, and perineum are optimally

NAME _____ WARD _____ NUMBER _____ DATE _____
AGE _____ ADMISSION WEIGHT _____

LUND AND BROWDER CHARTS

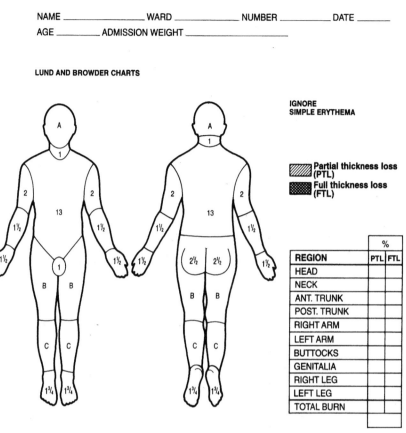

IGNORE
SIMPLE ERYTHEMA

Partial thickness loss (PTL)

Full thickness loss (FTL)

REGION	PTL	FTL
HEAD		
NECK		
ANT. TRUNK		
POST. TRUNK		
RIGHT ARM		
LEFT ARM		
BUTTOCKS		
GENITALIA		
RIGHT LEG		
LEFT LEG		
TOTAL BURN		

RELATIVE PERCENTAGE OF BODY SURFACE AREA
AFFECTED BY GROWTH

AREA	AGE 0	1	5	10	15	ADULT
A = ½ OF HEAD	9½	8½	6½	5½	4½	3½
B = ½ OF ONE THIGH	2¾	3¼	4	4½	4½	4¾
C = ½ OF ONE LEG	2½	2½	2¾	3	3¼	3½

Figure 2.6 Lund and Browder chart.

managed at a regional burn centre. Major inhalation injury, associated trauma, and chemical or electrical injuries are also indications for transfer.

Clinical history

The history must be thorough but concise. The time of the incident and type of burning materials must be determined. Some fuels such as petrol produce especially severe burns (Williams et al., 1990). Vapours from burning plastics cause a chemical pulmonary injury, especially if the fire occurred in an

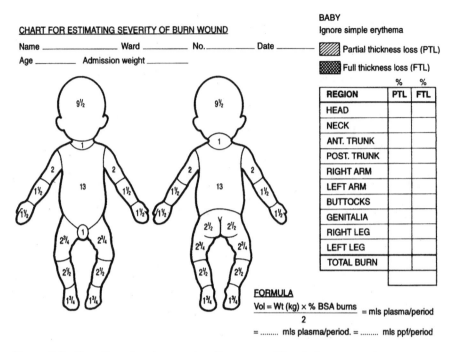

Figure 2.7a Chart for estimating severity of burn wound for a baby.

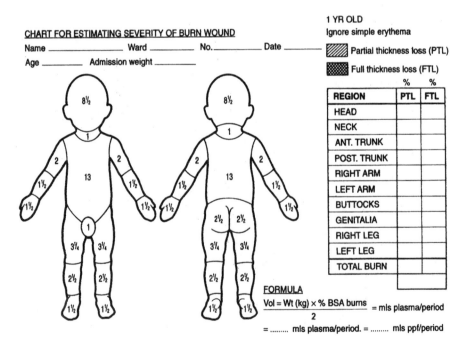

Figure 2.7b Chart for estimating severity of burn wound for a 1-year-old.

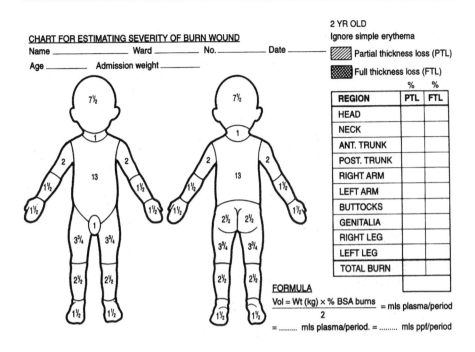

Figure 2.7c Chart for estimating severity of burn wound for a 2-year-old.

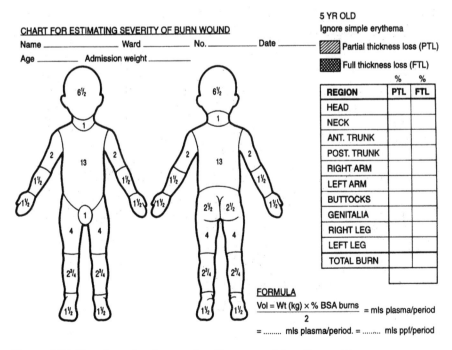

Figure 2.7d Chart for estimating severity of burn wound for a 5-year-old.

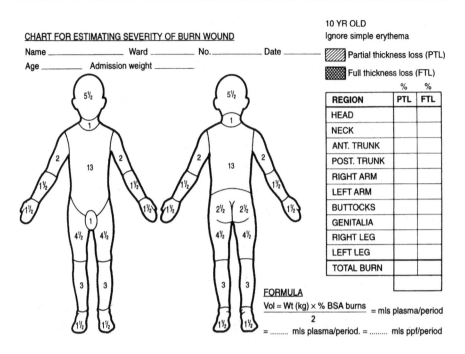

Figure 2.7e Chart for estimating severity of burn wound for a 10-year-old.

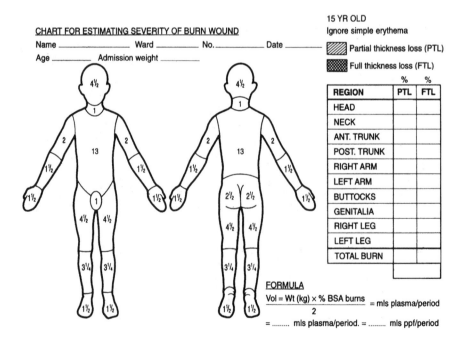

Figure 2.7f Chart for estimating severity of burn wound for a 15-year-old.

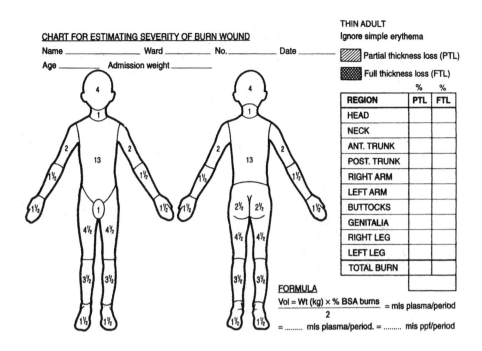

Figure 2.7g Chart for estimating severity of burn wound for a thin adult.

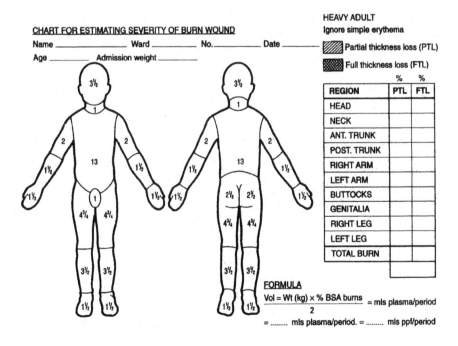

Figure 2.7h Chart for estimating severity of burn wound for a heavy adult.

CORNWALL COLLEGE
LIBRARY

enclosed space (Prien and Traber, 1988). The risk of blunt or penetrating injury is increased if there was an explosion, if the patient jumped or fell from a burning building or was burned in a motor vehicle accident.

A history of tobacco use increases the risk of pulmonary complications. A surprising percentage of patients sustain thermal burns as a result of alcohol or drug abuse (Parks et al., 1989). Acute substance withdrawal may complicate fluid resuscitation.

Mortality

Survival or death following a burn is highly dependent on the age of the victim and the extent of the injury. Other factors play lesser though important roles, and ultimate survival depends on successful management of the patient both initially and through the course of a number of potential complications. Bull (1971) devised a table of statistical values of mortality based on the patient's age and percentage area of body burned (see Table 2.3) and Tobiasen et al. (1982) developed the Abbreviated Burn Severity Index (ABSI).

Since Bull's first publication, a number of workers have identified additional characteristics of burned patients which have significant bearing upon their survival. Although it is universally agreed that age and percentage body surface area burned are two of the most important,

Table 2.3 Statistical values of mortality with age and percentage area of body burned (Adapted from Bull (1971) and reproduced with kind permission of *The Lancet* Ltd.)

Area of body burned	Age (years)								
	0–4	5–14	15–24	25–34	35–44	45–54	55–64	65–74	75+
93+	1.0	1.0	1.0	1.0	1.0	1.0	1.0	1.0	1.0
83–92	0.9	0.9	0.9	0.9	1.0	1.0	1.0	1.0	1.0
73–82	0.7	0.8	0.8	0.9	0.9	1.0	1.0	1.01	1.0
63–72	0.5	0.6	0.6	0.7	0.8	0.9	1.0	1.0	1.0
53–62	0.3	0.3	0.4	0.5	0.7	0.8	0.9	1.0	1.0
43–52	0.2	0.2	0.2	0.3	0.5	0.6	0.8	1.0	1.0
33–42	0.1	0.1	0.1	0.2	0.3	0.4	0.6	0.9	1.0
23–32	0	0	0	0.1	0.1	0.2	0.4	0.7	1.0
13–22	0	0	0	0	0	0.1	0.2	0.4	0.7
3–12	0	0	0	0	0	0	0.1	0.2	0.4
0–2	0	0	0	0	0	0	0	0.1	0.3

0.1 = 10% mortality; 0.9 = 90% mortality.

there are a variety of factors involved in the burned patient which may affect the final prognosis (Tejero-Trujeque, 2000).

Age

It is now well established that, for a given size of burn the prognosis worsens with advancing years after early adult life. Age related burn death has been explored by Bull and Fisher (1954). While some studies have minimised the importance of age on the outcomes of older patients with burns (Linn, 1980), Raff et al. (1996) and Covington et al. (1996) disagree. There is some controversy over survival rates in early life.

Sex

Most studies have reported mortality being higher in females (Moores et al., 1975).

Medical History

The pre-existing health of the individual has a crucial bearing on the outcome of the burn injury. A number of factors markedly increase the mortality of thermal injury, including diabetes mellitus, atherosclerosis, chronic renal failure, cirrhosis, collagen vascular disease, steroid use, malignancy, leucopoenia secondary to chemotherapeutic agents, and immunodeficiency states (Zawacki et al., 1979).

Total Body Surface Area

The percentage of total body surface area burned remains as one of the factors most closely associated with predicting mortality and morbidity (Raff et al., 1996). Due to the increased risk of sepsis and the demands placed upon the patient by surgery for wound closure, greater nutritional needs, and higher blood loss, a deep burn represents a considerably more severe injury in terms of prognosis than a partial thickness burn of the same area.

Site

The part of the body burned may have some bearing on prognosis, if for instance it is associated with a higher risk of infection, or on the other hand reflects the external injury related to a respiratory burn. Moores (1975) found that perineal burns had a significantly higher mortality. Burns to the face may also be associated with a poorer prognosis (Berry et al., 1982).

Type of Burn

There is little evidence that the mechanism of burning injury affects subsequent prognosis, provided that other factors, such as percentage of deep burn and respiratory injury are held constant.

Respiratory Injury

Inhalation injury or direct thermal damage to the respiratory lining confers a reduced prognosis to the burned patient (Clark et al., 1986). Many of the fatalities in house fires occur as the result of inhalation of hot smoke and other toxic fumes from the conflagration, particularly with the burning of certain foams used for the construction of modern furniture. Deaths from smoke inhalation have increased in recent years and are now the most important single cause of death in burns patients, (Muir et al., 1987).

Other Injuries

Concomitant injury may markedly influence survival or recovery from the burn injury.

Very few deaths occur purely as a result of the burn itself: most are from complications following the injury. Irreversible early shock with renal shutdown still occurs and is the cause of death in about 15% of cases (Curreri et al., 1980). The majority of deaths 60–80%, however, are due to one or more complications relating to infection. The principal infective complications are related to the respiratory system: either acute, from the injury itself, or delayed, as in pulmonary oedema (Rylah, 1992).

References

Berry CC, Wachtel TL, Frank HA (1982) An analysis of factors which predict mortality in hospitalised burns patients. Burns 9: 38.

Bull JP (1971) Revised analysis of mortality due to burns. Lancet ii: 1133.

Bull JP, Fisher AJ (1954) A study of mortality in a Burns Unit: a revised estimate. Annal of Surgery 139: 269.

Clark CJ, Reid WH, Gilmour WH et al. (1986) Mortality probability in victims of fire trauma: revised equation to include inhalation injury. British Medical Journal 292: 1303.

Covington DS, Wainwright DJ, Parks DH (1996) Prognostic indications in the elderly patient with burns. Journal of Burn Care and Rehabilitation 17(3): 222–30.

Curreri PW, Luterman A, Braun DW et al. (1980) Burn injury analysis of survival and hospitalisation time for 937 patients. Annals of Surgery 192: 472.

Dyer C (1988) Burn wound management: an update. Plastic Surgery Nursing (Spring): 6–12.

Dyer C, Roberts D (1990) Thermal trauma. Nursing Clinics of North America 25(1): 85–117.

Hobbs CJ (1986) When are burns not accidental? Archives of Disease in Childhood 61: 357–61.

Jackson D McG (1953) The diagnosis of the depth of burning. British Journal of Surgery 40: 588.

Kemble JVH, Lamb BE (1987) Practical Burns Management. London: Hodder and Stoughton.

Lund CC, Browder NC (1944) Estimation of areas of burns. Surgery, Gynecology and Obstetrics 79: 352–8.

Moores B, Rahman MM, Browning FSC et al. (1975) Discriminant function analysis of 570 consecutive burn patients admitted to the Yorkshire Regional Burns Centre 1966–1973. Burns 1: 135.

Muir IFK, Barclay TL, Settle JAD (1987) Burns and their Treatment. 3rd edn. London: Butterworths.

Parks JG, Noguchi TT, Klatt EC (1989) The epidemiology of fatal burn injuries. Journal of Forensic Science 34: 399–406.

Prien T, Traber DL (1988) Toxic smoke compounds and inhalation injury – a review. Burns 14: 451–60.

Purdue GF, Hunt JL, Prescott PR (1988) Child abuse by burning – an index of suspicion. Journal of Trauma 28: 221–24.

Raff T, Germann G, Barthold H (1996) Factors influencing the early prediction of outcome from burns. Acta Chirurgiae Plasticae 38(4): 122–27.

Rylah LTA (1992) Critical Care of the Burned Patient. Cambridge: Cambridge University Press.

Tejero-Trujeque R (2000) How effective is the abbreviated Burn Severity Index in predicting patient mortality. Journal of Wound Care 9(10): 475–78.

Tobiasen J, Hiebert JM, Edlich RF (1982) A practical burn severity index. Journal of Burn Care and Rehabilitation 3(4): 229–32.

Wallace AB (1951) The exposure treatment of burns. Lancet i: 501.

Wardrope J, Smith JAR (1992) The Management of Wounds and Burns. Oxford: Oxford University Press.

Westaby S (1989) Trauma – Pathogenesis and Treatment. Oxford: Heinemann Medical Books.

Williams JB II, Ahrenholz DH, Solem LD et al. (1990) Gasoline burns: the preventable cause of thermal injury. Journal of Burn Care and Rehabilitation 11: 446–50.

Wilson GR, Fowler CA, Housden PL (1987) A new burn area assessment chart. Burns 13(5): 401–5.

Zawacki BE, Azen SP, Imbus SH et al. (1979) Multifactorial probit analysis of mortality in burned patients. Annals of Surgery 189: 1–5.

CHAPTER 3

Nursing Children following Burn Trauma

DEBORAH BEEBY AND CHRISSIE BOUSFIELD

The last decade has witnessed several changes in the health and welfare of children in the UK. This has been reflected in Government reforms covering health, welfare and education intended to meet the changing needs of children and their families, and as a result all aspects of children's lives have continued to improve. At last the needs of children have been highlighted as being distinct to those of adults, while care has been taken to respect their rights. In the current climate, the care of children in hospital has been transformed by the greater provision of children's nurses with the knowledge and skills to provide a family-centred approach to care, in an environment where parents are always welcome and considered part of the team in caring for their child (Davies, 2000). Before discussing the management of care for children following a burn injury, it is appropriate to mention in this chapter some of the changes in child health that have occurred.

Child Health

With a government committed to monetarism and NHS reform, the passing of the NHS Community Care Act 1990 was destined to occur, with the establishment of internal market competition and consumerism well under way. Important health targets, following on from the publication by the Department of Health of *The Health of the Nation* (DoH, 1992) were established in child surveillance and accident prevention. Hospitals had to comply with the Patients' Charter of 1991 (DoH, 1991), further updated in 1995 to take account of waiting times for operations, outpatient services and Accident and Emergency departments. The publication of *Welfare of*

Children and Young People in Hospital in 1991 (DoH, 1991) reaffirmed the need for a 'child and family service'. As with the Platt Report (Ministry of Health, 1959) it recommended that children should only be admitted to hospital if care could not be provided at home. It also recommended that children admitted to intensive care units should be nursed separately from adults. The Allitt Inquiry (Clothier Report) of 1991 (DoH, 1994) laid the foundations for nurse staffing for children in hospital and, as a result, helped by government funding, the number of RSCN entrants increased (House of Commons, 1997). In addition, the report *Bridge for the Future* (DoH, 1997) addressed the issue of nurse staffing and specialist qualifications in relation to paediatric intensive care services.

The election of a Labour Government in 1997 meant a change of direction for the NHS, which has now been described as 'based on partnership and driven by performance' (Secretary of State for Health, 1997). The findings of the Acheson report (1998) into health inequalities reflect those of the Black Report, and government policy is now aimed at a reduction in health inequalities and eradication of child poverty within 20 years. In the community, GPs and other health care professionals, representatives from social services and voluntary agencies will commission services based on local need. Targets set by Action for Sick Children will also provide invaluable guidance to those who wish to ensure the needs of sick children are met in hospital and the community in the future (Action for Sick Children, 1999/2000).

Burn Care

The thoughtful, knowledgeable, sensitive nursing care that the burn-injured child receives has a profound impact on his survival and quality of life (Trofino, 1991). This chapter highlights the differences between children and adults, the causes of burn injury in children and the associated risk variables. Non-accidental injury and the importance of family-centred care is outlined. The treatment of the burn injury is mentioned (it is covered in more detail in Chapter 4), complications of burns encephalopathy and toxic shock syndrome are identified, and signs, symptoms and management are discussed. Psychological care is also alluded to.

Differences between Children and Adults

The management of care for a child with a burn injury is similar to that of an adult. However, there are significant differences between children and adults. With respect to children, these include:

- differing size and body proportions
- differing social and economical development
- the thickness of the skin
- an increased surface-area to weight ratio
- an increased metabolic rate
- increased evaporative losses
- increased heat loss
- an increased risk of developing hypothermia
- smaller airways, and other anatomic differences
- altered blood volume
- an increased proportion of extra-cellular fluid
- decreased renal tubular concentrating ability
- increased fluid loss
- excess fluid less easily handled
- risk of cerebral oedema and fluid overload

Causes of Burns and Scalds in Children

Seventy per cent of burns occur in children under 5 years of age, the most common age being 1 to 2 years, and the boy:girl ratio being 3:2. Flame burns can affect all ages, whereas contact burns are only a problem in the very young. Scalds occur mainly in the under-four age group, both sexes being affected equally. The boy:girl ratio for serious scalds is approximately 1.3:1. Older boys are also more likely than girls to suffer a burn injury because of risk-taking behaviour, for example, with fireworks and flammable liquids (Coleshaw, Reilly and Irving, 1997).

In 1998 in England and Wales, there were 39 fatalities resulting from fire and flames, and 3 from scalds. Over 35 000 under-fives and almost 14 000 children aged 5–14 went to hospital after a burn or scald, at home or in the garden, in the UK in 1997 (Child Accident Prevention Trust, 1999). Serious burns are noted to be slightly less common in the summer months.

There is a strong link between house fires and burns and scalds and poverty. Children in social class V are 15 times more likely to die in a house fire than children in social class 1 (Child Accident Prevention Trust, 1999). Poor housing, overcrowding and family stress contribute to the likelihood of injury in young children at risk from inadequately guarded fires and cookers and trailing electric flexes (Coleshaw, Reilly and Irving, 1997). However, deaths from burns are decreasing. This is partly due to:

- the increasing use of smoke detectors
- a reduction in clothing burns because of low flammability requirements for night-dresses
- a gradual move away from open fires to central heating

A downward trend has also been noted in scald fatalities, owing to
improved treatment and management. The kitchen, living/dining rooms
and bathrooms are the most common locations for burn and scald
injuries to occur. The main causes of injury are:

- babies and toddlers reaching and grabbing to get near unguarded
  fires
- hot liquids within easy reach
- irons standing on the floor
- parents holding a baby and a hot drink
- unsupervised baths (parents may go to answer the telephone and the
  child turns on the hot tap)
- pulling the flexes of kettles that have been left dangling (coiled flexes
  help to reduce this)
- overhanging pan-handles on the cooker

Among older children, especially boys aged between 9 and 14 years,
severe burns can occur as a result of their ignorance of the danger of
flammable liquids, such as petrol or those used to light bonfires, experimenting with matches or fireworks or cigarette lighters, or sniffing glue or
aerosols followed by smoking. The products involved (not in order of
importance) are:

- matches and smokers' materials
- bonfires and open coal-fires
- cookers, saucepans and chip pans
- heaters such as electric fires
- cups and mugs containing hot liquids
- hot fat and oils
- kettles
- flammable nightwear
- toxic fumes from non-combustion, modified foam-filled furniture
- irons
- curling tongs
- live wires

- baths and showers
- oven-cleaners
- fireworks
- motorbikes
- sunshine

Prevention

Removal of all possible causes of burn injuries is an unrealistic target. However, increasing the awareness of the general public, and manufacturers of equipment such as kettles, to the hazards of uncoiled long flexes should achieve a considerable reduction in accidents (Reid, 1996). It is envisaged the future will see a continued reduction in the number of burn and scald injuries through changes in laws and continuing health education. One of the objectives in the Government's White Paper *The Health of the Nation* is to reduce the death rate for accidents among children by at least 33% by 2005 (DoH, 1992). This has led to the promotion by health visitors of accident prevention education to parents.

Non-Accidental Injury

Hobbs (1989) gives the following definitions:

- *Accident* – a lapse in usual protection given to the child
- *Neglect* – inadequate or negligent parenting; failing to protect the child
- *Abuse* – deliberately inflicting injury

About 2% of children who suffer from burns are the victims of non-accidental injury, and 10% of abused children suffer from burns (Jones et al., 1993). All staff working with burn-injured children must be constantly alert for any signs of child abuse and ensure that immediate and effective action is taken in all suspected cases as hospital policy:

> All those working in the field of health care have a professional responsibility to protect children, and their participation in inter-agency support to social services departments is essential if the interests of children are to be safeguarded.
>
> (DoH, 1995)

The assessment should be multidisciplinary, involving medical staff, paediatricians, nurses, health visitors and social workers. The 'at risk' register should be checked immediately following admission if there is a suspicion of non-accidental injury. Photographs should be taken on admission and accurate diagrams drawn. Both medical and nursing documentation must be detailed, with relationships and reactions of the family also being recorded. Parents must be kept informed of everything that is going on and the guidance of the Children's Act (1989) as well as hospital policies and legal requirements must be adhered to.

Neglect – for example, a child sustaining a burn or a scald on a paralysed limb or after being left unattended in a bath – is much more common than is non-accidental injury. Improbable accidents do occur: for example, a strange burn to a child's back was the result of a faulty paddling pool melting onto the child in the sun.

The parents and child need a lot of support if a non-accidental injury is suspected, and care must be taken not to show adverse feelings to the person who has abused. It is also very important not to wrongly accuse or judge.

The peak age of children being deliberately burned is during the third year of their life, and the following injuries may be encountered.

- *Scalds* – for example, from dipping a child into boiling water, causing scalds to the perineum and genitalia – may be used to punish the child.
- *Cigarette burns* – a circular mark is unlikely to be caused by a child brushing past a lit cigarette (Jones et al., 1993). Additional scars may also be found on other parts of the body.
- *Hands* – the dorsal aspect is affected, whereas in accidents the palmar surface is usually affected. The hand may be held onto a hot object or in hot water.
- *Feet* – burns in a sock/stocking distribution, with no splash marks and a clear demarcation line from dipping into hot water. A contact burn to the sole – from an iron, curling tongs, etc. – may also occur.
- *Mouth* – from having hot food forced into the mouth.
- *Contact burns* – the injury resembles a brand mark, bearing the shape of the object that caused it. The burn is usually dry and of uniform depth.

The history is not usually consistent with the story, although some parents will admit to causing the accident. They may not know how the accident happened or may deny it is a burn or a scald, the accident may be unwitnessed, the parents may say the child did not cry, and the child's and the parents' stories may conflict. Parents may be abusive and hostile to staff, and refuse treatment for their child. Mothers may be withdrawn, depressed and seeking help and may show lack of concern or guilt (Hobbs, 1989). The reaction is usually not what is expected from parents of children with an accidental injury. The abused child may be passive, very withdrawn and not complaining about pain, or very anxious, angry or rebellious. If older children refuse to state the cause of their injury this may be significant (Hobbs, 1989).

According to Jones et al. (1993), common factors found in non-accidental injury families include:

- a high incidence of personality disorders
- maternal/paternal deprivation in parental, social, or family histories
- rigid parental attitudes to discipline
- a distorted perception of the child
- ignorance of normal childhood behaviour and development
- impulsive parental behaviour
- low tolerance of stress
- adverse social circumstances
- poor health
- low social class
- younger than average parents
- frequent changes of home
- larger than average family size
- an atypical family structure
- frequent marital upsets
- a high unemployment rate
- a high rate of general criminality

The children as a general group, have the following characteristics:

- they are more likely to be premature or of low birthweight.
- boys are more at risk than girls until adolescence, after which the trend reverses.
- the most serious injuries are on the youngest child.
- they are more likely to be illegitimate.
- injuries are reported more in older children.

Burns Unit Environment

The environmental needs of children in hospital are very different from those of an adult and while provision of a separate paediatric Burns Unit is desirable this is not always practical. However, providing facilities for parents to stay with the child, ample space for toddlers to run around and play in and the furniture scaled down to appropriate size is essential. Apart from play, social interaction such as contact with family members, friends, relatives and the school teacher helps to normalize the stressful situation of being burned or having a child who has experienced this type of trauma (Reid, 1996).

Burn Team

The Burns team has essential key members for the management of care for children. These include a burns surgeon and a burns anaesthetist experienced in caring for children, a liaison paediatrician, trained children's nurses, nursery nurses, play leaders/play therapists, the school teacher, and a clinical psychologist with a particular interest in children. All are invaluable and form the mainstay of the team from the child's admission to discharge from hospital.

Family-centred Care

Caring for the parents and the family is an essential part of caring for the child. As well as being upset and anxious, parents may feel guilty about the cause of their child's injuries. They may blame the person who was with the child at the time of the accident. If one was not there, he or she may take their anger out on the partner, at a time when they need each other's support most of all.

It is important to encourage parents to participate in caring for their child, and to involve them in any decisions regarding their child's care. To make these decisions, they need to be given unbiased and complete information in an appropriate and supportive manner (Cambell, 1993). Participating in care will help them to overcome feelings of guilt, anger and rejection.

The presence of parents has been shown to be beneficial to children, both physiologically and psychologically. Parents thus need to be made to feel welcome and relaxed, because if they are nervous or uneasy, the child may sense this and become frightened himself (Muller et al., 1992).

In 1959 the Platt report recommended that parents should have unrestricted access to their child in hospital (Ministry of Health, 1959). Numerous pieces of research since then have stated the importance of parents staying with their child and participating in care (Cambell et al., 1993). Parents should be made to feel part of the team caring for their child. The Department of Health (1991b) states that the provision of care for hospitalized children has to centre firmly on the recognition of the child as a member of a family – a family whose support during the hospital stay is essential to the child's well being. Parents need comfortable accommodation so that they can unwind and rest, and access to regular drinks and meals; information about the hospital, shops and the local area should be given to parents, so they feel as well equipped as possible, both mentally and physically, to help support their child.

Some parents may feel they are unable to participate in the care of their child or to be resident with them, and they must be offered support and not made to feel guilty – a single parent with other children at home, and no one to help, would not find it possible to be resident. Especially in cases such as this, the health care system needs to be flexible, accessible and responsive to a family's needs; for example, if parents are not resident, but would like to be there when their child's wound dressings are changed, arrangements should be made to choose a time suitable for all concerned.

It is important to implement appropriate policies and programmes that are comprehensive and provide emotional, spiritual, cultural and financial support to meet the needs of the family. Research by Goulding (1992) has shown that financial difficulties are not well catered for. As Burns Units cover a wide geographical area, cost can be a real problem when a child is in hospital. Multidisciplinary teams would do well to remember that the family is constant in the child's life, while the other teams caring for the child come and go (Cambell et al., 1993).

Treatment of the Burn Injury

Assessment of the type, depth and percentage body surface areas of the burn injury are the same for a child as an adult. However, when estimating the percentage of the burn injury it is important to use a chart which takes into account age-related differences (Wilson, Fowler and Housden, 1987). The significance of these differences can be illustrated using the example of a baby's head: for an infant, the head is 20% of total body surface area, whereas for a five-year-old the head represents only 13%. Accurate assessment is important as it informs subsequent management (Coleshaw, Reilly and Irving, 1997).

Once the severity of the burn injury has been assessed in the Accident and Emergency department, a decision is made regarding the environment of care for future management. This may involve transfer to a Burns Unit, or for severe cases and/or if an inhalation injury is suspected a Paediatric Intensive Care Unit. The criteria for transferring a child to a specialist Burns Unit are as follows:

- burns to more than 10% total body surface area
- full thickness burns over 5% total body surface area
- circumferential burns of the limbs, neck, trunk
- burns to specific areas of the body: hands, face, feet, perineum
- burns caused by chemicals or electricity
- burns with associated trauma
- burns suspected of being a non-accidental injury
- burns associated with inhalation injuries
- children with pre-existing medical conditions

The general resuscitation programme of a child with a burn injury differs little from that of an adult (Reid, 1996). In children with burns of less than 10% body surface area, oral resuscitation is usually adequate. Due to the risk of burns encephalopathy developing, it is best to use oral fluids in the form of salt containing solutions such as Dioralyte or milk for maintenance fluids and to avoid salt-free solutions such as fruit juice/squash (Carvajal, 1980). For children with burns over 10% intravenous fluid resuscitation is required (see Chapter 4).

The treatment of the burn wound is the same for a child as it is for an adult, although sometimes the dressings are problematical due to the site of the wound and/or the size of the child. Early excision and grafting of the burn wound is advantageous and a well-organized theatre technique goes a long way to minimize blood loss, accurately assess the skin graft requirement, excise the burn and apply the skin (Reid, 1996).

In the acute stage of the burn injury an intravenous infusion of morphine or oral Oramorph is paramount. Pain assessment and oral analgesia prior to wound care and physiotherapy should be planned in advance and evaluated after the procedure to ensure maximum benefit is achieved to minimize pain and discomfort for the child. In the operating theatre department the potential for local anaesthetic infiltration, peripheral nerve blocks and local application of agents such as bupivacaine to donor sites to minimize pain should be taken into consideration (Reid, 1996). The use of intravenous sedation or general anaesthesia may be used for some children to undertake dressing changes or painful procedures. It must also be born in mind that the child will feel distressed and frightened and will be subjected to potentially painful procedures throughout hospitalization. Distraction therapy and coping strategies can give the child some control during procedures which will enhance cooperation and reduce anxiety (Royal College of Paediatrics and Child Health, 1997).

Respiratory problems can arise in children with severe burns and may be due to airway compression due to oedema of the neck, thermal injury (direct heat), hypoxia due to carbon monoxide poisoning and respiratory distress due to smoke inhalation (Young, Manara and Burd, 1995). When exposed to high air temperatures a child's respiratory system will become inflamed or oedematous and there is a risk of airway obstruction for up to 24 hours post-inhalation injury (Coleshaw, Reilly and Irving, 1997). The heat also causes plasma and some of the cells to move into the interstitial spaces causing oedema and thickening of the walls of the alveoli, thus reducing gaseous exchange (Settle, 1996). Thermal injury can also result in damage to the cilia and deficiency of surfactant. Insufficient surfactant increases the surface tension of the walls of the alveoli causing resistance to air entry, collapse of the alveoli and decreased lung expansion. As a result of inhalation of toxic fumes the lower respiratory tract becomes inflamed and an obstruction may occur. If clinical observations reveal the presence of blistering or swelling inside the mouth, loss of or hoarseness of the voice, stridor and nasal flaring tracheal intubation should be performed immediately and the child transferred to the Paediatric Intensive Care Unit for respiratory monitoring and support (Coleshaw, Reilly and Irving, 1997).

Early enteral feeding is as important in children as it is in adults (see Chapter 10). Children who have sustained a burn injury often require additional support to meet the metabolic demands. Early enteral feeding within four hours of the burn injury occurring is necessary to prevent complications such as paralytic ileus and stress ulceration as well as meeting increased energy demands (McDonald, Sharp and Deitch, 1991). Henley (1989) implies that children with a burn injury often require normal daily requirements plus additional calories and protein to meet metabolic demands. A referral to the dietitian, regular calculation of requirements, supplements of vitamins, iron, continuous assessment of feeding regimes, identifying likes and dislikes and active encouragement ensures requirements are met and normal patterns of eating are quickly restored.

The use of prophylactic antibiotics is somewhat controversial. Children tend to carry streptococcus and staphylococcus in the nose and throat and are susceptible to developing toxic shock syndrome. Therefore it may be policy within the Burns Unit to prescribe all children with a burn injury a 5-day course of oral flucloxacillin, of an appropriate dose for their age and weight.

Complications

Burns Encephalopathy

Cerebral oedema is an infrequent but life-threatening complication of a burn or a scald in a child, generally under five years of age, with any percentage of burn or scald, usually 3–4 days after the injury. A possible cause of burns encephalopathy is cellular overhydration and hyponatraemia following the administration of excess poor salt fluids during the resuscitation phase. Clinical signs include cerebral oedema, altered conscious levels and fitting. Strict monitoring of fluid intake and output is essential, therefore, and the use of salt-free solutions is not recommended when treating children following a burn injury (Carvajal, 1980).

Toxic Shock Syndrome

Burned children are susceptible to developing toxic shock syndrome, which is not related to the percentage of body surface area burned, and once 'shock' has occurred, a 50% mortality rate has been reported (Frame et al., 1985). It is thought the cause may be absorption into the circulation of toxins released by a specific phage type of staphylococcus aureus which colonizes the burn wound (McAllister et al., 1993), although blood cultures are usually negative. Adults are rarely affected as they have often been exposed to the toxin and have appropriate antibodies. Diagnosis is mainly clinical and may be confirmed by investigations.

The clinical manifestations of toxic shock syndrome develop rapidly and one of the first signs is a pyrexia >39°C. So, both core and peripheral temperatures should be recorded, a difference of more than 3°C giving a poor prognosis. The temperature difference may also be caused by hypovolaemia; urine output, blood pressure and pulse must therefore be monitored hourly. If a child's temperature reaches 39°C, the medical staff should be informed immediately and a full bacteriological screen commenced. Other clinical signs include tachycardia, tachypnoea, decreased white blood cell count, platelets and red blood cells, (some children develop neutrophilia and disseminating intravascular coagulation), non-specific rash, vomiting, diarrhoea, oliguria, neuro-disturbances, and can progress to complete circulatory collapse and death.

Investigations include blood cultures, swabs from burn wounds, ear, nose and throat, and urine and stool specimens should be obtained. Blood samples are taken for full blood count, urea and electrolytes, creatinine/osmolarity and a clotting screen. A urine sample is sent for sodium, urea creatinine and osmolarity.

Treatment should be started early if the condition is suspected as the progression is very rapid. Oral paracetamol and ibuprofen are given as antipyretics to help reduce the child's temperature, to maintain comfort and prevent febrile convulsions. The child's level of consciousness needs to be carefully monitored; it may become impaired due to a convulsion or the need for ventilation. Appropriate treatment should be given to correct the signs and symptoms at each stage of the process. This usually involves intravenous infusion of Fresh Frozen Plasma 10–20mg/kg (which contains antibodies), and antibiotic therapy – it is recommended that all children who have burns or scalds (however small) are prescribed a 5-day course of oral flucloxacillin of appropriate dose for their age and weight. Other supportive measures may be implemented and close monitoring of the child's clinical condition is vital throughout.

Psychological Needs

Children have needs different from those of adults, and these vary according to their age (Kemble and Lamb, 1987). Children also need to be cared for in an appropriate environment and by appropriately trained staff.

It is important to learn as much about the child's normal stage of development, what and whom they like and dislike, their hobbies and personality, etc., so that any changes can be detected and the child's routine can be continued as much as possible. Play is necessary for a child's normal development, and a wide range of toys is needed to cater for all ages. Play can be used to educate children about their care, and as a way for them to express their feelings about the accident and work their way through fears and worries. Play – for example videos, blowing bubbles, and imagination – can be used to distract children during procedures. It can also be useful for physiotherapy: a child may not perform standard finger exercises, but will push buttons on a computer or pick up toys. Blowing bubbles can also be used as a breathing exercise. The provision of a playroom perceived as a safe environment by the child, where no medical or nursing interventions are undertaken, is essential. A nursery nurse/play specialist also fulfils a very important role during a child's stay in hospital.

Explanations to children must be at the appropriate level according to the child's stage of development (Piaget and Inhelder, 1969). Children under two years of age need someone familiar with them, as they like to explore but have no concept of safety. At all ages, it is important to provide information for parents so that they are able to understand and help explain to their child what is happening. Regression can occur at any age to any hospitalized sick child: for example, a toilet-trained toddler may start wetting the bed, or an older child may want his parents around, whereas at home he prefers his friends (Swanwick, 1990).

Age 2–6 years

Explanations need to be immediate and related to the present environment. Time can be explained in relation to something familiar to the child – mealtimes, for example. Parents should be encouraged to leave personal items to show that they are returning whenever they leave the child, even if only for a few minutes. In a child's view, illness is caused by external factors, as children are unable to conceive internal illness; they feel that they are ill because they are bad and are being punished – reassurance, therefore, is needed to overcome this (Swanwick, 1990).

Age 7–11 years

At this age, children can start to apply thinking and reasoning to real objects and events and begin to understand cause and event: they can understand that something external can be caused by internal problems. They can name and draw people, so uncomplicated drawings and explanations can be useful for teaching (Swanwick, 1990).

Adolescents

Adolescents understand that illness can be caused by a variety of factors, and that their organs can malfunction, but they may worry unduly as a result of incomplete knowledge of internal processes (Swanwick, 1990). Psychological problems are not immediately resolved on discharge. The child and family have to come to terms with scarring and aftercare, as the damage is visible and permanent. Problems such as nightmares and sleepless nights are usually resolved by three months; if they are not, or if there are other problems, the child can be referred to a child psychologist for help and support (Forshaw, 1990). Some families find support by discussing their problems at the Outpatients Department when they attend for their follow-up appointments, or by meeting other people who have been through a similar experience. Different people find different ways of coping, but support from the Burns Unit should always be available.

It has been found that families from low social-economic classes cope better, as there are other more pressing problems to deal with (Forshaw, 1990), but the family must never be forgotten, as they may also require psychological help in order to cope with the injury.

Aftercare

Aftercare involves rigorous physiotherapy, washing, moisturizing and massaging scar tissue (see Chapter 13). Some children will need to wear pressure garments to increase the cosmetic appearance of scarring, while others may require splints to prevent contractures developing. Accepting inevitable scarring and a degree of altered body image will undoubtedly be a difficult process, particularly for the child. Support services and networks are available to allow children and their families/carers to discuss problems and share solutions with others in similar circumstances.

Summary

Caring for a child with a burn injury differs from that of an adult due to a variety of factors. These may include different physical responses and needs, decreased cooperation, increased psychological needs and different emotional needs (Kemble and Lamb, 1987). Meeting the needs of the child's parents and family is an essential part of caring for the child and should be considered carefully during the course of hospitalization and following the child's discharge from the Burns Unit. A burn injury is a traumatic experience for any individual irrespective of age. However, in caring for children the burns team needs to acknowledge that the thoughtful, knowledgeable and sensitive care that a child receives following burn trauma has a profound impact on survival and quality of life.

References

Action for Sick Children (1999/2000) Millennium targets. Paediatric Nurse 1(10): 6–8.
Acheson D (1988) Independent enquiry into inequalities in health. London: The Stationery Office.
Cambell S (1993) Keeping it in the family. Child Health 1(1): 17–20.
Cambell S, Kelly P, Summergill P (1993) Putting the family first. Child Health 1(2): 59–60.
Carvajal HF (1980) A physiological approach to fluid therapy in severely burned children. Surgery, Gynaecology and Obstetrics 150: 379–84.
Child Accident Prevention Trust (1999) Burns and Scalds. Milton Keynes: CAPT
Coleshaw S, Reilly S, Irving N (1997) Management of burns. Paediatric Nursing 9(7): 29–36.
Davies R (2000) A celebration of 100 years' achievement in child health. British Journal of Nursing 9(7): 423–28.

Death A, Brignall J (1999) Back to normal. Nursing Times 95(39): 54–56.

Department of Health (1989) The Children Act. London: HMSO.

Department of Health (1991a) The Patients' Charter. London: HMSO.

Department of Health (1991b) Welfare of Children and Young People in Hospital. London: HMSO.

Department of Health (1992) The Health of the Nation. London: HMSO.

Department of Health (1994) The Allitt Enquiry. London: HMSO.

Department of Health (1995) Child Protection: Clarification of Arrangements Between the NHS and other agencies. London: HMSO.

Department of Health (1997) Bridge for the Future. London: HMSO.

Department of Trade and Industry (1997) Home accident surveillance system: report on 1995 accident data and safety research. London: Department of Trade and Industry Consumer Safety Unit.

Forshaw A (1990) Proven methods. Paediatric Nursing 2(8): 20–21.

Frame JD, Eve MD, Hocked ME (1985) The toxic shock syndrome in burned children. Burns 11: 234.

Goulding J (1992) The Costs of Visiting Children in Hospital. London: Action for Sick Children.

Henley M (1989) Feed that burn. Burns 15(6): 351–61.

Hobbs CJ (1989) ABC of child abuse. British Medical Journal 298: 1304–8.

House of Commons (1997) Health Services for Children and Young People in the Community, Home and School. London: The Stationery Office.

Jones DN, Pickett J, Oates MR et al. (1993) Understanding Child Abuse. Basingstoke: Macmillan.

Kemble JVH, Lamb B (1987) Practical Burns Management. London: Hodder and Stoughton.

Marsh T, Kendrick D (1996) Childhood burns and scalds. Community Nurse 1(12): 11–14.

McAllister RMR, Mercer NSG, Morgan BDG et al. (1993) Early diagnosis of staphylococcal toxaemia in burned children. Burns 19: 22–25.

McDonald WS, Sharp CW, Deitch EA (1991) Immediate enteral feeding in burn patients is safe and effective. Annals of Surgery 213: 177–83.

Ministry of Health (1959) Report of the Committee on the Welfare of Children in Hospital (Platt Report). London: HMSO.

Muller DJ, Harris PJ, Wattleys L et al. (1992) Nursing Children – Psychology and Research in Practice. 2nd edn. London: Chapman and Hall.

Pearce S (1989) Researching burns and scalds. Paediatric Nursing 1(10): 13.

Piaget J, Inhelder B (1969) The Psychology of the Child. London: Routledge and Kegan Paul.

Reid C (1996) Paediatric Burns. In Settle JAD, (Ed) Principles and Practice of Burns Management. Edinburgh: Churchill Livingstone. pp 377–84.

Royal College of Paediatrics and Child Health (1997) Prevention and control of pain in children. London: British Medical Journal Publishing.

Secretary of State for Health (1997) The New NHS: Modern, Dependable. London: The Stationery Office.

Settle JAD (1996) Principles and Practice of Burns Management. Edinburgh: Churchill Livingstone.

Swanwick M (1990) Knowledge and control. Paediatric Nursing 2(5): 18.

Trofino RB (1991) Nursing Care of the Burn Injured Patient. Philadelphia: FA Davis.

Wilson GR, Fowler CA, Housden PL (1987) A new burn area assessment chart. Burns 13(5): 410–15.

Young A, Manara A, Burd DA (1995) Intensive care management of the child with burns. Care of the Critically Ill 11(3): 93–97.

CHAPTER 4

Management in the first 48 hours following Burn Trauma

DAVID WILSON

Introduction

An estimated 2 000 000 people are burned each year. Of these 70 000 require hospitalization and 6–9000 die of their injuries. Until the middle of the twentieth century a massive burn was universally fatal, death being due to 'burns toxaemia'. It is only in the last 50 years that the pathophysiology of burns 'shock' has been appreciated, and appropriate treatment regimes established. The chances of surviving massive burns today are much improved, but without appropriate treatment the outlook is no better than at the turn of the century.

This chapter outlines the management necessary in the first 48 hours including the initial assessment and history taking. Fluid and electrolyte management will be discussed, as well as the systemic effects on the patient, and methods of monitoring and minimizing potential complications during the resuscitation phase.

Although much of the treatment starts, and complications may arise in the first 48 hours, there is no natural break in the clinical situation. Treatment continues until the wound is closed and beyond, and complications can occur anywhere along the way.

First Aid

If you should be unlucky enough to be the first at the scene of a burn injury, the initial step is to prevent further injury to the casualty. This may simply mean removing them from the source of the heat, or extinguishing burning clothes. Clothing soaked in hot fluid acts like a hot poultice and should therefore be removed if not adherent to the wound, or cooled with cold water. Cooling in other circumstances is of debatable value, and although it may soothe the burn may also induce hypothermia. However, prompt application of cold water to a burn eases pain (Davies, 1982) and according to Lawrence (1986) quenches residual heat thus reducing tissue damage caused by the burning or scalding agent. The current first aid treatment recommended by the British Burn Association is prompt cooling of the burn with copious amounts of tap water for 10–20 mins (Lawrence, 1987; Lawrence, 1996). The application of a temporary dressing, e.g. cling-film, may then be appropriate in preparation for transfer of the individual to the Accident and Emergency Department. However, initiating these measures should certainly not delay the transport of the patient to hospital.

The Accident and Emergency Department

As with any other trauma patient, initial management in the Accident and Emergency Department should be interlinked with the guidelines laid down by advanced trauma and life support (ATLS) courses.

- *Airway.* Ensure that the patient has a patent airway and no breathing difficulties. Severe facial burns and/or a history of inhalation injury should raise the question of ventilatory support and an anaesthetic review should be requested. High flow oxygen by a non-rebreathing face mask should be applied as an interim measure.
- *Circulation.* The circulatory state should be checked with pulse and blood pressure readings, and signs of shock should be elicited. Clinical signs of shock in the first few hours after injury are more likely to be due to other injuries than the burn.
- *History.* A brief history of the events should be obtained including the time and nature of the accident.
- *Examination.* A brief general examination should be performed, assessing the conscious state, presence of other significant injuries or illnesses and the extent of the burn injury. From this the need for admission and/or intravenous fluids can be obtained. Children with a burn of 10% or more body surface area and adults with 15% or more require intravenous fluids, but smaller burns may need admission because of the site or severity.
- *Intravenous access.* If intravenous fluids are required, good access is essential. Large bore peripheral cannulae, which can be inserted through burned skin if necessary, are preferable. Cut-downs onto large

veins may be necessary if the patient is peripherally shut down, but central vein cannulation is best avoided if possible. In children, and occasionally in adults, intraosseous access may be necessary which will allow initial resuscitation until definitive access is obtained. Fluid infusion may then be commenced with either plasma or a suitable plasma expander.

- *Blood samples.* These can often be taken at the same time as the intravenous access is being established. Urea and electrolytes, full blood count and a haematocrit should be requested. In large percentage burn injuries the patient should also be blood grouped, and if there is a possibility of an inhalation injury, carboxyhaemoglobin levels and arterial blood gases should also be taken. In children, consider the blood glucose.
- *Analgesia.* Intravenous opiates are the analgesics of choice as they can be titrated against the patient's pain. Oral or intramuscular drugs will have erratic absorption during the 'shock' phase and will give poor pain control. Inhalational agents such as Entonox may also be helpful.
- *Catheterization.* If the burn area is in excess of 10% of body surface area in children, 15% in adults, or involves the perineum, the passage of a urinary catheter should considered. The volume of urine drained at this time should also be measured.
- *The individual's general condition* should be reassessed, looking for any change in the general state of the patient and ensuring that the airway is still patent and the infusions running. Other injuries should also be reassessed.
- *The burn* should be assessed using the Lund and Browder (1944) chart or the percentage by age charts (Wilson et al., 1987) to determine its size, and an attempt should be made to differentiate partial and full thickness burns. The need for escharotomies should also be evaluated when circumferential burns are evident on the neck, trunk or limbs.
- *Wound dressing.* If the patient is to be transferred to a Burns Unit, a temporary wound dressing should be applied. Ideally, this should be easy to apply and remove, painless on removal, non-stick, sterile and water-proof. Cling-film, as advocated by Wilson and French (1987), fulfils most of these criteria and is also very cheap. If the patient is to be discharged, a definitive dressing should be applied.
- *Transfer* should be arranged if required, but only once the above measures have been taken and the patient is fit for transfer. The Burns Unit is often some distance away, so the patient's condition should be stable and all intravenous lines carefully secured for the journey. If the

patient is intubated, an anaesthetist will have to accompany them and the availability of an intensive care bed at the receiving hospital should be checked before departure.

The Burns Unit

The immediate aspects of management should all have been commenced in the Accident and Emergency department (unless the patient is admitted directly) and need to be continued by the burns team. The first priority is to check:

- the airway
- that the intravenous infusion is running
- the urinary catheter
- analgesia
- blood samples
- the patient's weight

If any of these matters have not yet been addressed, now is the time to do it. Once this has been completed, a more detailed history and examination can be performed and the fluid requirements calculated.

History

Probably the first step in treating any trauma patient is to establish the history of the event. The treatment of the burns patient is no different.

The main points to establish are the time of the accident (as all the resuscitation formulae start from this point, rather than the time the patient is first seen), and the causal agents. These may be roughly divided into four groups: wet, dry, chemical or electrical. Knowing the causal agent will often help in estimating the severity of the burn.

- **Wet** burns are generally scald injuries from hot fluids or steam, and account for a large proportion of burn injuries, especially in the under-5-year-olds.
- **Dry** burns occur from flame or hot objects, which may be from direct contact or radiated heat, and are more common in adults.
- **Chemical** burns arise from a variety of substances, usually acid or alkali, which may continue to burn long after the initial exposure. The severity of the injury depends on the strength of the chemical involved, duration of exposure and any first aid that was given. The main treat-

ment for most chemicals is removal of the agent by copious irrigation, but some have specific treatments, e.g. phosphorus burns and hydrofluoric acid burns. If there is any doubt about the type of chemical involved, specialist advice should be sought from the manufacturer or Guy's Hospital Poisons Unit, London.

- **Electrical** injuries may have an element of thermal damage, either from direct contact or from a flash injury, as well as an electrocution injury. Where an electrocution injury is suspected, entry and exit wounds should be sought and an ECG performed to check for arrhythmias. If there is any abnormality on the ECG they should be admitted for 24-hour cardiac monitoring. If the ECG is normal and the burn small, they may not require admission.

Not only is the type of burn important, but the length of exposure will also determine the severity. A flash of intense heat may only produce erythema or superficial damage, whereas prolonged exposure to relatively low heat can still cause full thickness damage. Removal of clothing soaked in hot liquid is important as it may retain heat and thus increase the depth of the burn.

Having established the nature and timing of the burn, it is important to establish the circumstances of the accident. Fires in enclosed spaces carry a significant risk of inhalation injuries. Accidents at work may be open to negligence claims if safety measures were not enforced. There may be predisposing factors either at the place of the accident or in the patient themselves, e.g. epilepsy and diabetes. Not all burn injuries are accidental, and this applies equally to adults as well as children, with increasing numbers of reports of abuse of the elderly. In adults, self-harm and assault victims form a significant number of admissions, and it may be necessary in these cases to involve other agencies such as the police or psychiatric services.

Non-accidental injury (NAI) in children should always be suspected where the injury and history do not tally. A past history of injuries and signs of old injuries such as bruising, healed burns, etc. should also raise suspicion. If there is any doubt, the child should be admitted whilst the social services are alerted, the 'At risk' register checked, and review by a paediatrician arranged. Any injuries found should also be photographed at this stage for future reference. If at all possible, all this should be done without arousing the suspicions of the parents, who can be unnecessarily distressed by unfounded claims of NAI when already feeling guilt over the accident.

As with any other trauma patient we should not be tempted to concentrate only on the obvious problem. It is all too easy to miss other injuries or medical conditions unless they are specifically elicited. These may predate the accident or have occurred at the same time, often playing a role in the cause of the injury; examples are fractures sustained while escaping from the fire or from a road traffic accident, the elderly patient who collapses with a myocardial infarction or cerebrovascular accident while cooking. These other conditions may be more serious than the burn injury, which may well take secondary importance, and treatment should be tailored appropriately.

A full history of the patient's past medical problems is also relevant as this may well influence their subsequent treatment. Any medications taken should be fully documented, along with any allergies and their tetanus status (if the patient is not covered, immunization is required).

Assessment

The initial assessment of the burn injury is performed in the Accident and Emergency Department and is mainly a form of triage. Burns of over 10% total body surface area in children and 15% in adults require admission for intravenous resuscitation. The British Burn Association criteria for referral to a Burns Unit also include the following:

- burns of the face, hands, feet, perineum or major joints
- full thickness burns over 5% total body surface area
- electrical burns
- chemical burns
- burns with associated inhalation injury
- circumferential burns of the limbs or trunk
- burns with associated trauma
- patients with pre-existing medical conditions that may complicate management

Assessment of the burn injury involves assessment of both the body surface area and depth of the burn. Depth may be classified as erythema, superficial partial thickness, deep partial thickness, or full thickness burns as described in Chapter 2. In some countries 'degrees' of burn are used, but this can be confusing as definitions vary. Estimating depth takes into account the appearance of the burn, capillary return and sensation. Erythema is generally ignored as it does not require treatment and does not affect the fluid losses (unless very extensive). Superficial partial thickness burns are often blistered, painful and pink, with a good capillary return. Deep partial thickness burns may be blistered, have a deeper red or mottled appearance which does not readily blanch, and may have reduced sensation. Full thickness burns are pain-free, feel tough and leathery with no capillary function at all (Kemble and Lamb, 1987).

Various methods have been described for assessing the area of the burn injury, and, as several studies have shown, the area is often miscalculated by as much as 60% or more. The simplest guide to area is to use the patient's hand which, from the distal wrist crease to the finger tips, represents 1% of the body surface (Kirby and Blackburn, 1987). This is useful when estimating small areas, however it is not practical when dealing with large ones.

The Rule of Nines was advocated by Wallace in 1951 (Kyle and Wallace, 1951) and is accurate enough for most practical purposes as well as being easy to remember. The body is essentially divided into parts that represent 9%, or multiples thereof, of the total body surface area, leaving 1% for the genitalia (see Figure 2.5: p20). However, it cannot be applied to children under 10 years old unless modified to account for their differing body proportions.

More accurate estimations can be gained by using the Lund and Browder charts (Lund and Browder, 1944) available in most Accident and Emergency Departments (see Figure 2.6: p21) or the Percentage by Age charts (Wilson et al., 1987; see Figures 2.7a–h: pp22–25). Both rely on accurate drawing of the burn onto a chart, the areas then being added up. The latter charts are more accurate, as they come in a range from baby to adult sizing, adjusted for the changing ratios of head to body and limbs.

Not only should the area and depth of the burn be assessed, but the site of the burn may well be relevant to the admission. Burns of certain areas such as the hands, feet, face and genitalia require specific treatment as detailed in Chapter 6. Involvement of the eyes may require a specialist opinion, and fluorescein staining to exclude corneal damage should be carried out early before the lids swell. Where there has been extensive or deep burns of the eyelids, temporary tarsorrhaphy and/or early skin grafting may be necessary to prevent exposure of the cornea.

Where there are circumferential full thickness burns on a limb or the trunk, escharotomies may be needed. Areas of full thickness burn where the skin elasticity has been lost will not stretch as the underlying tissues swell following the injury. Where this is circumferential it will lead to a tourniquet effect, raising tissue pressure and reducing blood flow distally.

This may then lead on to necrosis and loss of the distal part. Where the burns affect the chest, they may interfere with ventilation.

To allow the areas to swell without these problems requires release of the burned area by splitting the burnt tissue down to normal tissues, a technique known as escharotomy. As full thickness burns are anaesthetic, little analgesia is required. The incision should be made through the burnt skin along the entire length into unburned skin (which may require local anaesthesia) and down to healthy tissues avoiding major cutaneous and digital nerves. Often the patient will gain considerable relief from this process as ischaemic tissues are extremely painful.

Evidence of inhalation injury should again be assessed, especially if there are facial burns. Singeing of nasal hairs, soot in the mouth or throat, hoarseness or stridor are all significant signs and indications for intubation. The marked swelling of the face and neck following injury may in itself lead to airway obstruction and be an indication for early intubation. If there is any doubt, an anaesthetic opinion should be sought earlier rather than later. Inhalational injuries are dealt with in more detail in Chapter 7.

Having fully assessed the burn wound itself, a full medical examination of the patient should be made looking for any associated illnesses as outlined earlier.

Fluid Requirements

Fluid loss occurs both from the burn surface as exudate and blister fluid, and into the surrounding tissues as oedema. This loss is mainly of plasma and is greatest over the first 8 hours following injury, but continues until the capillaries recover at about 36 hours. Overall, these losses can be predicted fairly accurately and this forms the basis of the various fluid replacement regimes.

Fluid loss as the cause of 'burns shock', rather than toxins released from the burned tissue, was first proposed by Underhill et al. (1923), but it was not until 20 years later that this theory was widely accepted. Various formulae were subsequently described to calculate the volumes of fluid replacement necessary (Figure 4.1: Harkins et al., 1942; Cope and Moore, 1947; Baxter, 1981). Evans et al. (1952) produced the first widely publicized formula, relating fluid requirement to the size of the burn and the size of the patient. Equal parts of plasma and saline were used, giving two thirds of the total in the first 24 hours, and the remaining third in the second 24. The Brooke formula (Reiss et al., 1953) gives 3ml/kg/% BSA burn, but uses less plasma and an increased rate of infusion. This trend continued in America with Moyer in 1965 (Moyer et al., 1965) and Baxter in 1968 (Baxter and Shires, 1968). This formula used 4ml/kg/% BSA burn of Ringer's Lactate in the first 24 hours with no colloid at all, giving half in the first 8 hours and half over the next 16 hours. In the UK, Muir and Barclay (1962) continued to use plasma in the Mount Vernon Formula, and this is still widely used today in many units in the UK.

$$\text{Volume/period} = \frac{\text{Total \% area of burn} \times \text{weight (kg)}}{2}$$

Brooke	Day 1	- 0.5ml/kg/% colloid + 1.5ml/kg/% crystalloid - half in first 8 hours, half in next 16 hours.
	Day 2	- 0.25ml/kg/% colloid + 0.5ml/kg/% crystalloid Maintenance - 2000ml/m2 of 5% Dextrose.
Modified Brooke		No colloid. No maintenance.
	Day 1	- 2ml/kg/% for adult or 3ml/kg/% for children - half in first 8 hours, half in next 16 hours.
	Day 2	- 0.3-0.5ml/kg/% of colloid. No crystalloid.
Parkland	Day 1	- 4ml/kg/% Ringers Lactate. No colloid or maintenance - half in first 8 hours, half in next 16 hours.
	Day 2	- 700-2000ml colloid to maintain urine output. No crystalloid and 5% Dextrose maintenance fluids.
Evans	Day 1	-1ml/kg/% colloid + 1ml/kg/% Ringers Lactate half in first 8 hours, half in next 16 hours. plus 5% Dextrose 2000ml/m²
	Day 2	- 0.5ml/kg/% colloid + 0.5ml/kg/% Ringers Lactate.
Bull & Jackson	Day 1	- 1-1.5 litres/10% plasma (1952) half in first 8 hours, half in next 16 hours.
	Day 2	- half this volume over 24 hours. Children - one plasma volume/15% given as above.
Sorensen (1971)		120ml/% Dextran 70 in adults. Half in 8 hours, quarter in next 16 and quarter in next 24 hours. Plus 50ml/kg 5% Dextrose maintenance.
Monafo		250mEq Na, 150mEq Lactate, 100mEq Cl titrated to (1970) urine flow + liberal 'free water' by mouth.

Figure 4.1 Burn Formulae.

The 36 hours is divided into periods of 4, 4, 4, 6, 6, and 12 hours and the calculated volume is infused in each period, starting from the time of the injury, not the time the infusion started (Figure 4.2).

There is still debate over the best fluids to use and the best formula (Demling, 1987). In general there are three schools of thought: (a) protein should be given from the start along with crystalloid; (b) protein should not be given in the first 24 hours as it is no more effective than salt water during this time; and (c) protein infusion should be started between 8 and 12 hours, using crystalloid or non-protein colloid in the first 8 to 12 hours as most of the fluid shifts occur during this time (Moncrief, 1972). In general, during the first 48 hours the patient needs about 0.5mmol Na/kg/% BSA burn and 2–4ml fluid/kg/% BSA burn, at least half of which is given in the first twelve hours (Settle, 1982).

In America crystalloids are mostly used, while in the UK it is mainly colloids in the form of albumin solutions, Human Albumin Solution (HAS) or Human Plasma Protein Fraction (HPPF). Both methods are equally successful, but it is claimed there is less oedema with colloids and thus fewer complications with ulcers, paralytic ileus, pulmonary problems and compartment syndrome. However, colloids are expensive and carry the theoretical risk of all blood products for infection transmission

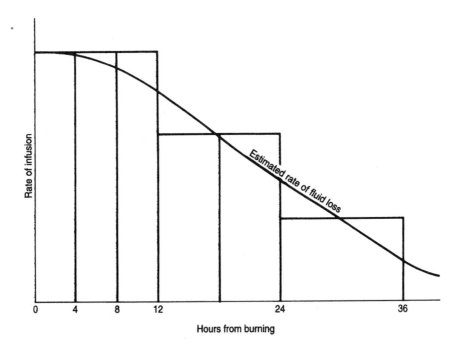

Figure 4.2 Estimated rate of fluid loss.

although HAS is heat treated to destroy infective particles. The viability and transfer of prion particles which cause CJD in humans is also a cause for concern. The Cochrane report of 1998 has also thrown the use of albumin in to debate (Cole, 1999).

All the formulae are only guidelines and a point from which to start. Frequent reassessment and adjustment is required for an uneventful resuscitation. At any time during the resuscitation period, the plasma deficit can be calculated from the following formula:

$$\text{deficit} = \text{blood vol.} - (\text{blood vol.} \times \text{normal haematocrit/observed haematocrit})$$

Blood volume (ml) is regarded as being approximately 70 × weight (kg) for adults, and 80 x weight (kg) for children.

Thus, if at any stage the calculated fluid volumes do not seem to be adequate, the plasma deficit can be calculated and this amount added to the fluids being given to correct the deficit.

Maintenance fluids

As well as to compensate for fluid losses from the burn wound, the patient needs fluids for normal metabolic requirements. This requirement is related to extra renal and evaporative losses, and is increased if the wound is exposed or the patient pyrexial. In the first 24 hours, there will be antidiuretic hormone secretion as part of the 'stress response', and it may be wise to restrict water intake during this time to about 100ml/hour for adults (starting at about 60ml/hour and increasing to 100ml/hour if there are no problems; Baxter, 1974); children's needs will be considered below.

Burns of more than 25% of total body surface area are often accompanied by some degree of paralytic ileus, so that absorption from the gut is greatly reduced, and vomiting often occurs. It may be better to keep these patients nil by mouth initially until normal gut function is restored. However, in many units a policy of early feeding is being advocated; this will be discussed further in Chapter 10. In burns greater than 20% surface area, it is advisable to pass a nasogastric tube and to aspirate hourly.

Patients with burns between 10% and 15% of total body surface area should be able to tolerate fluids orally, but if there is vomiting, the maintenance fluid should be given intravenously. Sodium-free solutions should be avoided, especially in children, as there is a significant risk of hyponatraemia and water intoxication (Batchelor et al., 1961). This leads to cellular overhydration, which may play a role in burns encephalopathy, where there is cerebral irritability, increased temperature, vomiting, fits and eventual coma. In children, it is thus best to use salt-containing solutions such as Dioralyte or milk for maintenance fluids and avoid salt-free solutions such as fruit juice/squash (Carvajal, 1980).

Maintenance requirements for children are:

<10kg	100ml/kg/hr
10–15kg	90ml/kg/hr
15–20kg	80ml/kg/hr
20–25kg	70ml/kg/hr
25–30kg	60ml/kg/hr

If intravenous resuscitation is also in progress, this maintenance volume should be reduced to 75% of the total and this maintenance fluid restriction should continue for the first five days post-burn.

Oral resuscitation

In burns of less than 10% of surface area in children and 15% in adults, oral resuscitation is usually adequate. However, unless the burn is trivial, input and output should still be monitored and, if the burn is near the critical level, the patient should be regularly reassessed. Also, some areas such as the face lose fluid out of proportion to the size of the burn.

Hypotonic solutions are tolerated better than isotonic solutions by mouth and are thus used for this group of patients. Moyer's solution of 3g salt + 1.5g sodium bicarbonate per litre ($\frac{1}{2}$ teaspoon salt + $\frac{1}{2}$ teaspoon bicarbonate in 2 pints) is a suitable solution (Moyer, 1953), and this can be flavoured to make it more palatable.

Requirement for Blood

Muir (1961) showed the relationship between red cell destruction and the extent of the full thickness burn. Some cells are actually destroyed by the heat of the burn, and, if this happens in significant numbers, it will be manifest by haemoglobinuria. Others are rendered fragile, so that they are removed from the circulation during the next few hours. However, even in burns of more than 50% of surface area, this loss does not exceed 10% of the total red cell volume. During the main part of the shock phase, further loss continues, for reasons that are not entirely clear.

In general, where there is a large area of full thickness burn there will
be a significant fall in haemoglobin concentration, and the patient will
require transfusion. Where the area of full thickness loss exceeds 10%, the
blood requirement is 1% of the patient's normal blood volume for each
1% of full thickness burn. For an adult this works out at about one unit of
blood for every 10% full thickness burn over and above 10% BSA burn.
This is usually given in the sixth period so that it does not interfere with
the monitoring during the early stages.

Monitoring

Monitoring of the burns patient is mainly aimed at detecting the signs of
shock so that it can be treated appropriately to avoid more serious
complications (Demling, 1987).

- **Restlessness** is often a sign of oligaemia and is especially useful in
  children, although it may have other causes.
- **Skin colour** is also of use. Pink skin indicates dilated arterioles and an
  adequate circulation, whereas pallor indicates constricted arterioles. A
  bluish tinge indicates stagnation of blood in capillaries that are dilated,
  and is a bad sign in the severely shocked patient.
- **Pulse and blood pressure** are recorded routinely. Many factors
  affect the pulse rate, so that trends in the rate are more important than
  hourly fluctuations. A fall in the blood pressure is a late sign, and
  monitoring of blood pressure is of less value than other parameters.
- **Skin and deep body temperature** can be recorded, a difference in
  the two shows a degree of vasoconstriction. As the patient's condition
  improves, the gap narrows (normally 1–4°C). The skin temperature is
  relatively easy to measure, whilst the core temperature is measured
  either rectally or using probes attached to the catheter or in the external auditory meatus.
- **Urine output** reflects the perfusion of the kidney and is thus a useful
  measurement. However, in the early stages, the output will be affected
  by antidiuretic hormone (ADH), catecholamines and angiotensin,
  which are secreted as part of the 'stress response'. Thus, there may be
  wide variation in hourly volumes, so that it is important to note the
  concentration as well to make sense of the readings. ADH is present
  for the first 24 hours after injury, so the urine is more concentrated
  than the filtrate, and the osmolarity will be 2–3 times higher than that
  of the plasma (approximately 300mOsmol/litre). An adequate flow is

0.5–1.0ml/hour per kg body weight. Low flow with concentrated urine indicates inadequate resuscitation, whereas reduced concentration and a high flow indicates overtransfusion (Settle, 1974).

- **The haematocrit** is a measure of the proportion of red cells to plasma volume expressed as either a percentage or a fraction. A raised haematocrit almost always indicates a low plasma volume, but a normal or low reading does not necessarily mean adequate resuscitation (other factors, such as anaemia, may play a role). Again, absolute values are less relevant than the trend over several readings. Measurements can be made from a skin prick and collecting the blood in a capillary tube, which is then centrifuged. The haematocrit can then be measured directly.

- **Central venous pressure** (CVP) readings are used extensively in the treatment of major trauma where there are rapid changes in the haemodynamic state of the patient. In burns shock, the changes are more gradual so that this type of invasive monitoring is seldom necessary and has been shown to be inaccurate. There is also the risk of infection in the burn patient as well as the other risks from placement of the cannula. Where this type of monitoring is needed, pulmonary artery pressure is probably a better guide than CVP, but requires placement of a Swann-Ganz catheter.

- **Gut absorption** is affected by the circulatory state, and burns of 20% total body surface area or greater are more likely to have a degree of paralytic ileus. This may present as vomiting or large amounts of aspirate if a nasogastric tube has been passed. Once adequate resuscitation is under way, gut function will return and many people advocate early feeding to reduce the risk of bacterial translocation and subsequent sepsis.

Analgesia

Adequate analgesia is essential in the treatment of burns and is dealt with more fully in Chapter 8. As most people know, even a small burn can be excruciatingly painful, but where the burn is deep, it will be relatively pain free. In the initial stages of treatment, an analgesic is required which gives good pain control, is easily adjustable, and has some sedative effects. Oral and intramuscular drugs will have an erratic absorption during the resuscitation period, so that the intravenous route is the route of choice. An ideal method of pain control is the Diamorphine infusion, which can be titrated against the patient's symptoms and increased or reduced as necessary.

Entonox is a useful adjuvant, and can be used in both adults and children by self administration.

Dressing the burn wound reduces much of the discomfort from the injury, and is often quite soothing once the dressings are in place. The types of dressings used and their management are discussed in Chapter 6.

Complications

Complications can arise at any stage in the treatment of the burn patient, and may loosely be divided into early and late complications. At this stage, we will deal mainly with those complications arising in the first few days after injury. However, many of the problems occurring later have their roots in the early management of the patient.

Renal Failure

Renal failure is largely preventable with adequate resuscitation, and acute tubular necrosis due to hypovolaemia should rarely be seen. However, patients with a burn of 20% or more of total body surface area often have a degree of renal impairment, due to mixed tubular and glomerular damage which manifests itself as proteinuria in the first few days after injury. The severity of the damage varies from minor with no adverse effects, to severe with acute oligaemic renal failure where there is low flow, fixed osmolarity, low urinary urea: blood urea ratio, low urinary creatinine with rising blood creatinine and urea.

Occasionally high output renal failure occurs which is harder to detect as there is a good flow of urine. However the blood urea rises, with a urine concentration of 350–400mOsmol/litre, and a urinary:blood urea ratio of less than 10.

Treatment of renal failure in the burns patient can be complicated and often requires CVP monitoring to assess the fluid balance, as the urine output cannot be used. Overtransfusion is relatively easy to do and can lead to pulmonary oedema unless there is careful monitoring. In nonoliguric failure it may be possible to promote a diuresis with osmotic diuretics, but if this fails then dialysis will be necessary. Haemodialysis, peritoneal dialysis, or haemofiltration may be used depending on the patient's condition and the skills available.

Where there are large areas of full thickness burns or electrical burns, haemoglobinuria or myoglobinuria may occur and will be detected by discolouration of the urine. If this occurs, it is essential to maintain a good urine flow to clear these substances. If this is not done, they will precipitate in the renal tubules leading to tubular damage and renal failure. If simple measures such as increasing the resuscitation fluids are not successful, alkalinization of the urine or the use of Mannitol (an osmotic diuretic) may be considered. However, only one dose of Mannitol should be used as it may precipitate pulmonary oedema if not excreted.

Respiratory Complications

Respiratory complications in the early stages of care may arise from inhalational burns and the toxic products of combustion, or respiratory distress syndrome may develop later. These will be dealt with in greater depth in Chapter 7.

Electrolyte Disturbances

Electrolyte disturbances are not uncommon in the burns patient during the first few days and, with the volumes of fluid transfused over this time, not entirely unexpected (Baxter, 1974). The main emphasis at this time should be on maintaining adequate volume replacement, as once the patient is taking a normal diet, and providing that renal function is normal, any imbalance will soon be corrected. In some patients, however, there is an abnormality of the cell membranes which allows potassium to leak out and sodium to leak in to the cell in abnormal quantities – the so-called 'sick-cell syndrome' – in which the patients become restless, disorientated and overbreathe. This may be difficult to detect, as plasma levels of electrolytes are often normal, but the sodium:potassium ratio in the urine may be reversed. The first step in treatment is to correct any cause of tissue hypoxia, such as unrecognized anaemia, and the administration of glucose and insulin has been shown to be beneficial.

Infection

Infection is a serious problem and in large burns may lead to overwhelming sepsis. The burn wound is a large open area rich in nutrients and devoid of bodily defences in the eschar, which makes it ideal for colonization once contamination has occurred. Infection only occurs when there are enough organisms present to invade healthy tissue which will lead to sepsis and septicaemia.

In large burns, there is a degree of immunosuppression with a temporary failure of the local cellular defences, leading to reduced phagacytosis and clearance by the reticulo-endothelial system and impaired response to antigens. The loss of immunoglobulins is transient, but lymphocyte and T-cell activity is reduced by substances released by damaged tissue and bacteria, which allows organisms such as *Staphylococcus aureus,* haemolytic *Streptococcus, Pseudomonas* and *Acinetobacter* to thrive.

The main way to avoid these problems is prevention, using aseptic techniques at all stages. The burn wound is initially sterile, and the aim should be to keep it that way. Wound dressings should be performed in a clean environment, with gloves and gowns being worn; dead tissue removed and the wound irrigated before the dressings are applied. Ideally, single cubicles with positive pressure ventilation should be used, with care in hand-washing, etc. to prevent contamination. The use of prophylactic antibiotics is not generally recommended as this encourages the emergence of resistant strains of bacteria, but Flucloxacillin is often used in children to prevent staphylococcal colonization and the potential development of toxic shock syndrome. Early surgery, with the removal of the eschar and skin grafting before colonization occurs, is a good ideal, but is not always possible to achieve.

The maintenance of adequate nutrition is essential, as is regular bacterial surveillance, wound swabs being taken at every dressing change. The treatment of established infection involves the use of topical and systemic antibiotics, and surgical excision of the eschar.

Gastric and Duodenal Ulceration

Gastric and duodenal ulceration has been described in burn patients and can lead to serious complications. Superficial erosions are common in the first few days and may be related to vasoconstriction with reduced blood flow to the mucosa in the shock phase. True duodenal ulceration (Curling's ulcer) usually develops 10–14 days post burn. Treatment is again aimed at prevention, with the use of sucralfate (a coating agent), H_2 antagonists, e.g. cimetidine or ranitidine, and early feeding regimes.

Red Cell Destruction

Red cell destruction occurs to some degree in all deep burns but seldom leads to a loss of more than 10% of red cells. In some cases, there is a rapidly increasing loss due to increased red cell fragility, which shows as a failure to respond to treatment despite a falling haematocrit. There will also be haemoglobinuria occurring after 12 hours, either for the first time or after a period of clear urine. Treatment is to replace the losses which may mean massive transfusion.

Glycosuria

Glycosuria is not uncommon, and is usually transient, lasting about 48 hours, and with no associated ketonuria. There may be exacerbation of pre-existing diabetes with glycosuria, ketonuria and raised blood sugar levels which should be treated symptomatically.

Occasionally, gross hyperglycaemia and glycosuria develop several days after the injury, as a result of adrenal cortical overactivity. This pseudo-diabetes of burns is insulin resistant and treatment is supportive with high calorie intake to reduce the muscle wasting until normality returns.

Liver and Pancreas

Liver failure, liver necrosis and pancreatitis have all been described in severe burns, and are probably due to oligaemic problems and subsequent ischaemia.

Toxic Shock Syndrome

Toxic shock syndrome has been described in burnt children and is not related to the burn size (Frame et al., 1985). It is due to toxins released by a specific phage type of *Staphylococcus aureus* which colonizes the burn wound. Adults are rarely affected, as they have usually been exposed to the toxin and have the appropriate antibodies. The syndrome develops very rapidly, from the first signs of pyrexia, rash, diarrhoea and vomiting, to complete circulatory collapse and death. There is also a falling platelet and white cell count, although blood cultures are negative. Treatment is the administration of fresh frozen plasma (which contains antibodies), antibiotics and supportive measures until the child recovers. Treatment should be started early if the condition is suspected as the progression is very rapid.

Burns Encephalopathy

Burns encephalopathy has also been described in burnt children and again may develop rapidly. It is thought to result from cellular overhydration and hyponatraemia following the administration of excess salt-poor fluids during the resuscitation period. This can lead to cerebral oedema, with reduced levels of consciousness and fitting. For this reason the use of water or salt-free solutions is not recommended when treating burned children.

Metabolic Effects of Burns

After any serious injury, including burns, there is a change from the normal anabolic storage state to one of catabolic breakdown. There is a greatly increased energy expenditure, leading to increased nutritional requirements, which are further increased by, for example, stress, anxiety, heat loss, dressing changes and anaesthetics. In a burn of 50% body surface area, the basal metabolic rate may double, this change persisting until the patient is virtually healed. To maintain the energy supply, the body draws on all the available stores, including muscle.

Any trauma leads to a release of catecholamines, which act to increase the levels of circulating glucose, leading in turn to raised levels of insulin, glucagon, growth hormone and glucocorticoids. Glucagon acts to increase gluconeogenesis, which is largely from the substrates of muscle breakdown and proteolysis, as fat is a relatively poor source of substrates. The excess nitrogen released is then excreted in the urine and can be used as a measure of protein breakdown. Maintaining adequate nutrition and calorie intake can reduce the amount of protein lost and prevent the gross wasting seen in some burns patients. Early feeding regimes and the nutritional aspects of treatment are discussed in greater depth in Chapter 10.

References

Batchelor ADR, Kirk J, Sutherland A (1961) The treatment of shock in the burnt child. Lancet (Jan): 123–27.

Baxter CR, Shires T (1968) Physiological response to crystalloid resuscitation of severe burns. Annals of the New York Academy of Science 150: 874.

Baxter CR (1974) Fluid volume and electrolyte changes in the early post-burn period. Clinics in Plastic Surgery 1: 693.

Baxter CR (1981) Guidelines for fluid resuscitation. Journal of Trauma 21: 667.

Carvajal HF (1980) A physiological approach to fluid therapy in severely burned children. Surgery, Gynaecology and Obstetrics 150: 379–84.

Cochrane Injuries Group Albumin Reviewers (1998) Human albumin administration in critically ill patients: systematic review of randomised controlled trials. British Medical Journal 317: 235–40.

Cole RP (1999) The UK albumin debate. Burns 27(7): 565–68.

Cope O, Moore FD (1947) The redistribution of body water and the fluid therapy of the burned patient. Annals of Surgery 126: 1010–45.

Davies JWL (1982) Prompt cooling of burned areas. A review of the benefits and the effector mechanisms. Burns Journal 9: 1–6.

Demling RH (1987) Fluid replacement in burned patients. Surgical Clinics of North America 67: 15–22.

Evans IE, Purnell OJ, Robinett PW et al. (1952) Fluid and electrolyte requirements in severe burns. Annals of Surgery 135: 804–17.

Frame JD, Eve MD, Hackett MEJ et al. (1985) The toxic shock syndrome in burned children. Burns 11: 234–41.

Harkins HN, Lam CR, Romence H (1942) Plasma therapy in severe burns. Surgery, Obstetrics and Gynaecology 75: 410.

Kyle MJ, Wallace AB (1951) Fluid replacement in burnt children. British Journal of Plastic Surgery 3: 194.

Lund CC, Browder NC (1944) Estimation of areas of burns. Surgery, Gynaecology and Obstetrics 79: 352.

Monafo WW (1970), The treatment of burns shock by intravenous and oral administration of hypertonic lactated solution. Journal of Trauma 10: 575.

Moncrief JA (1972) Burn formulae. Journal of Trauma 12: 538.

Moyer CA (1953) An assessment of the therapy of burns. Annals of Surgery 137: 628–38.

Moyer CA, Margraf HW, Monafo WW (1965) Burn shock and extravascular sodium deficiency – treatment with Ringer's solution with lactate. Archives of Surgery 90: 799–811.

Muir IFK (1961) Red cell destruction in burns. British Journal of Plastic Surgery 14: 273.

Muir IFK, Barclay TL (1962) Treatment of burn shock. In Muir IFK, Barclay TL, (Eds) Burns and their Treatment. London: Lloyd Luke.

Reiss E, Stirman JA, Artz CP et al. (1953) Fluid and electrolyte balance in burns. Journal of American Medical Associates 152: 1309–13.

Settle JAD (1974) Urine output following severe burns. Burns 1: 23–42.

Settle JAD (1982) Fluid therapy in burns. Journal of the Royal Society of Medicine 75(1): 1–11.

Wilson GR, French G (1987) Plasticised polyvinyl chloride as a temporary dressing for burns. British Medical Journal 294: 556–57.

Wilson GR, Fowler CA, Housden PL (1987) A new burn assessment chart. Burns 13: 401–5.

Underhill FP, Carrington GL, Kapsinow R et al. (1923) Blood concentration changes in extensive superficial burns, and their significance for systemic treatment. Archives of Internal Medicine 32: 31–48.

Further reading

Cason JS (1981) Treatment of Burns. London: Chapman and Hall.

Clarke JA (1992) A Colour Atlas of Burn Injuries. London: Chapman and Hall.

Emergency Management of Severe Burns. Course manual: British Burn Association.

Kemble JVH, Lamb B (1987) Practical Burns Management. London: Hodder and Stoughton.

Kirby NG, Blackburn G (1987) Freid Surgery Pocket Book. London: HMSO.

Lawrence JC (1986) The causes of burns in burncare. A teaching symposium. Hull: Smith and Nephew Ltd.

Lawrence JC (1987) British Burns Association recommended First Aid for burns and scalds. Burns Journal 13: 153.

Lawrence JC (1996) First aid measures for treatment of burns and scalds. Journal of Wound Care 5: 319–22.

Muir IFK, Barclay TL, Settle JAD (1987) Burns and their Treatment. London: Butterworths.

CHAPTER 5

Ethical Decision-making in Burn Care

TINAZ POCHKHANAWALA

Modern burn care often leads to the dilemma of what should or should not be done for patients who have been severely burnt. The questions are, 'When is enough enough?' and 'Who decides?'. All ethical dilemmas vary according to the nature of the situation, the individuals involved and the many differing rules that may apply. Inevitably, decision-making will be complex and require confidence.

To be severely burned is a devastating experience, both physically and emotionally (Noyes et al., 1971), and the individual concerned may experience extreme psychological reactions. Warden (1996) suggests that advances in burn therapy during the past 25 years in terms of decreased mortality and decreased length of hospital stay have been truly outstanding. As a result, Platt et al. (1998) argue that successive improvements in burns care have steadily increased the survivability of many major burn injuries. Half a century ago, an individual who had sustained a burn injury was one of the most neglected in surgery (Bosworth, 1997). Today, in specialized Burns Units, the patient is the object of keen, competitive, multidisciplinary care (Marvin, 1991). Consequently, the management of care for an individual following severe burn trauma has changed dramatically, leading to decreased morbidity and improved survival, function, and cosmetic result in the long term (Marvin, 1991). However, Ward et al. (1987) argue that a consequence of reduced mortality is a new type of morbidity: the physical and psychological problems experienced by burn survivors. Furthermore, the increased likelihood of physical survival of a burn victim heightens concern for potential psychological morbidity for the burn survivor (Blakeney and Meyer, 1996).

For patients with the most severe burn injuries, Platt et al. (1998) believe comfort care rather than active resuscitation has been acknowledged as the correct course of action. While modern intensive care is capable of keeping burned patients alive for substantial periods of time despite burn severity (Watchel et al., 1987), more sophisticated medical knowledge and practice may contribute to suffering, since it helps to prolong life even in conditions when life's further sustenance has ceased to be a categorical imperative (Konigova, 1976).

To survive a severe burn but never to regain a meaningful quality of life is not a desirable goal, although some would say that there is no quality of life if a person is dead. In some severe burns cases, 'survival' appears to be worse than death (Birnbaum and Kraft, 1996). If one could predict with certainty when aggressive curative therapy would be futile, there would be no dilemma, but this is not possible (Wachtel et al., 1987). The result, therefore, is a dilemma, and one may question if there is any ethical justification for performing rigorously the entire medical treatment in the care of patients whose condition has been diagnosed as hopeless and whose suffering is not only made worse but prolonged by the treatment (Konigova, 1976).

For health care professionals, this dilemma is an issue which must be addressed in the clinical setting, as they are involved in decision-making on a daily basis and these decisions may have an ethical component to them. According to Grant (1999), ethical decision-making is the bread and butter of burn care. While the ethical issues seen in burns nursing care are similar in some respects to those in other areas of nursing, they are different in relation to aspects surrounding severe, disfiguring disability which will often require major emotional adjustment (Schumann, 1991).

As a result, health care professionals are faced with issues of impending death, severe disfiguring burns, and physical and emotional dysfunction, that impair an individual's daily living activities and quality of life.

The practices of nurses (and other members of the multidisciplinary team) need, therefore, to remain dynamic, sensitive, relevant and responsive to the changing needs of patients (UKCC, 1992). The management of care for a severely burned patient is a specialized area that requires a wealth of knowledge and clinical skills from a large multidisciplinary team. Nurses, as a part of this team, are involved in making judgements about what constitutes the best care for patients. Such professional judgements often contain moral judgements, and lead us into ethical debates (Melia, 1989) dealing with important questions of human conduct that have great relevance to us both as individuals and as health care professionals (Davis et al., 1997). Because of their training and experience, nurses have a great deal to offer in terms of judgement in these matters, and a significant contribution to make in arriving at such decisions which is all part of the management of care.

Comfort Care or Active Treatment

In a severely burned patient with a poor prognosis, family, friends and members of the medical team need to respect the wishes of the individuals concerned and do everything possible to preserve that person's dignity. Some people request that only 'comfort care' be given (i.e. withdrawal of treatment while maintaining patient dignity, leading to a comfortable and dignified death). Recognizing the likelihood of death they choose to be allowed to die and only want treatment that is designed to manage the pain (Munster, 1993). However, other patients request active resuscitation (i.e. fluid therapy and all possible treatment), as they have decided to fight for survival against the odds. No burn is certainly fatal until the patient dies. According to Imbus and Zawacki (1977) the most severely burned patient may speak of hope with his last breath.

If the patient understands his or her medical situation and the various therapies available, and if the decision is the patient's own, then either of these decisions is acceptable within our understanding of informed consent. However, severely burned patients with little or no likelihood of survival present a difficult ethical and practical problem for medical decision-makers (Wachtel et al., 1987). In this chapter, the aim is to discuss issues surrounding comfort care and active treatment that make ethical judgements for patients with critical burns difficult and troubling.

In the United States, patients with burn injuries greater than 80–90% of their total body surface area routinely survive (Warden, 1996). This success is questionable – while it is evident that more patients such as these are surviving, are these patients returning to society to become productive citizens, and is survival really the measure of productivity for our specialty? The real measurement of an effective service is a patient who can successfully interact socially within a community. Although more patients with larger and more severe burns are surviving, this has created new problems relating to such patients' quality of life. The results of improved technology and surgical procedures are impressive, but for some patients the ability to survive may have outstripped the progress being made to reconstruct and rehabilitate them in the long term (Grant, 1999). As a result, Warden (1996) suggests we may be returning our patients to a society which is not ready financially, psychologically or socially to accept them. It is fortunate that scientific and technological advances in medicine have allowed us to develop strong weapons against illness and injury, but they must not be abused to prolong an agonizing process and dying should remain a natural process (Vincent, 1996).

The premise that one should do all one can is no longer accepted as universally valid (Grant, 1999). Being faced daily with a patient who is screaming 'Let me die!' may make nurses question their own purpose in caregiving. When faced with an individual who has major disfiguring burns the nurse may question the intense push to keep that patient alive (Schumann, 1991).

For victims of major burn injuries there is a relatively well established relationship between the severity of the injury and the chance of survival. Grant (1999) suggests the burns doctor can with reasonable confidence identify a group of patients for whom medical intervention would be futile and would be associated with no precedent of survival. However, this raises the question of whether one should give active resuscitation to a patient whose burn is of sufficient severity to render the intervention futile.

Opinion is divided on the issue. It is argued by Zawacki (1996) that to initiate resuscitation on the grounds of medical futility is paternalistic, as however benevolent one's motives are, the patient is deprived of control of his or her own destiny. In 1979 the National Institute of Health Consensus exercise in the USA (cited by Grant, 1999) concluded that physicians have a duty always to give resuscitation and have the authority to do so without obtaining informed consent.

Advocates of absolute patient autonomy would justify resuscitation on the grounds that, even if the patient does not eventually survive, resuscitation may restore the patient to his or her decision-making capacity (Grant, 1999). Proponents of active interventions in severe injuries would argue that without an active approach to the severely injured the boundaries of burn care would not have been pushed forward (Platt et al., 1998). Herndon (1993) argues to the contrary. He implies that physicians have a duty not to treat burn shock in patients with no established precedent for survival, and that treatment beyond the point of futility merely prolongs a difficult dying process, thus making continuation of therapy a prolongation of death rather than a prolongation of life. This view is also supported by Imbus and Zawacki (1977).

To see a severely burned individual discharged home is a touching, rewarding accomplishment. Yet accomplishing the goal of discharge loses its rewards when one acknowledges that some of these individuals have severe emotional scars and have not adjusted to their disfigurement and impaired mobility (Schumann 1991).

Quality of Life

Quality of life is an important issue that needs to be considered when dealing with the dilemma of what should or should not be done for patients with severe burns. The attainable quality of life if a severely burned patient does survive is difficult to predict (Wachtel et al., 1987). According to Birnbaum and Kraft (1996) it is much more difficult to measure the quality of life than it is to measure mortality. Unlike the objectivity of mortality, quality of life is subjective: there are many shades of survival. Each person has an individual concept of what defines a meaningful existence. A frail 80-year-old will have a different view of what constitutes a good quality of life than a robust 25-year-old.

In addition, the patient may have a different concept of what is meant by a quality and meaningful life than their family, the health care professional, or nursing staff providing care in a Burns Unit. But who is to say what is in the patient's best interest (Melia, 1989)? We are often left with the most simple litmus test of all: how would I like it if that was me? Even this 'Do as you would be done by' approach is not foolproof. Mackie (1977) refers to Bernard Shaw's comment on the golden rule: 'Do not do unto others as you would have that they should do unto you, their tastes may not be the same.'

It is impossible to know in advance how patients will accept or adjust to an impaired quality of life. For these reasons, it can be argued that quality of life decisions should carry limited weight in decisions made by surrogate decision-makers unless the anticipated quality is profoundly reduced (Wachtel et al., 1987). However, although it is difficult to measure satisfaction with life, it may be the most important measure of the benefits associated with the process of critical care medicine. Some would argue that simply to 'survive' is not enough. According to Birnbaum and Kraft (1996), patients should be able to survive and then rehabilitate to achieve a level of health that allows them to have a meaningful life. Furthermore, Blakeney and Meyer (1996) suggest that burns treatment extends beyond patient survival to include recovery of optimal function of the whole person. Although medical factors are always involved, the final issues invariably prove to be primarily ethical. Thus one should ask the question: 'Which is better for this patient – maximum therapy or comfort care and upon whose value system should the judgement be based?' (Imbus and Zawacki, 1977).

Ethical Concepts

Many publications emphasize concern and insistence on the patient's right to decide upon his or her treatment. This element is directly related to the ethical principle of autonomy, i.e. ethical principles that oblige one to allow individuals to self-determine their own plans and actions. It entails respecting the personal liberty of individuals and the choices they make based on their own personal values and beliefs (Fry, 1994).

Each human being of adult years and sound mind has the right to determine what shall be done with his or her own body (Urwin, 1996). In 1868, Abraham Lincoln (cited by Imbus and Zawacki, 1977) stated: 'No man is good enough to govern another without the other's consent'; thus no physician is so skilled that he may treat another without the other's consent.

In addition to uncertainties in prognosis, there is always an uncertainty as to the degree of autonomy in decision-making which a severely burned patient is capable of exercising (Wachtel et al., 1987). It is common for patients on Burns Units to have compromised autonomy and decision-making capacities due to critical illness and its management. Researchers have argued that, for some patients, shock, denial and lack of knowledge of burns injuries have precluded their effective participation in the decision-making process, always (McCrady and Khan, 1980) or sometimes (Zawacki, 1981). However, during the first few hours of hospitalization, even the most severely burned patient is usually alert and mentally competent but often has only a few hours of mental clarity in which to respond to his or her predicament (Imbus and Zawacki, 1977).

Although patients' autonomy demands respect, their ability to make autonomous, competent decisions is often compromised because they have a variety of physiological derangements that are compounded by treatments with analgesics and sedatives (Fratianne et al., 1992). As a result, surrogate decision-makers are sometimes asked to help decide. However, one must consider that close family and surrogates are often subject to shock, denial, guilt and ignorance, as well as self-interest, which may impair their decision-making processes (Wachtel et al., 1987). Imbus and Zawacki (1977) argue that turning to the family for decision-making when death seems imminent for an incompetent patient is rarely satisfactory: guilt-ridden families often find it very difficult to be objective and unselfish in their decision-making. However, in circumstances when patients are unable to respond due to the severity of their injuries the burns team and family will need to make a decision and determine what outcome the patient would be most likely to want if he or she were able to communicate (Imbus and Zawacki, 1977).

Kubler-Ross (1969) points out that when a patient is severely ill he or she is often treated like a person with no right to an opinion. Yet it is the patient's life and rights that are at stake. Statistics may describe past experience with a given type of injury receiving maximal therapy or comfort care; physicians may cite such an experience and are experts in carrying out programmes of active treatment or comfort care: but only the patient may choose between them, because only he or she has the right to consent to one or the other (Imbus and Zawacki 1977). If asked, the physician may offer an opinion about the choice, but it will merely be a *personal* opinion about whether it is better to accept death or fight to make history as the first survivor in such an injury (Imbus and Zawacki, 1977).

Bioethicists Fletcher and Ramsey (cited by Imbus and Zawacki, 1977) urge that unselfish love for the patient, and regard for his or her full stature as a person, should be the criteria upon which to base our answers to bioethical questions. According to Hudak et al. (1997), respect for people is the overriding principle under which respect for autonomy falls.

Imbus and Zawacki (1977) first drew attention to the possibility of offering the patient an opportunity to make an autonomous decision whether or not to receive curative or comfort care in cases where survival is unprecedented. While still lucid, and with sufficient information, the patient is asked if he or she wishes to choose between a full therapeutic regime or comfort care. Some research studies relating to withholding intensive care seem to ignore issues of obtaining the patient's informed consent, i.e. ensuring that sufficient information is given in terms readily understandable to the patient and ensuring that this information has been understood – with all its risks and ramifications – so as to enable patients to make a truly informed decision.

In other studies, authors simply assign to the physician what they believe to be the patient's ultimate right – to decide whether or not a particular form of therapy will be received (Imbus and Zawacki, 1977). Their approach, developed over several years, is based on the conviction that the decision to begin or to withhold maximal therapeutic effort is more of an ethical than a medical judgement. The physician and the burns care team present to the patient the appropriate medical and statistical facts together with authoritative medical opinion about available therapeutic alternatives and their consequences. The Patients' Charter (Department of Health, 1991) requires that a patient be given 'a clear explanation of any treatment including any risks or alternatives'. Thus informed, a patient may give or withhold consent to receive a particular form of therapy, but it is his or her own decision, based on his or her own value system, and it is reached before communication and competence are impaired by intubation or altered states of consciousness.

To allow the patient maximum clarity of thought in decision-making, several points should be communicated to health professionals involved with the patient immediately after injury (see Figure 5.1). One point is that the patient must not be administered narcotics before arrival at the Burns Unit. However, this practice may be deemed to be unrealistic, in view of the pain and discomfort a severely burned patient may be suffering. Such an approach is said not to have changed the mortality rate of patients but to have increased both the self-determination they exercise and the empathy they receive. The more voiceless and vulnerable the patient, the more easily we find ourselves slipping into a paternalistic role, using terms such as 'hopeless' which Imbus and Zawacki (1977) describe as prejudicial (literally, judging before the fact). Experience continues to convince us that 'truth is the greatest kindness'. It seems inevitable that more effective and earlier communication with the patient will prove to be the most honest and compassionate answer to many of the remaining problems of ethical decision-making in the Burns Unit (Imbus and Zawacki, 1977).

---

1. Prompt fluid resuscitation
2. Oxygen administration for possible carbon monoxide intoxication
3. No administration of narcotics before arrival at the Burns centre
4. Avoidance of tracheostomy or endotracheal tube insertion unless absolutely necessary to preserve airway and maintain ventilation
5. Rapid transportation to Burns centre

Figure 5.1 A protocol for the decision and administration of comfort care (Imbus and Zawacki, 1977).

According to Grant (1999) the accepted rights of an individual patient include:

- Autonomy – the patient should be able to think and act without influences or control by others.
- Nonmalificence – the patient should come to no harm.
- Beneficence – the patient should receive the benefit of an intended treatment.
- Justice – treatments should be implemented in a fair and impartial manner.

Decision-making – Who Decides?

Wachtel et al. (1987) emphasized that patients and/or close relatives should also be presented with the option of changing the treatment regimen from curative to comfort care when curative treatment is clearly futile. As with the approach of Imbus and Zawacki (1977), Wachtel et al. came up with a process for reaching such decisions and a protocol (see Figure 5.2) for administering comfort care that is designed to decrease the patient's suffering as much as possible while promoting pain relief and sedation to calm fears and anxieties during the dying process. Similar decisions, both for the burns team to suggest and for the patient to accept comfort care, in cases where survival is marginally possible – or possible but with exceptional disfigurement and disability – are even more difficult (Wachtel et al., 1987). It is important to evaluate such research to see which findings can be validated and how they might be incorporated into clinical practice (Polit and Hungler, 1997).

---

1. Consider writing an order that no 'codes' or cardiopulmonary resuscitation efforts be instituted.
2. Consider the removal of unneeded intravenous and arterial catheters, nasogastric tubes, and bladder catheters.
3. Consider that anxiety may be alleviated with tranquillizers and that pain may be controlled with analgesic medications, including those which might possibly, as a side-effect, somewhat shorten life. One need not fear addiction in a patient whose death is imminent.
4. Consider discontinuing antibiotics. Other medications may be administered as needed to enhance patient comfort.
5. Consider whether continuation of respiratory support and artificial airways are beneficial to the patient or in keeping with the patient's expressed desires.
6. Consider whether the patient will benefit from further blood sampling.
7. Consider whether the patient will benefit from aggressive surgical procedures.
8. Consider modifying nursing procedures such as the frequency of monitoring vital signs, bathing, turning, and, dressing changes.
9. Consider making psychological and spiritual support (by physicians, nurses, social worker, psychologist, psychiatrists and clergy) available to the patient, family and health-care team as required and as resources permit.
10. Consider that the continued assessment of moribund patients is necessary for optimization of their comfort.
11. Consider the personalization of visiting privileges to accommodate the special needs of patients, families and friends.
12. Consider discussing with patients and families the need for organs for transplantation. Many families find comfort in the knowledge that some benefit to others may be salvaged from their loss.

Figure 5.2 Points to consider in obtaining consent to receive therapy (Wachtel et al., 1987).

The difficulty in defining the point at which further treatment is futile undoubtedly results in continuation of aggressive therapy in patients because physicians generally err on the side of doing more for the patient rather than less (Fratianne et al., 1992). Studies such as the one by Civetta (1981) recognize that the futility point is difficult to identify and that such identification always contains an element of uncertainty and inherent error. This study clearly demonstrates such uncertainty and error, since five patients did survive after all those around them (Burns team and relatives) had made the judgement that they would not. Most troubling is the case of one patient who, having originally accepted comfort care, then had second thoughts and ultimately survived. He was severely disfigured and deformed, remaining severely depressed for months after discharge, and despite continuing psychiatric support he was not convinced that either he or the Burns team had made the right decision. He later committed suicide.

It must be stressed that the protocol of Wachtel et al. (1987) for foregoing life-sustaining treatment is not a decision to abandon care but is, rather, a change in goals (Jonsen et al., 1982). The new goal is to enhance the quality of life remaining and to support the patient's autonomy, while ensuring as much comfort as possible. This goal precludes unduly prolonging the dying process. Thus, implementing the comfort care programme seems to address these goals. However, when adopting such a programme it is important to be careful that one does not accept inevitable death so readily as to deny any patient a reasonable chance of survival and recovery, or to develop a defeatist attitude which might inhibit research and efforts to improve burns care and rehabilitation for future patients.

Zawacki (1981) suggests that, regardless of what may be tolerated conventionally or required legally, free, competent, comprehending, and adequate informed consent to treatment is becoming a widely prized moral ideal. The policy of Wachtel et al. (1987) represents a significant step in the pursuit of this ideal and probes deeply into its implications. The pursuit of this ideal challenges us to face honestly the limits of our knowledge about the past and the impossibility of knowing the future.

Judgement that survival is 'impossible' or 'hopeless' implies that one can read the future. A statement that further treatment would be futile expresses not a fact but a value judgement and should be identified as such. Reports of past experience expressed in terms of probability values are far more objective and serve to open or continue dialogue rather than stop it, and that is the core of the ideal we seek to approximate (Zawacki, 1981).

CORNWALL COLLEGE
LIBRARY

As part of the Code of Professional Conduct (UKCC, 1992) registered nurses have a responsibility to keep abreast of and to evaluate research reports and literature on this subject area, and by accurate evaluation have the capability of changing and improving nursing practice (Morrison, 1991).

In response to the dilemma of 'When is enough enough, and who decides?' Fratianne et al. (1992) developed a structured process which would address these issues and help to decide whether to recommend continued invasive diagnostic and therapeutic intervention or to allow the patient to 'die with dignity'. This process can be requested by any member of the Burns team who feels uncomfortable with what is being done for and to the patient. It involves a meeting of the entire multidisciplinary Burns team and its purpose is to discern the judgement of the group. When the consensus is to forego additional therapy, the decision is then presented to the patient (if the patient is able to understand and respond) and to the patient's family. The group decision removes an individual's responsibility for making a stressful decision. Fratianne et al. (1992) believe that patients who accept this decision exhibit a peaceful calm that invariably reaffirms the group dynamics. Family members often experience a great relief, because they are not forced to make the decision even though they wanted it made. Attending staff may perceive this process as an abdication of responsibility; in the experience of Fratianne et al. (1992), however, the consensus conference has led to a conviction that wisdom of the team is always best.

In comparison, Imbus and Zawacki (1977) oppose decision-making by a select committee convened 'to explore what the best interests of the patient and his relatives require' without necessarily asking or respecting the opinions of either. They argue that dealing with an alert, competent patient, one need not struggle against distractions and prejudice to imagine what the patient wants, one needs only to ask. Who is more likely to be totally and lovingly concerned with the patient's best interest than the patient him- or herself? They argue that whenever caregivers in the past have tried to decide these matters on a patient's behalf issues such as what was best for the morale of the nursing team or for the solvency of the hospital have constantly clouded judgement. They advocate shedding a 'We know best' defence and promote actually asking the patient what he wants – on admission, when he is most competent to decide.

Despite the opposition of Imbus and Zawacki (1977), Fratianne et al. (1992) reported many positive reactions among all who participated in the consensus conference decision. Experience shows that when patients accept the consensus recommendation not to undergo active treatment, the decision leads to a peaceful and dignified death. By having the team make the recommendation, family members can continue a positive relationship with a dying loved one without carrying the guilt that may be experienced as a result of making the decision. Working in consensus with other health care professionals to address these difficult decisions is reassuring. The attitude of openness, trust and compassion among team members leads to openness, trust and compassion with patients and families. Patient care is best when the team functions best and excellent patient care is essential when deciding when enough is enough.

It must be appreciated that no study is perfect. Although limitations may exist in the above studies, sound, relevant evidence may be extracted and considered for potential use in clinical practice.

In reaching decisions regarding the treatment of severely burned patients, patient autonomy needs to be respected wherever possible (Wachtel et al., 1987). However, considerations of limited resources and of distributive justice need to be acknowledged. Some patients with severe burns, both survivors and non-survivors, have consumed many hundreds of thousands of pounds in resources, human and material. Although the limits of the resources used in the management of care of the burned patient have at times been stretched, there are severe implications in the case of a massive disaster with many burn patients requiring care at the same time. These limits are being lowered in the current climate in which there is a general effort to restrict the total portion of the societal resources available for health care. We may be entering an era in which rights and benefits available to individuals will be increasingly diminished in favour of those of society as a whole (Siegler, 1985). If this is true, decisions to forego life-sustaining treatment may, in future, have to include considerations of the cost to others. This would result in placing some patients on comfort care whether they wish it or not. Society has begun to accept such decisions for end-stage cancer patients but has not yet done so for victims of severe burn injuries. Physicians find it especially difficult to make triage decisions since it means abandoning hope and efforts to save some patients, contrary to our traditional ethic.

Economic analysis cannot replace clinical decision-making at individual patient level. It can merely provide a pointer and must be considered alongside many important factors including ethics (Dales, 1996).

The Future

Nursing is rife with difficult situations which will always raise moral issues and call for moral choices to be made (Melia, 1989). Ethical codes will take us some of the way but we have to accept that moral uncertainty is part and parcel of nursing practice.

In a society that values the individual, ethics has to be centred on individual patients and the maintenance of their individual rights. The Human Rights Act (1998), brought into force in 2000, has significant implications for the debate on burns treatment. Healthcare professionals working in burn care must be directed towards the best interests of the burn victim and to protect their fundamental rights (Grant, 1999). Individual choice must be uppermost. The Code of Conduct (UKCC, 1992) states that the nurse should 'always act in such a manner as to promote and safeguard the interests and well being of patients and clients' and 'recognize and respect the uniqueness and dignity of each patient'.

Arguably, for nurses one of the most rewarding aspects of care is being involved in the successful treatment of a severely burned patient who makes a full recovery. In stark contrast, inappropriate treatment can be very distressing for all involved, particularly when it is merely prolonging the process of dying.

The goals of critical care include saving the salvageable and allowing the dying to die with peace and dignity (Birnbaum and Kraft, 1996). As Virginia Henderson (1960) stated: 'The unique function of the nurse is to assist the individual sick or well in the performance of these activities contributing to health or recovery or to a peaceful death that he would perform unaided if he had the necessary strength, will or knowledge.' Balancing all considerations and participating in decision-making for individual patients requires maturity, expertise, and emotional as well as physical strength, and calls on each of us to give the best we have to offer of all of these to our patients (Wachtel et al., 1987).

When caring for burns victims, ethical decisions will require some deliberation, and consideration of the rights of the patient, the duties of professionals and the good of society, in order to achieve the goal of maximized human potential (Grant, 1999).

The very nature of ethical decision-making often means that there is no clear black or white solution to the problem (RCN, 1997). Ultimate agreement may be unobtainable but we should still, however, strive to obtain it (RCN, 1997). Ethics proves at times to be difficult, controversial and changing; at its best, it is about personal struggle and achievement – not passive acceptance of 'expert' opinions – and involves, finally, a recognition that the burden of ethical decision-making, while always personal, need not always be lonely (Zawacki, 1996).

References

Birnbaum ML, Kraft S (1996) Results of critical care and the quality of survival. In Tinker J, Browne D, Sibbald WJ, (Eds) Critical Care: Standards, Audits and Ethics. London: Arnold. pp 297–314.

Blakeney PE, Meyer WJ (1996) Psychological recovery of burned patients and reintegration into society. In Herndon DN, (Ed) Total Burn Care. London: WB Saunders, pp 556–63.

Bosworth C (1997) Burns Trauma: Management and Nursing Care. London: Baillière Tindall.

Civetta JM (1981) Beyond technology: intensive care in the 1980s. Critical Care Medicine 9: 763.

Couchman W, Dawson J (1995) Nursing and Health Care Research, 2nd edn. London: Scutari Press.

Dales J (1996) Establishing health care priorities. In Tinker J, Browne D, Sibbald WJ (Eds) Critical Care: Standards, Audits and Ethics. London: Arnold. pp 331–43.

Davis AJ, Arosker MA, Liaschenko J et al. (1997) Ethical Dilemmas and Nursing Practice. 4th edn. Stamford: Appleton and Lange.

Department of Health (1991) The Patients' Charter. London: Department of Health.

Fratianne RB, Brandt C, Yurko L et al. (1992) When is enough enough? Ethical dilemmas on the Burns Unit. Journal of Burn Care and Rehabilitation 13(5): 600–4.

Fry ST (1994) Ethics in Nursing Practice: a Guide to Ethical Decision Making. Switzerland: International Council of Nurses.

Grant I (1999) Ethical issues in burns care. Burns 25: 307–15.

Henderson V (1960) Basic Principles of Nursing Care. London: International Council of Nursing.

Herndon DN, Rutan RL, Desai MH et al. (1993) What size burn should be resuscitated? Proceedings of the Burn Association 25: 106.

Hudak C, Gallo B, Gonce Morton P (1997). Critical Care Nursing: a Holistic Approach. 7th edn. Philadelphia: Lippincott Raven Publishers.

Imbus SH, Zawacki BE (1977) Autonomy for burned patients when survival is unprecedented. New England Journal of Medicine 297(6): 308–11.

Jonsen AR, Siegler M, Winslade WJ (1982) Clinical Ethics. New York: MacMillan.

Konigova R (1976) The ethical problems associated with the treatment of severe burns. Burns 2(3): 137–39.

Kubler-Ross E (1969) On Death and Dying. New York: MacMillan.

Marvin J (1991) Cited in Trofino RB, (Ed) Nursing Care of the Burn Injured Patient. Philadelphia: FA Davis Company.

Mackie JL (1977) Ethics: Inventing Right and Wrong. Harmondsworth: Penguin Books.

McCrady VL, Kahn AM (1980) Life or death for burn patients. Journal of Trauma 20: 356.

Melia K (1989) Everyday Nursing Ethics. London: Macmillan Education Ltd.

Morrison P (1991) Critiquing Research. The Medicine Group (UK) Ltd. pp 20–22.

Munster AM (1993) Severe Burns – a Family Guide to Medical and Emotional recovery. London: The John Hopkins University Press:

Narayanasamy A (1997) An exploratory study into the effectiveness of the nurse education in meeting the spiritual needs of chronically ill patients. MPhil thesis, University of Nottingham.

Noyes R, Andreasen NJC, Hartford CE (1971) The psychological reaction to severe burns. American Journal of Psychosomatic Medicine 11: 416–22.

Platt AJ, Phipps AR, Judkins K (1998) Is there still a place for comfort care in severe burns. Burns 24: 754–56.

Polit DF, Hungler BP (1997) Essentials of Nursing Research – Methods, Appraisal and Utilization. 4th edn. Philadelphia: Lippincott-Raven.

RCN (1997) Ethical Dilemmas. London: Royal College of Nursing.

Schumann L (1991) History of Burn Care. In Trofino RB, (Ed) Nursing Care of the Burn Injured Patient. Philadelphia: FA Davis Company. pp 10–11.

Siegler M (1985) A review of who should decide? Paternalism in health care. Perspectives in Biology and Medicine 28: 452.

UKCC (1992) Code of Professional Conduct for the Nurse, Midwife and Health Visitor. London: HMSO.

Urwin J (1996) Medico-legal aspects of critical care. In Tinker J, Browne D, Sibbald WJ, (Eds) Critical Care: Standards, Audit and Ethics. London: Arnold. pp 372–90.

Vincent JL (1996) Withholding and withdrawing. In Tinker J, Browne D, Sibbald WJ, (Eds) Critical Care: Standards, Audit and Ethics. London: Arnold. pp 344–49.

Ward HW, Moss RL, Darko DF et al. (1987) Prevalence of post burn depression following burn injury. Journal of Burn Care and Rehabilitation 9(4): 376–84.

Wachtel TL, Frank HA, Nielsen JA (1987) Comfort care: an alternative treatment programme for severely burned patients. Burns 13(1): 1–6.

Warden GD (1996) Functional sequelae and disability assessment. In Herndon DN, (Ed) Total Burn Care. London: WB Saunders, pp 523–28.

Zawacki BE (1981) Ethical and practical considerations in decision making in burn care. Topical Emergency Medicine 3: 1.

Zawacki B (1996) Ethically valid decision making. In Herndon DN, (Ed) Total Burn Care. London: WB Saunders, pp 575–82.

CHAPTER 6

Wound Care

SARAH PANKHURST AND TINAZ POCHKHANAWALA

In a healthy individual, the healing process and the immune response are natural occurrences and are completely automatic. They do not depend upon medical care; on the contrary, medicine depends on being able to facilitate this physiological process.

When one imagines a patient suffering from severe burns, it is difficult to comprehend that the body has the ability to repair itself. In these cases, without medical intervention, the complications caused by hypovolaemia and septicaemia would be fatal long before the stages of the healing process were able to take place. According to Cason (1981), it would take months or even years for a 30% full thickness burn to heal spontaneously, and the patient would have succumbed to infection or complications long before.

However, patients suffering from less extensive injuries are able to heal naturally, which is well demonstrated by a partial thickness burn. Deeper burns will also be capable of the physical and biochemical processes of healing, but at a prolonged rate and with a poor cosmetic appearance.

Scientific knowledge has allowed surgeons to save lives by the excision of necrotic tissue and the application of skin grafts. This reduces the risks of infection, promotes healing and returns the skin's natural protective function. Surgical intervention also offers an improved cosmetic appearance over that of a deep burn left to heal by its own devices.

Research into the processes of wound healing has resulted in the development of wound care products that facilitate the body's natural healing action. Therefore, whether a wound is to be treated surgically or conservatively with dressings, the best method of healing can be achieved. The wound care market is constantly developing new products; these continue to be clinically evaluated in Burns Units today.

This chapter outlines the normal processes of wound healing and how the ability of the skin to repair itself following a burn injury depends on the depth of skin damage. The initial care and treatment of the burn wound are described, with particular attention to certain anatomical areas. Infection control procedures are briefly considered throughout. Finally, the care of less extensive/minor wounds is discussed.

The Stages of Wound Healing

Wound healing can be defined as the physiology by which the body replaces and restores function to damaged tissues (Tortora and Grabowski, 1996). The following stages are based upon the phases described by Westaby (1985).

It must be remembered that these processes take place concurrently and do not always follow one another in an orderly sequence (Bale and Jones, 1997).

Stage 1: Inflammation (0–3 days)

The phase of traumatic inflammation begins within a few minutes of injury and lasts for about 3 days. The features of this phase are similar to those caused by a wound infection, and care must therefore be taken not to confuse the two.

There are five classic signs of inflammation:

• heat
• redness
• swelling
• pain
• loss of function

The signs of infection are as those given above, but with the addition of malodour, purulent exudate, green slough and extending cellulitis (Morison, 1994).

When tissue is damaged, the redness and heat are caused by the increased blood supply and cellular activity in the affected area. Injured blood vessels bleed into the defect until clotting occurs. Damaged tissue and mast cells secrete histamine and other enzymes that cause vasodilatation and increased capillary permeability. The capillary walls then allow inflammatory exudate (containing plasma, antibodies, white blood cells and a few red blood cells) to infiltrate the surrounding tissues, resulting in swelling and oedema.

During this phase, two important cell types arrive at the wound site: polymorphonucleocytes and macrophages. These defend against bacteria, and clear debris, damaged tissue and blood clots, thus leading to Stage 2.

Stage 2: Destruction (2–5 days)

The wound is cleaned of devitalized tissue by the polymorphonucleocytes and macrophages. Macrophages are large mobile cells that can engulf and digest bacteria and dead tissue. They play a crucial role in the process of wound healing, for if they are removed healing ceases (Westaby, 1985). This is because they attract further macrophages to the wound site, where they are responsible for stimulating the development and multiplication of fibroblasts. Fibroblasts synthesize collagen, which is the supportive fibrous protein of the skin.

Macrophages are also known to initiate angiogenesis, the process by which new blood vessels are formed: these vessels grow into the wound from the edges, and fibroblasts follow them to assume their role. This is the beginning of Stage 3. The natural degradation of devitalized tissue is known as autolysis and requires a moist environment to promote its occurrence (Davis et al., 1993).

Stage 3: Proliferation (3–24 days)

Fibroblasts begin to produce strands of collagen, the main constituent of connective tissue. The optimum environment for this to occur is one of slight acidity (Westaby, 1985). The production of collagen increases the tensile strength of the wound; early collagen is, however, irregularly constructed, and its synthesis depends upon the vascularity and perfusion of the wound. Vitamin C, zinc, copper and iron are crucial stimulators for this stage (McLaren, 1992) and collagen synthesis is inhibited if the nutritional intake is insufficient. Most of the factors that impair healing during this phase are systemic: they include age, anaemia, hypoproteinaemia and zinc deficiency (Westaby, 1985; Flanagan, 1997).

The activity of the healing process at this stage produces granulation tissue, consisting of new and fragile capillary loops supported in scaffolding of collagen fibres. The granulation tissue is moist, red and fragile, and it fills the wound, allowing it when combined with the processes of epithelialization and contraction to heal. The wound will, at the end of this stage, have the appearance of being healed but will remain red, raised and itchy.

Stage 4: Maturation (24 days–1 year)

During this phase, the structure of the new scar is extensively remodelled. There is a progressive decrease in the vascularity of the scar, and its red appearance fades. The amount of collagen initially increases but, after several months, reduces, flattens and softens. The strength of the scar gradually grows, although only 50% of the normal tensile strength of a skin wound is regained in the first 6 weeks (Westaby, 1985). Davis et al. (1993) state that the scar will reach a strength comparable to that of normal tissue. However, Flanagan (1997) suggests that the tensile strength of scar tissue is never more than 80% of that of non-wounded skin.

The time scales described at the beginning of each stage act only as a guide for a wound undergoing a simple healing process without complication. The time taken for many wounds to heal depends on a multitude of intrinsic and extrinsic factors, including their depth, size and chronicity, but they will still pass through these phases. Wounds can also have different stages of healing occurring at the same time. In addition to the four phases described above are the processes of epithelialization and contraction, which are of greatest importance when there has been tissue loss or destruction, as in a burn injury.

Contraction

Contraction is the process by which large wounds become small without the need for a skin graft or secondary closure (Westaby, 1985).

The mechanism of contraction is not yet fully understood, but certain facts are known (Westaby, 1985):

- Collagen is not essential.
- Myofibroblasts supply the motive force.
- Interference with the viability of cells at the wound edge inhibits the process.
- Contraction can begin on the fourth day after injury. Contraction is evident in full thickness wounds which appear to 'shrink', pulling in the surrounding skin: this is one cause of the poor cosmetic appearance if full thickness burns are left to heal spontaneously.

Epithelialization

The skin has a covering of squamous epithelial cells that are constantly being shed and replaced from below. When an injury causes a defect in this squamous covering, the cells at the wound edges multiply, flatten and migrate towards the area of cell deficit (Westaby, 1985). This mechanism is of vital importance after a burn injury, as it is the major factor in deciding whether or not the burn will require a skin graft.

Wounds epithelialize not only from the wound edges but also from deep dermal appendages that are lined with epithelium, such as hair follicles (Figure 6.1). Partial thickness burns, therefore, which have hair follicles intact, have the ability to epithelialize from these appendages and so the wound surface will be covered faster, in approximately 10–14 days (Settle, 1996). Full thickness burns have no deep dermal appendages left in situ, so epithelialization can only occur from the wound edges (Figure 6.2). Epithelialization can begin within hours of injury during the inflammatory phases, but the cells will only migrate over live granulation tissue and will move into the layer below debris, blood clots or eschar, which form a mechanical obstruction in the wound bed.

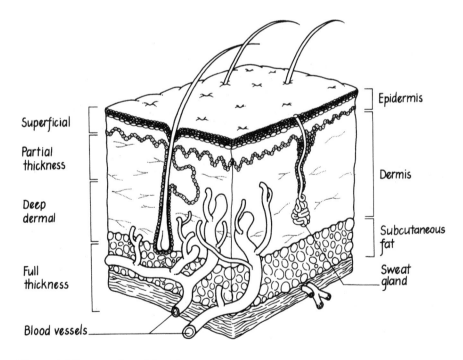

Figure 6.1 Cross-section of the skin.

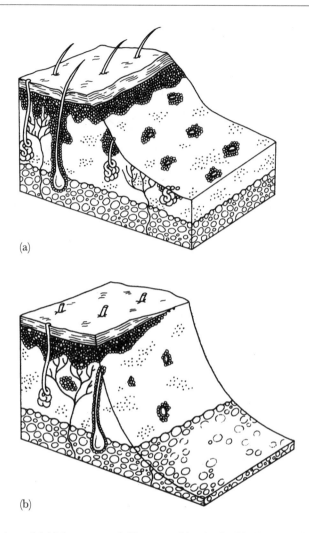

(a)

(b)

Figure 6.2 (a) A partial thickness wound. Numerous islands of epithelium remain around the hair shafts and glands, each being a source of regeneration. (b) A full thickness wound. No viable epithelium remains in the wound area; dermis heals slowly by granulation and a skin graft may be needed.

In the wounds allowed to heal by this method the protective influence of dressing prevents physical trauma, drying, haemorrhage and invasion from micro-organisms. In order for the fragile epithelial cells to migrate across the wound surface, a moist environment under a non-adherent dressing is preferable, as it facilitates the process (Davis et al., 1993; Westaby, 1985). Owing to the intense cellular activity in the area, the wound edges have a raised hyperplastic zone, which disappears once epithelialization is complete. The process ceases when the epithelial cells meet across the wound surface, by 'contact inhibition' (Pape, 1993).

Local Pathophysiology of the Burn Wound

Heat causes injury to the cells, resulting in tissue destruction and seriously impairing the normal functioning of the skin. The interruption of the protective barrier that the skin provides leaves an accessible route for micro-organisms to enter the body's internal environment. Life is then threatened by this vulnerability to infection and the overall systemic effects to the circulation (Rylah, 1992).

The burn wound has been described as having three zones (Dyer and Roberts, 1990), which are three-dimensional, as demonstrated by Figure 6.3 (Rylah, 1992).

- The zone of *coagulation* – usually in the centre of the wound, comprising non-living tissue.
- The zone of *stasis* – tissue is viable but, having decreased perfusion is at risk of ischaemic damage.
- The zone of *hyperaemia* – normal skin with increased blood flow as a response to injury.

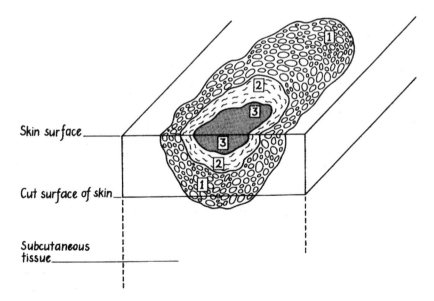

Figure 6.3 Pathophysiology of a burn wound. 1: zone of hyperaemia; 2: zone of stasis; 3: zone of necrosis.

When a burn injury occurs, the body responds by initiating the inflammatory process, as described above. Burn oedema formation is rapid and produces copious amounts of exudate. In order to stop the burning process, immediate care of the burn is to cool it with cold water. This reduces, and can even reverse, the total cellular damage and oedema formation (Clarke, 1992).

The inflammatory process is completed as the oedema subsides, followed by the series of events in the healing process described earlier. However, the ability of the skin to repair itself depends on the depth of skin damage, which is an important factor in determining treatment.

Burn Depth and the Healing Process

The assessment of the depth of tissue damage does not take place until 48 hours post-burn injury, when the oedema has subsided. Wound healing and management will vary, depending on the type of burn, and many injuries will be a combination of different depths. Superficial burns, involving only the epidermis, and partial thickness burns, involving the upper layers of dermis, have the ability to heal spontaneously in approximately 7 to 14 days respectively (Clarke, 1992). This is possible because the damage only extends to the mid-dermis, and the deep dermal appendages, such as hair follicles and sweat glands, remain intact. As described above (Figure 6.2a), because these are encapsulated by a layer of epithelial cells that can regenerate, the wound can heal by itself and the result is only minimal scarring.

Deep partial thickness/deep dermal burns involve the majority of the dermis, leaving only the deepest layers intact. Some of the dermal appendages will remain, but epithelialization will be slow, healing will be prolonged over 3–4 weeks and poor-quality skin cover will result (Parker, 1993).

Full thickness burns involve all the layers of the skin and may extend to fat, muscle, tendon and bone. Granulation and contraction are the processes by which these wounds heal, with epithelialization only occurring from the edges in the latter stages (Figure 6.2b). This can take weeks or months and will leave unsightly scarring.

Deep partial thickness and full thickness burns will therefore benefit from excision and skin grafting (see Chapter 9).

Care of the Burn Wound

At the scene of the injury, the first aid measures should be followed by application of a clean, non-fluffy material to protect the burned area from further contamination. Plasticized polyvinyl chloride film (cling film) has proved itself to be an ideal first aid cover for burned areas (Wilson and French, 1987) despite little being published on its use as a temporary dressing for wounds. It is cheap, thin and, being pliable, moulds to the contour of the wounds, forming an impermeable, non-adherent barrier screening raw nerve endings from air and reducing pain (Settle, 1996). Its transparency permits inspection through the film. Application and removal is easy, painless and promotes patient comfort (Wilson and French, 1987). It adheres to itself not to the wound surface or intact skin.

Cling film is not supplied as a sterile dressing. However, it is acceptable for use as a temporary dressing (Wilson and French, 1987; Flanagan et al., 1994; Nottingham Hospital Trusts, 1996) since proliferation of bacteria is minimal on smooth, clean surfaces (Thompson and Bullock, 1992; Nottingham Hospital Trusts, 1996). Laboratory studies have demonstrated that the film is sterile within the roll: the first few inches, however, should be discarded (Settle, 1996). Although Flanagan et al. (1994) support this, Aycliffe et al. (1992) argue that anything coming into contact with wounds should be sterile.

Disadvantages of its use are that the wound may be visible to the patient, an exudating wound may result in leakage, and surrounding skin may become macerated if cling film is left for prolonged periods (Nottingham Hospital Trusts, 1996). Cling film can be routinely used in the Burns Unit for wound dressings before ward rounds, surgery and during transfer from Accident and Emergency departments to the Burns Unit.

Otherwise, a clean sheet can be used. Elaborate dressings are inappropriate, and ointments should not be applied as they hamper subsequent wound assessment (Settle, 1996).

On arrival to the Accident and Emergency Department, although the appearance of the damaged skin is most shocking, priority over any wound procedure must go to treatment of the airway, breathing, circulation and pain.

Once these functions have been stabilized and the body surface area covered by the burn has been assessed, care of the wounds can then begin. It is essential that the dressing technique incorporates strict asepsis to try and prevent any contamination of an already immunocompromized patient. The wearing of an apron and sterile gloves for the nurse and the use of sterile towels to surround and cover the patient assist in maintaining a clean environment.

Management of the wound

The burn wound is irrigated with isotonic saline 0.9% solution applied at room temperature. It is non-toxic to healing tissues, has no detrimental side effects, is cheap and cost-effective (Morison, 1989; Hateley, 1993).

Tap water is often not considered as a wound cleansing solution because it is not sterile and many health care professionals express unease at the prospect of using non-sterile solutions in wound cleansing for fear of introducing bacteria from solutions into wounds and thereby delaying wound healing. The absence of controlled clinical trials has served to exacerbate this uncertainty (Ferguson, 1988).

However, a randomized clinical trail on 705 patients compared sterile saline with tap water for the cleansing of acute traumatic soft tissue wounds (Angeras et al., 1992). The study indicated that use of tap water had no detrimental effect on healing in comparison with saline. Less infection was found in wounds cleaned with tap water. Furthermore, even if bacteria were present in the tap water used for wound cleansing, they were not present in the wound. However, tap water should be allowed to run for 10–15 seconds before use (Angeras et al., 1992), and it would be prudent to ensure that it is taken from a fast running supply.

Although the study by Angeras et al. was specific to traumatic wounds, it has become accepted practice to use tap water in many clinical areas specialising in the treatment of wounds (Oliver, 1997).

In contrast to the wound infections described by Lowry and Tompkins (1993), Chrintz et al. (1989) demonstrated that there was no increase in wound infection when patients showered as early as one day after surgery, and the use of tap water in the early management of burns has been advocated for many years (Lawrence, 1987).

Tap water is easy to use and effective in removing excessive wound exudate and foreign particles. It promotes patient comfort and hygiene. Its use has both practical and economic advantages (Angeras et al., 1992) and it may therefore be viewed as a satisfactory wound cleansing agent.

However, Griffiths-Jones and Ward (1995) argue that if cleaning is required all fluids used should be sterile, but provide no research evidence in support of this opinion. It is argued that water is a major vector for *Pseudomonas aeruginosa* which is naturally resistant to many disinfectants and antibacterial drugs and is categorized as one of the major pathogens leading to hospital-acquired infections (Meers et al., 1992).

Legionella pneumophilia can also be present in tap water and warrants consideration. Lowry et al. (1991) describe three cases of sternal wound infection with *Legionella pneumophilia* together with evidence that the infections may have been caused by early post-operative bathing in tap water, or skin cleansing around sternal wounds with tap water. However, legionella is of low virulence, and wound infection due to these organisms is rare except in high risk patients (Meers et al., 1995). The degree of risk must therefore be assessed on an individual basis (Hollinworth, 1998).

Any fears concerning bacterial contamination from non-sterile water supplies and subsequent effects on wounds appear to be unfounded (Angeras et al., 1992)

In many Burns Units today, the use of plain tap water for irrigating and cleansing of burn wounds has already been adopted and has a positive effect on patient well-being (Gilchrist, 1994). Optimum wound healing is achieved by using only non-toxic solutions for cleaning (Flanagan, 1997). Often, the practice is to bath patients, but care should be taken, however, not to soak wounds for long periods: open tissues have a tendency to absorb water, which increases the amount of exudate produced and often necessitates more frequent dressing changes (Flanagan, 1997).

The temperature of a wound directly affects the rate of healing (Ferguson, 1988; Hollinworth et al., 1993; Flanagan, 1997) and biological processes are temperature-dependent (Johnson, 1988). Research has shown that all solutions used for wound cleansing or irrigation should be warmed to body temperature (37°C) prior to use to avoid lowering the temperature of the wound site and the patient and thereby delaying the healing process (Lock, 1980; Turner, 1985; Thomas, 1990; Fletcher, 1997). Any discomfort to the patient is also prevented (Clarke, 1992).

A constant temperature of 37°C promotes both macrophage and mitotic activity during granulation and epithelialization (Dealey, 1994). Saline at room temperature could cause local vasoconstriction and impair wound resistance (Angeras et al., 1992). Lock (1980), Myers (1982), and Miller and Dyson (1996) noted that when wounds were cleaned with solutions at room temperature and not warmed it took 40 minutes for a wound to return to normal temperature after cleansing and three hours for mitotic cell division to commence. The same was noted for leucocyte activity. Thomas (1990) also stated that a decrease in the temperature of a wound can have a significant effect on the availability of oxygen within a wound.

Cooling of the wound, perhaps by lengthy dressing change, may reduce the surface temperature by several degrees (Dealey, 1994; Fletcher, 1997; Williams and Young, 1998). Extended exposure of wet wounds may reduce the temperature to 12°C. The use of a cold cleansing agent has the potential to reduce the temperature even further to 3°C (Williams and Young, 1998). Hollinworth et al. (1993) advocate that exposure of the wound is kept to a minimum; therefore the practice of taking down dressings prior to the doctor's round should be discontinued.

Consequently, in the Burns Unit saline or tap water must be warmed before cleansing so as not to reduce the wound temperature, and warm dressing change conditions must be enforced (Westaby, 1985).

Dead epithelium is trimmed away using sterile scissors and forceps, and blisters are deroofed.

There has been controversy regarding whether to evacuate blisters following burns or leave them intact (DuKamp, 2000; Flanagan and Graham 2001). There is no uniform agreement on their management (Hartford, 1996). Most physicians choose to evacuate and debride blisters covering large burns because the fluid contained in the blister may increase the risk of infection by serving as a culture medium for bacteria (Rockwell and Ehrlich, 1990).

Rockwell and Ehrlich (1990) suggest that blister fluid retards healing by impairing local immunity at the wound site, thus increasing the inflammatory response and retarding the rejuvenation of the dermal vascular patency. They state that small blisters may be left intact. However, evidence suggests that, with large blisters, leaving blister fluid on the wound can have detrimental effects (Rockwell and Ehrlich, 1990), and this is supported by Deitch et al. (1987). Publications as early as 1969 recommend evacuation of fluid from large blisters to reduce potential for bacterial growth. Rockwell and Ehrlich (1990) supports this. Furthermore, a significant burn may need a topical antibiotic such as flamazine to be applied on skin that is viable, not on top of a blister that is going to slough off. In addition, blisters impede the assessment process, and restrict movement if located over joints. Based on these considerations, the case can be made that blistered skin should be removed to facilitate healing.

However, Settle (1996) disagrees, stating that blisters form a biological dressing, protecting the burn from contamination, and advocates leaving them until they burst or, if they become very large, can be aspirated. 'Deroofing' blisters causes unnecessary pain, may be harmful, delays healing and increases the risk of infection. Lawrence (1989) supports this as does Hartford (1996), who notes that blisters form in the stratum spinosum layer of the epidermis so an intact blister usually indicates a superficial partial thickness wound which heals spontaneously within three weeks. If the blister is removed, the wound is converted from an absolutely painless one to a painful, open wound exposed to colonization by bacteria (Hartford, 1996); Hartford therefore recommends leaving this protective layer.

Arturson (1993) states that, although the fluid contained in blisters facilitates healing and the roof of the blister provides effective cover to protect new structures forming underneath, the size and weight of the blister creates a risk of traumatic shearing, increasing the extent of the wound. To remove this risk, blisters could be treated as devitalized tissue and deroofed (Settle, 1996).

Other recommendations include needle aspiration of blister fluid, leaving the blister roof acting a as natural dressing (Dziewulski, 1992). Hartford (1996) disagrees, arguing that blistered skin violated by needle aspiration has the potential for bacterial contamination and infection. Attempts to use loose skin as a protective dressing are generally ineffective (Hartford, 1996).

Current practice in the Burns Unit is to leave small blisters undisturbed, but large ones are burst and deroofed, thereby implementing the research findings of Rockwell and Ehrlich (1990).

Any foreign material, such as clothing and debris, will need gently removing from the wound, and it may be necessary to wash away any soot or dirt with tap water and non-perfumed soap (Parker, 1993). Hair in the close vicinity of the wound may also require clipping, as it will become encrusted with exudate and act as a focus for bacterial colonization. When the wound has been assessed, further treatment can take place if necessary.

Circumferential burns

An important consideration before the wound dressing is applied is whether or not the burn appears to be circumferential around the neck, trunk, limbs or fingers, particularly if it already appears to be full thickness (Settle, 1986). As the burn oedema develops, the inelastic eschar acts as a tourniquet and has the potential to cause fatal ischaemia of the extremities, or respiratory difficulty if the chest or neck is constricted. If this complication arises, the tension created by the restricting eschar must be released by an escharotomy. This is a longitudinal excision through the burned skin along its full extent, and, because the skin is dead, little analgesia is required (Settle, 1986). An alginate dressing with haemostatic properties is applied to the escharotomy site, as the relief of tension causes the wound to gape open and some bleeding will occur when viable tissue is reached.

Dressing the burn wounds

Each patient's wound needs assessing within a holistic framework, an appropriate plan of wound care needs to be implemented to promote wound healing, and the effects of wound management need to be evaluated (Hateley, 1993)

The ideal burn dressing (Turner, 1985; Muddiman, 1989; Settle, 1996) must:

- protect the wound from physical damage and micro-organisms
- be comfortable, compliant, and durable
- absorb exudate
- be non-toxic, non-adherent, and non-irritant
- allow gaseous exchange
- allow high humidity at the wound
- be compatible with topical therapeutic agents
- be able to allow maximum activity for the wound to heal without retarding or inhibiting any stage of the process

Each wound needs individual assessment (Oliver, 1997). The principles of moist wound healing should be used at all times (Williams and Young, 1998) and have long been incorporated into clinical practice. This criterion is based on the work of George Winter (1962). His research has had a profound effect on wound management. He compared the effect of leaving superficial wounds exposed to form a scab with the effect of applying a vapour-permeable film dressing, using an animal model. Epithelialization was twice as fast in those wounds covered with a film dressing. This was because the dressing maintains humidity on the wound surface. The net result of this has been an explosion in the range of new wound management products available for use (Westaby, 1985; Dealey, 1994). However the search for an ideal burn wound dressing continues (Dziewulski, 1992) There is no single dressing suitable for all types of wound, and often a number of dressing types will need to be used during the healing of a single wound (Courtenay, 1998). It is important to remember that it is not the dressing that heals the wound. The dressing only promotes the ideal healing environment (Flanagan, 1997; Williams and Young, 1998).

The surface, depth and location of the burn have to be considered when choosing the appropriate dressing cover (Fowler, 1994).

Initial dressings focus around the inflammatory stage, where copious exudate is present, and the destructive phase, where autolysis demands a moist environment (Holt, 1998). Paraffin gauze is the primary dressing of choice when initially covering a large area of burn (Settle, 1996). Conventional dressings are the most widely used as they are easy to use (Dziewulski, 1992) and relatively inexpensive, and Settle (1996) argues that when several layers are placed upon heavily exudating wounds, they have a low adherence to the wound surface and remain moist. This is supported by Hollinworth et al. (1993). Westaby (1985) argues that it partially insulates the surface against heat loss. Layers of gauze followed by gamgee pads are then applied to the wound to absorb the prolific amounts of exudate. Crêpe bandages are used to hold the dressings in place. 'Strike-through' is a problem because burn wounds produce copious exudate (Settle, 1996). As soon as any leakage occurs there is a route by which micro-organisms can enter the wound from the environment and repadding is required (Dealey, 1994; Flanagan, 1997; Parker, 1993). When lengths of paraffin gauze and cotton gauze are applied to the limbs or chest, they should not be wrapped around in spirals, as they will act as a tourniquet when the oedema is maximal.

Crêpe bandages are used because they will stretch to accommodate for swelling, but the patient should be regularly checked for any discomfort. Paraffin gauze has traditionally been used as a primary dressing for burns for many years but Williams and Young (1998) argue that this does not make it the best dressing. They outline several disadvantages associated with such a dressing.

The dressing is used as primary wound contact layer and the paraffin is present to reduce the adherence of the product to the surface of a granulating wound. However, paraffin gauze is known to adhere to the wound surface, dry out (Hollinworth et al., 1993) and damage newly formed epithelial and granulation tissue, all of which delays wound healing (Lawrence, 1989; Hollinworth et al., 1993; Williams and Young, 1998). This may lead to renewed inflammatory response (Dealey, 1994) and delayed epithelialization (Westaby, 1985).

Removal of adherent paraffin gauze is tedious and time consuming (Muddiman, 1989; Settle, 1996). Granulation tissue can also grow through the mesh of the dressing, and is pulled off during removal (Williams and Young, 1998). Fibres can also shed into the wound (Hollinworth et al., 1993; Settle, 1996; Flanagan, 1997). Because the constituents of the dressing are water-repellent, removal is not facilitated by soaking in warm saline (Flanagan, 1997; Williams and Young, 1998). Terrill et al. (1991), Dziewulski (1992), and Dealey (1994) argue that these conventional dressings are too bulky for use in the hand and seriously affect mobilization, restricting finger/joint movement thus leading to increased stiffness (Muddiman, 1989; Dziewulski, 1992). Mobilization also contributes to a reduction in oedema (Muddiman, 1989). These dressings are not waterproof and soil readily (Lawrence, 1989) requiring frequent changing (Dziewulski, 1992; Holt, 1998). During the inflammatory phase, which is when these dressings are initially applied, it is important to ensure they are not too constrictive, and patient analgesia should be considered as tissues become very oedematous and uncomfortable (Flanagan, 1997).

There is now no place for the traditional and often painful alternatives (Young, 1995) and there is little point in using a dressing to promote healing only to find it causes secondary trauma on removal (Dealey, 1994).

It is strongly suggested by implication (Hollinworth et al., 1993) that paraffin gauze has no role in wound management. However, this can be viewed as overly simplistic. Despite the variety of disadvantages, this traditional dressing is almost invariably used for burn injuries (Settle, 1996) and indeed initially in many Burns Units today. There seems to be no other readily available product to match the convenience and capability for dressing burn wounds exceeding about 2% body surface area (Settle, 1996).

The neck is a difficult area to apply dressings to and it is unable to have a bandage applied, so a paraffin gauze collar can be made and held in place by a rolled-up gamgee in a tubular gauze stocking or a physiotherapy collar, to keep the chin elevated.

Burn injury elicits oedema in the tissues immediately subjacent to a wound (Herndon, 1996). Burned limbs and extremities should therefore be elevated to help gravity overcome oedema (Settle, 1996; Clarke, 1992), promote venous return (Trofino, 1991) and minimize swelling that will occur from the accumulation of fluid; for the same reason, patients with burned faces should be nursed in an upright position. The most efficient position for an injured part is just slightly above the level of the heart. To elevate higher above the heart does not further enhance removal of excess tissue fluid (Herndon, 1996). One of the most effective ways to reduce the incidence of infection is to eliminate oedema from a burned part (Herndon, 1996).

In the Burns Unit, the type of dressings described above are applied for the first 48 hours of treatment, until the assessment of the wound depth is made. No creams should initially be applied: because of their tendency to 'mask' the wound, causing it to appear deeper than it actually is, it makes the assessment of the depth of burn extremely difficult (Settle, 1996). Assessment of burn depth is of great importance at this time, as it influences the decision of whether surgical intervention will be necessary.

There are five anatomical areas that are an exception to this treatment: the face, ears, hands, feet and perineum.

Face

Burned faces are regularly cleaned with warmed saline and are then left exposed until they are dry and the exudate has coagulated. Soft paraffin may be applied over any crusted areas to facilitate easy removal of dead skin and to moisturize the new epithelium. Partial thickness burns treated by exposure should start to shed their coagulum after 12 days, revealing healed skin underneath. Attempts to remove any scabs before they are loose will damage the developing epithelium underneath. When the surface of a full thickness burn separates, a dressing or skin graft may be required (Settle, 1986). Soft white paraffin is applied to the lips to prevent cracking and soreness, which may inhibit nutritional intake, and oral hygiene must be attended to with regular mouth and dental care. A patient who has suffered facial burns will usually have shut their eyes during the accident as an automatic reaction, except in extreme circumstances. Eyelashes will be singed, diminishing the protection that they normally provide, and the eyes will be susceptible to infection. The eyes are initially checked for damage with fluorescein eye drops (Cason, 1981); they are then kept clean and moist with regular applications of normal saline. It is imperative that the patient is warned that his eyes will close as a result of the oedema, and emphasis should be placed upon the fact that this is only temporary.

Ears

When ears are burned, it is important that the cartilage is not allowed to dry out, as this can lead to deformity. If any infection occurs to the ears, this can cause internal damage and result in complications and defects of hearing. For these reasons, silver sulphadiazine cream is applied (after the ears have been gently plugged with paraffin gauze), and paraffin gauze and cotton gauze padding is held on by a head bandage of netting bonnet.

Hands and feet

The inflammatory reaction means that an individual with burns to the hands and feet will present with oedematous, blistering hands and feet oozing a protein-rich exudate (Muddiman, 1989). Partial thickness burns of the hands and feet can be treated successfully by the use of hand bags containing flamazine (Clarke, 1992; Settle, 1996).

An alternative to the use of occlusive dressings was proposed by Slater and Hughes (1971) and Sykes and Bailey (1975) who put patients' hands in plastic bags. Early mobilization is essential when healing is taking place (Gairns and Martin, 1990) to help prevent stiffening of the joint by preservation of active hand and foot function, reducing the incidence of contracture (Dealey, 1994; Settle, 1996). Morale and independence is increased if patients are able to freely mobilize digits in the bag (Muddiman, 1989; Dealey, 1994) compared to conventional dressings (Terrill, 1991).

The environment is found to be more conducive to healing for epidermal growth and dermal presentation than occlusive dressing (Muddiman, 1989; Clarke, 1992) as it prevents drying out of the wound and contamination from the environment (Muddiman, 1989; Clarke, 1992). Bags are changed daily or more frequently if leakage occurs (Settle, 1986).

Dealey (1994) and Muddiman (1989), however, outline several disadvantages with the use of plastic bags.

They cause maceration of all burned and non-burned skin (supported by Bache, 1988; Terrill, 1991; Settle, 1996), as large quantities of exudate accumulate in the bag (Muddiman, 1989; Dealey, 1994). Clarke (1992) argues that burns are surprisingly painless because they are kept macerated.

When used for hand burns, the bag becomes heavy, and pulls the wrist into flexion, making hand movement which is already compromised more difficult (Muddiman, 1989; Gairns and Martin, 1990; Terrill, 1991).

As unburned skin becomes 'soggy', it is difficult to tell which area is burned and which is merely macerated, making early accurate assessment difficult (Gairns and Martin, 1990). Frequent bag changes may be necessary, to cope with accumulation of unpleasant looking exudate, and it is liable to leak or tear (Muddiman, 1989; Gairns and Martin, 1990; Dealey, 1994). This takes up nursing time and increases the likelihood of infection (Muddiman, 1989).

Gore-tex bags have replaced the use of plastic bags. It is based on a semi-permeable membrane and has the property of water vapour permeability, so excessive fluid content can evaporate, acting as a barrier to airborne particles and bacteria (Muddiman, 1989). Gaseous exchange takes place through it and a good wound healing environment is retained (Muddiman, 1989).

Martin et al. (1990) and Terrill et al. (1991) undertook trials comparing gore-tex bags with conventional plastic bags. Results showed gore-tex bags to be superior. Clinically, hand and foot maceration and accumulation of exudate are significantly reduced, so there is no need for frequent bag changes, and less pain, and improved hand movement was noted. Ease of burn assessment was allowed, and the bags' durability and nonslip nature increased patient independence. The potential risk of infection is reduced since the bags do not tear, and it is less distressing for patients not to see their burned hand. Witchell and Crossman (1991) conducted a randomized trial of the use of Gore-tex bags in the treatment of hand burns in children compared to the use of paraffin gauze, and reported similar findings.

The bag lends itself to parental or patient home care (Muddiman, 1989; Gairns and Martin, 1990). One limitation is that where vascularity needs to observed for circumferential burns to arms, legs or digits, the plastic bag will need to be used so that the hand or foot can be observed for signs of decreased circulation such as pallor, coolness, numbness and lack of pulse. Terrill (1991) suggests removal of Gore-tex bags to assess vascularity as lack of maceration makes circulatory assessment easier; however, this seems impractical, and frequent exposure of the wound encourages contamination (Clarke, 1992), drying of the wound and reduction in temperature (Johnson, 1988).

Another factor is the initial high cost which over a one-year period has been estimated to be higher than that incurred using paraffin gauze (Witchell and Crossman, 1991). This is offset, however, by a reduction in the number of dressings, nursing time and length of hospital stay, and the reusable nature of the bag (Muddiman, 1989; Gairns and Martin, 1990; Terrill, 1991; Hall, 1997).

The semi-permeable membrane has been used in one Burns Unit for 12 years as a safe, reliable way of treating hand burns (Hall, 1997), allowing easy access to wounds while never delaying wound healing (Gairns and Martin, 1990). The bag has a definite place in the management of hand burns (Muddiman, 1989), as the system presented here appears to meet the requirements of an ideal burn dressing.

Perineal burns

In both males and females, the oedema resulting from a burn to the perineum may obstruct or impede the passing of urine. Catheterization of the bladder may consequently be required in the initial stages of treatment before swelling occurs. The perineum is a site with an increased risk of infection, owing to the close proximity of the anus and the urethra. The area may be dressed with paraffin gauze and padding, which is changed each time the patient uses the toilet, with meticulous attention being paid to hygiene.

These dressings are all continued until the 48-hours 'check'. When the wounds have been properly assessed, silver sulphadiazine cream may then be applied to all the areas, in conjunction with the paraffin gauze.

Silver sulphadiazine cream

In the management of many burns and scalds antibacterial creams such as 1% silver sulphadiazine (flamazine) may be recommended to assist in the desloughing process and to reduce wound colonization (Hoffman, 1984), bacterial contamination (Dealey, 1994; Gairns and Martin, 1990; Britto and Phipps, 1995; Dealey, 1994) and preserve dermis. It has a broad spectrum antibacterial effect (Britto and Phipps, 1995) and is particularly effective against Gram-negative organisms such as pseudomonas aeruginosa (Settle, 1996).

The cream needs to be applied every 24 to 48 hours to achieve its therapeutic effect (Holt, 1998) and to achieve a moist environment conducive to wound healing (Parker, 1993). It is active in the presence of blood, pus and exudate and has no effect on wound healing (Britto and Phipps, 1995; Nottingham Hospital Trusts, 1999). It is expensive but is the usual choice of topical medication in many Burns Units (Lawrence, 1989; Herndon, 1996). Because flamazine impedes epithelialization, it should be discontinued when healing partial thickness wounds are devoid of necrotic tissue and evidence of epithelialization is seen (Herndon, 1996).

Sykes and Bailey (1975) found the application of flamazine in hand bags seemed to favour wound healing.

Silver is rapidly absorbed and distributed throughout the body when applied to open wounds, but appears safe when used in the treatment of moderate burns. Coombs et al. (1992) and Settle (1996) argue that therapeutically it has a low solubility which results in a gradual release of silver so the antibacteriological activity is prolonged.

However the widespread effect use of flamazine on burns can have a cytotoxic effect on leucocytes and may contribute to local immune dysfunction with an adverse effect on wound healing (Zapata-Sirvent and Hansbrough, 1993; Gbaandor et al., 1987). In addition, flamazine can cause kernicterus and therefore should not be used on infants under three months, during pregnancy or where there is hepatic or renal dysfunction (MIMS, 1996; Herndon, 1996).

It should not be used on patients with sulphonamide sensitivity (Herndon, 1996; Nottingham Hospital Trusts, 1999). However, instances of sulphonamide sensitivity are rare (Settle, 1996). The study by Wilson et al. in 1986 appears to be the first report of sulphadiazine levels in a profoundly neutropenic burned patient. Absorption is greatest through partial thickness burns (Wilson et al., 1986) and in particular through areas from which blisters have been removed.

In a study of the side effects of flamazine, Lockhart et al. (1983) concluded it is an extremely effective topical antimicrobial agent for the treatment of burns but that it is constituently absorbed in small amounts. Such absorption may lead to hypersensitivity reactions but seems reversible.

Another concern is neutropenia in patients with extensive injuries, particularly when burns are of deep partial thickness (Settle, 1996). However, profound neutropenia occurs rarely in burned patients treated with flamazine (Jarrett et al., 1978; Lockhart et al., 1983).

Spontaneous recovery occurs without discontinuing the use of flamazine (Herndon, 1996) and should not inhibit further use of this otherwise well tolerated and effective medication (Wilson et al., 1986). No morbidity has been accountable to this transient neutropenia (Settle, 1996). However it has been shown to be toxic to human fibroblasts (McCauley et al., 1990).

As the risk of septicaemia is so great in patients suffering from major burns, wound swabs are obtained for micro-biological culture and sensitivity at each dressing change. However, when the wounds have almost healed, and in the case of minor burns, it is only necessary to take a wound swab if signs of infection are present or if infection is suspected (Flanagan, 1997). Many wounds are swabbed routinely if the presence of erythema and or oedema is noted, despite the fact that these signs are normally seen during the inflammatory phase of healing (Flanagan, 1997). Wound infection should always be treated with a systemic antibiotic rather than topical preparations (Morison, 1994).

Wound Care of Minor Burns

The admission of an individual to a Burns Unit for management of care will depend upon the size, cause, depth and location of the burn wound, the age of the patient and social circumstances. Any wound which requires regular or specialized dressings or close observation, i.e. to the face, perineum, ears or neck; any circumferential or electrical burn; and, often, wounds to the hands and feet, will require admission. All burn wounds covering more than 5% of the body will usually be admitted: however, after the initial period of maximal exudation is over (at around 48 hours) the wound, if it is small enough to be managed in the outpatients department, may be dressed accordingly and the patient discharged home.

Wounds not falling into the aforementioned categories, and also patients requiring surgery for smaller full thickness burns, may be managed as outpatients from the time of the accident, until any necessary surgery will take place. Fowler (1999) states that issues to assess prior to considering a patient for outpatient management include:

- the patient's ability to keep the wound clean and manage own dressing
- the patient's ability to recognize complications
- the patient's ability to act on information given
- the patient's ability to learn and perform care required
- the patient's ability to return regularly for review (if required)
- potential social problems/issues arising from the incident
- the patient's previous medical history/coping skills

Uncontrollable pain may also be a presenting problem, which results in admission for management.

All minor burns can be cared for with modern wound care products, which facilitate moist wound healing as desired by Winter (1962), and which possess the properties of the ideal dressing (Turner 1985) stated earlier in this chapter.

The choice of dressing will depend upon the assessment of the wound, which should take account of size and depth, site, type of tissue present in the wound, amount of exudate, pain, odour and whether the signs of infection are present (Bennett and Moody, 1995).

A variety of dressings are available to manage the presenting symptoms of a burn wound, according to the criteria described above. The management of wounds, in general, largely depends upon exudate control and non-adherence to the wound surface, which is of particular importance in burn wounds as dressing changes can be extremely painful. In the initial stages of a burn injury, because exudate production is excessive, dressings with absorbent properties are required. Traditionally, paraffin gauze dressings, for their perceived non-adherent properties, with gauze and gamgee for absorbency, have been used for all wounds major or minor, and for reasons stated earlier, due to the adherent nature and painful removal of paraffin gauze this has had to be reviewed, particularly for use in minor wounds.

With the plethora of wound care products now available the choice of dressings for burns, along with all other wound types, has led to many alternatives being available to the traditional dressing types. These are now categorized in Table 6.1 and their appropriateness to burn wounds is described. Wound assessment should take into account whether the wound is necrotic, sloughy, granulating or epithelialising and also the condition of the surounding skin (Dealey, 1994; Flanagan, 1997). Due to the nature of burn injuries often the periwound area is erythematous and this can extend hours after the burn injury. Therefore care must be taken with adhesive dressings if the injury is seen soon after it occured or if the full extent is unknown. For this reason bandaging is often the preferred method of fixing dressings into place.

All the products in the table can be used on infected wounds if the manufacturers' guidelines are followed, the wound is observed more closely, and the patient is taking systemic antibiotics.

However, the characteristics of infected wounds may contra-indicate their usage, e.g. heavy exudate. If antimicrobial treatments are required to reduce bacterial colonization at the wound site, silver sulphadiazine cream, as discussed earlier, is usually the dressing of choice in burn wounds, but iodine-based dressings could also be considered. Debate regarding the use of antiseptics continues, but dressings such as Inadine and Iodosorb are regarded as safe and effective (Bennett and Moody, 1995; Flanagan, 1997).

One problem, which occurs frequently during the latter stages of the burn wound, is that of overgranulation. Overgranulation (or hypergranulation) can be described as a 'raised, red gelatinous mass that protrudes above the level of the surrounding skin' (Young, 1995). The cause of this is unknown. However, it is thought to be related to the inflammatory response of injured tissue. Dealey (1994) states that prolonged inflammation can result in excessive granulation, as can too much inflammation (Morison, 1992). Burn wounds do appear to have an exaggerated inflammatory response, which can be demonstrated by excessive exudate in the initial stages.

Table 6.1 Selection of wound care products for burns

Dressing type	Product names Examples	Advised usage in burn wounds
Non-/low-adherent dressings	NA N/A Ultra Mepitel	Alternatives to paraffin gauze. N/A Ultra and Mepitel are silicon-based. Mepitel can be left in situ for 7 days undisturbed, whilst secondary dressings are changed. Should not cause trauma to wound surface on removal.
Hydrogels	Intrasite Nugel	Rehydration of dry or dead tissue. Useful for debridement of necrotic or full thickness burns, which are not suitable for surgery. Require a secondary dressing to maintain moisture or absorb, depending upon amount of exudate. Contra-indicated in heavily exuding wounds and can macerate surrounding skin. Can be used throughout stages of healing. Require changing every 1–3 days.
Hydrocolloids	Comfeel Granuflex Tegasorb	Rehydration of sloughy/necrotic tissue promotes granulation throughout all stages of wound healing. Waterproof and does not require a secondary dressing. Can be left in situ 5–7 days. Contra-indicated in heavily exuding wounds.
Alginates	Sorbsan Kaltostate Tegagen	Absorbent dressings which produce a moist gel in presence of exudate. Gel then promotes autolysis and granulation. For moderate/heavily exuding wounds. Act as a haemostat. Contra-indicated on dry wounds. Can be left in situ 3–5 days. Require a secondary dressing.
Hydrofibre (Hydrocolloid)	Aquacel	Absorbent dressings which produce a moist gel in presence of exudate. Gel then promotes autolysis and granulation. For moderate/heavily exuding wounds. Can facilitate debridement. Contra-indicated on dry wounds. Can be left in situ 3–5 days. Require a secondary dressing.
Foam Dressings	Lyofoam Allevyn Tielle	Absorbent dressings which maintain a moist healing environment. Can facilitate debridement in the presence of large amounts of exudate. Contra-indicated in dry wounds. Can be left in situ up to 7 days. Useful secondary dressing. For moderate/heavily exuding wounds. Waterproof types available.
Film Dressings	Opsite Tegaderm	Cannot absorb exudate but can be used on very superficial, minimally exuding wounds, or as a secondary dressing to keep a primary dressing moist. Can be left in situ for up to 7 days.

Information taken from Flanagan, 1997; Miller and Glover, 1999; and the authors' experience.

A non-traumatic method of reducing overgranulation was trialled by Harris and Rolstad (1992) using Lyofoam, which proved successful. However some overgranulating wounds appear unaffected by this treatment. Resistant overgranulation can be treated with topical corticosteriod cream (Young 1995) under a non-adherent dressing. However, caution is advised, as corticosteroids are not indicated for this use and medical supervision is recommended (Thomas, 1990).

In conclusion, the aim of the overall treatment and care of the burn wound is to control the proliferation of bacteria on the burn surface, to provide a moist environment to promote healing, to encourage the separation of burn eschar, and eventually to achieve a clean, vascularized wound bed that will heal spontaneously or will accept a skin graft. Knowledge of the wound healing process and the functions of dressings are essential to help nurses improve patient understanding and facilitate participation in care where possible.

References

Angeras M, Brandberg A, Falk A, Seeman T (1992) Comparison between sterile saline and tap water for the cleaning of acute traumatic soft tissue wounds. European Journal of Surgery 158: 347–50.

Arturson G (1993) Management of burns. Journal of Wound Care 2(2): 107–12.

Aycliffe GAJ, Lowbury EJL, Geddes AM (1992) Control of Hospital Infection: a Practical Handbook. 3rd edn. London: Chapman and Hall.

Bache J (1988) Clinical evaluation of the use of Op-Site gloves for the treatment of partial thickness burns of the hand. Burns 14(5): 413–16.

Bale S, Jones V (1997) Wound Care Nursing: a Patient-centred Approach. London: Baillière Tindall.

Bennett G, Moody M (1995) Wound Care for Health Professionals. London: Chapman and Hall.

Britto J, Phipps A (1995) Major Burn Trauma: Pathophysiology and Early Management. The Medicine Groups (Journals) Ltd. pp 283–88.

Cason JS (1981) Treatment of Burns. London: Chapman and Hall.

Clarke JA (1992) A Colour Atlas of Burn Injuries. London: Chapman and Hall.

Chrintz H, Vibits H, Cordtz TO et al. (1989) Need for surgical wound dressing. British Journal of Surgery 76: 204–5.

Coombs CJ, Wan AT, Masterton JP et al. (1992) Do burn patients have a silver lining? Burns 18(3): 179–83.

Courtenay M (1998) Choosing wound dressings. Nursing Times 94(9): 46–47.

Davis H, Dunkley D, Harden R et al. (1993) The Wound Handbook. Dundee: Centre for Medical Education.

Dealey C (1994) The Care of Wounds: a Guide for Nurses. London: Blackwell Science.

Deitch EA, Bridges RM, Dobke M et al. (1987) Burn wound sepsis may be promoted by a failure of local antibacterial host defences. Annals of Surgery 119: 83.

DuKamp A (2000) Managing burn blisters. Nursing Times Plus 96(4): 19–20.

Dyer C, Roberts D (1990) Thermal trauma. Nursing Clinics of North America 25(1): 85–117.

Dziewulski P (1992) Burn wound healing: James Ellsworth Laing memorial essay for 1991. Burns 18(6): 466–75.

Ferguson A (1988) Best performer. Nursing Times 84(14): 52–55.

Flanagan M, Fletcher J, Hollingworth H (1994) Cling film as a temporary dressing. Journal of Wound Care 3(7): 339.

Flanagan M (1997) Wound Management. London: Churchill Livingstone.

Flanagan M, Graham J (2001) Should burn blisters be left intact or debrided? Journal of Wound Care 10(1): 41–5.

Fletcher J (1997) Wound cleansing. Professional Nurse 12(11): 793–96.

Fowler A (1994) Nursing management of a patient with burns. British Journal of Nursing 3(21): 1105–12.

Fowler A (1999) Burns. In Miller M, Glover D, (Eds) Wound Management: Theory and Practice. Nursing Times Books. London: Emap.

Gairns CE, Martin DL (1990) The use of semi-permeable membrane bags as hand bag dressings. Physiotherapy 76(6): 351–52.

Gbaandor BM, Policastro AJ, Durfee D et al. (1987) Transient leucopenia associated with topical silver sulfadiazine in burn therapy. Nebraska Medical Journal 72(3): 83–85.

Gilchrist B (1994) Treating bacterial wound infection. Nursing Times 90(50): 55–58.

Griffiths-Jones A, Ward K (1995) Principles of Infection Control Practice. Harrow: Scutari Press.

Hall M (1997) Minor burns and hand burns: comparing treatment methods. Professional Nurse 12(7): 489–91.

Harris A, Rolstad BS (1992) Hypergranulation tissue: a non-traumatic method of management. 3rd European Conference on Advances in Wound Management Proceedings. London: Macmillan Magazines.

Hartford C (1996) Care of out-patients burns. In Herndon DN, (Ed) Total Burn Care. London: WB Saunders, pp 74–75.

Hateley P (1993) Lotions and potions: a review of wound cleansing agents. Nursing Times 89(45) (Infection control nurses' supplement): viii–x.

Herndon DN (1996) Total Burn Care. London: WB Saunders.

Hoffman S (1984) Silver sulphadiazine cream, an antibacterial agent for topical use in burns: a review of the literature. Journal of Reconstructive Surgery 18: 118–19.

Hollinworth H, Fletcher J, Hallet A et al. (1993) Cleansing wounds with warm saline. Journal of Wound Care 2(5): 271.

Hollinworth H (1998) Using a non-sterile technique in wound care. Professional Nurse 13(4): 226–29.

Holt L (1998) Assessing and managing minor burns. Emergency Nurse 6(2): 14–16.

Jarrett F, Ellerbe S, Demling R (1978) Acute leucopenia during topical burn therapy with silver sulphadiazine. American Journal of Surgery 135: 818.

Johnson A (1988) Wound management: are you getting it right? Professional Nurse 3(8): 306–9.

Lawrence JC (1987) British Burns Association recommended first aid treatment for burns and scalds. Burns 13(2): 153.

Lawrence C (1989) Treating minor burns. Nursing Times 85(26): 69–73.

Lock PM (1980) Proceedings of the Symposium of Wound Healing. Gothenberg: Linden and Sonner.

Lockhart SP, Rushworth A, Azmy AAF et al. (1983) Topical silver sulphadiazine: side effects and urinary excretion. Burns 10: 9–12.

Lowry PW, Blankenship RJ, Grindley W et al. (1991) A cluster of legionella sternal wound infections due to postoperative topical exposure to contaminated tap water. New England Journal of Medicine 324(2): 109–13.

Lowry PW, Tompkins LS (1993) Nosocomial legionellosis: a review of pulmonary and extra-pulmonary syndromes. American Journal of Infection Control 21(1): 21–27.

Martin DL, French GWG, Theakstone J (1990) The use of semi-permeable membranes for wound management. British Journal of Plastic Surgery 43: 55–60.

McCauley RL, Poole B, Heggers JP et al. (1990) Differential in vitro toxicity of topical antimicrobial agents to human keratinocytes. Proceedings of the American Burn Association 22: 2.

McLaren SMG (1992) Nutrition and wound healing. Journal of Wound Care 1(3): 45–55.

Meers P, Jacobsen W, McPherson M (1992) Hospital Infection Control for Nurses. London: Chapman and Hall.

Meers P, Sedgwick J, Worsley M (1995) The microbiology and epidemiology of infection for health science students. London: Chapman and Hall.

Miller M, Glover D (1999) Wound Management: Theory and Practice. Nursing Times Books. London: Emap.

Miller M, Dyson M (1996) Principles of Wound Care. London: Macmillan Magazines Ltd.

MIMS (Monthly Index of Medical Specialities) (1996) London: Haymarket Medical.

Morison M (1992) A Colour Guide to the Nursing Management of Wounds. London: Wolfe.

Morison MJ (1989) Wound cleansing- which solution? Professional Nurse, Feb: 220–25.

Morison MJ (1994) Which wound care product. Professional Nurse Information Sheet. London: Austin Cornish.

Muddiman R (1989) A new concept in hand burn dressing. Nursing Standard, Sept: 1–3.

Myers JA (1982) Modern plastic surgical dressings. Health and Social Services Journal 92: 336–37.

Nottingham Hospital Trusts (1996) Wound Management Guidelines. Nottingham.

Nottingham Hospital Trusts (1999) Wound Care Formulary and Wound Management Guidelines. Nottingham.

Oliver L (1997) Wound cleansing. Nursing Standard 11(20): 47–56.

Pape SA (1993) The management of scars. Journal of Wound Care 2(6): 354–60.

Parker JA (1993) Burns Educational Leaflet 14. Northampton: The Wound Care Society.

Riyat MS, Quinton DN (1997) Tap water as a wound cleansing agent in accident and emergency. Journal of Accident and Emergency Medicine 14: 165–66.

Rockwell W, Ehrlich HP (1990) Should burn blisters be burst? Emergency Medicine 22(11): 57–59.

Rylah LTA (1992) Critical Care of the Burned Patient. Cambridge: Cambridge University Press.

Settle JAD (1986) Burns: the First Five Days. Hull: Smith and Nephew

Settle JAD (1996) Principles and Practice of Burns Management. London: Churchill and Livingstone.

Slater RM, Hughes NC (1971) A simplified method of treating burns of the hands. British Journal of Plastic Surgery 24: 296–300.

Sykes PJ, Bailey BN (1975) Treatment of hand burns with occlusive bags: a comparison of 3 methods. Burns 2: 162–68.

Terrill PJ, Kedwards SM, Lawrence JC (1991) The use of gore-tex bags for hand burns. Burns 17(2): 161–65.

Tortora GJ, Grabowski SR (1996) Principles of Anatomy and Physiology, 8th edn. New York: Harper Collins College Publications.

Thomas S (1990) Wound Management and Dressings. London: Pharmaceutical Press.

Thompson G, Bullock D (1992) To clean or not to clean. Nursing Times 88(34): 62–65.

Trofino RB (1991) Nursing Care of the Burn-injured Patient. Philadelphia: FA Davis Company.

Turner T (1985) Which dressing and why? In Westaby S, (Ed) Wound Care. London: Heinemann.

Westaby S (1985) Wound Care. London: Heinemann.

Williams C, Young T (1998) Myth and Reality in Wound Care. Salisbury: Mark Allen Publishing Ltd.

Wilson GR, French G (1987) Plasticised polyvinyl chloride as a temporary dressing for burns. British Medical Journal 292: 556–57.

Wilson P, Robert G, Raine P (1986) Topical silver sulphadiazine and profound neutropenia in a burned child. Burns 12: 295–96.

Winter GD (1962) Review of classic research: moist wound healing. Journal of Wound Care 4(8): 366–71.

Witchell M, Crossman C (1991) Dressing burns in children. Nursing Times 87(36): 63–66.

Young T (1995) Common problems in wound care: overgranulation. British Journal of Nursing 4(3): 169–70.

Young T (1995) Burns and scalds. Practice Nurse 6(18): 37–40.

Zapata-Sirvent RL, Hansbrough JF (1993) Cytotoxity to human leukocytes by topical antimicrobial agents used for burns. Journal of Burn Care and Rehabilitation 14: 132–140.

CHAPTER 7

Management of the Patient with an Inhalation Injury

DAVID KNIGHTS

Introduction

The literature concerning inhalation injury is extensive and confusing. Much of the confusion results from the use of differing terminology and a marked change in opinion and practice over the last 15 to 20 years. This chapter attempts to present a simple categorization of inhalation injury along with a distillation of the most recent and salient features of diagnosis and management.

Epidemiology and Prognosis of Inhalation Injury

Statistics vary widely but approximately 700–1 000 people die annually in the UK as a result of fire. Most deaths occur at the scene and three quarters of these victims have no cutaneous burn. They have died as a result of inhaling toxic substances contained in fire smoke, most commonly carbon monoxide (CO). By comparison, most patients who reach hospital alive with an isolated inhalation injury survive. In patients with a cutaneous burn who reach hospital alive, the presence of an inhalation injury increases their predicted mortality by a minimum of 20–40%. This increases markedly at the extremes of age and with the presence of significant co-morbidity. The development of pneumonia in addition to a cutaneous burn and an inhalation injury increases predicted mortality based on burn size by as much as 70%. Thus the combination of a cutaneous burn and an inhalation injury has a synergistic rather than a purely summative effect on morbidity and mortality.

While antimicrobial therapy and early surgery have both contributed to a reduction in mortality from cutaneous burns, little impact has been made on mortality associated with the inhalation injury. The full spectrum of lung injury can be seen, ranging from little evidence of impaired gas exchange to those patients who die rapidly of intractable hypoxia despite maximal therapy. Many patients who survive the early phase go on to develop the adult or acute respiratory distress syndrome (ARDS), which is seen in many other forms of major injury or illness.

Classification of Injury

The use of differing terminology causes confusion. The following classification is gaining favour and is used in both the Advanced Burn Life Support (ABLS) and Emergency Management of Severe Burns (EMSB) courses.

Inhalation injury can be divided into three categories:

• airway injury above the larynx
• airway injury below the larynx
• systemic intoxication injuries

Patients may sustain each type of injury in isolation or in any combination.

Airway Injury Above the Larynx

This is a thermal burn to the mucosa of the nose, mouth and pharynx and occurs when the patient has inhaled hot gas.

The injury is usually confined to the structures above the larynx for two reasons. Firstly, the nose, mouth and pharynx are well adapted as heat and moisture exchangers that normally warm and humidify inhaled air. In the fire environment, they cool the hot gases, protecting the lower airway but sustain burns as a consequence. Secondly, the highly irritant nature of hot smoke causes reflex closure of the larynx that protects the lower airway from injury for a short time. This may be long enough to allow escape from the fire environment and hence, lower airway injury may be avoided. In prolonged entrapment this protective reflex is overcome by the need to breathe and damage to the lower airway can occur.

The pathophysiological processes of injury above the larynx are identical to those of the cutaneous burn. Thus, oedema will occur relatively early and partial or complete upper airway obstruction is a very real danger.

Airway Injury Below the Larynx

This injury is very rarely due to heat for the reasons stated above. Most commonly, this injury is a chemical injury due to the irritant constituents of smoke. The constituents of smoke vary according to duration of the fire, the position of the patient in relation to the fire and the materials that are burning. Highly water-soluble substances will tend to exert their effects high in the respiratory tract while the less water-soluble will be able to reach much lower down the airway. The carbon particles in smoke have previously been thought to be relatively harmless but it is now known that they can carry heat energy down to the lower airways and, more significantly, have many chemicals adsorbed onto their surface, which subsequently cause airway injury. The variable nature of smoke content is the reason that symptoms and signs vary, and that they may present immediately or be delayed for several days.

Rarely, thermal injury below the larynx occurs in situations where steam or inflammable gases have been inhaled or hot liquids aspirated.

Systemic Intoxication Injuries

These occur because constituents of the inhaled gas are toxic to the body as a whole rather than causing damage localized only to the respiratory tract.

The level of oxygen in the fire environment falls because the combustion process consumes it. The same combustion process simultaneously produces carbon dioxide. Hypoxia and hypercarbia are both thought to be common causes of intoxication at fire scenes involving entrapment. The consequent confusion and impaired dexterity may reduce the victim's ability to escape from the fire environment.

Carbon monoxide (CO) is produced by fires that no longer have an adequate supply of oxygen to allow full combustion. CO poisoning is the most frequent intoxication injury seen in patients surviving to reach hospital. Toxicity occurs as CO binds to the oxygen binding sites on the haemoglobin molecule, forming carboxyhaemoglobin (COHb). It binds 250 times more readily than oxygen and therefore reduces the ability of the haemoglobin molecule to transport oxygen. It also binds to tissue myoglobin and to the mitochondrial cytochromes, reducing the ability of the cells to use any oxygen that may reach them.

Hydrogen cyanide (HCN) is produced in fires involving nitrogen-containing polymers, both natural and synthetic. HCN is an extremely potent cellular poison that blocks cytochrome function and thus cellular metabolism.

Management of Patients with Inhalation Injuries

In the UK, the majority of patients with inhalation injury are likely to receive treatment at three main sites:

- Pre-hospital
- Accident and Emergency departments
- Burns Units/Intensive Therapy Units (ITU)

Care in these three areas will be discussed separately in an attempt to provide clarity while recognizing that this is an over-simplification as there will be considerable overlap and local variation.

Pre-hospital Care

The priorities here are exactly the same as for any other major trauma:

- safety of rescuer and patient
- assessment of airway, breathing and circulation (ABC)
- appropriate treatment of problems found in the ABC
- transfer to an appropriate hospital

A history of the fire event including type of fire, occurrence of explosions, length of entrapment and mode of escape or rescue must be sought. This information will guide treatment and investigation at the scene and in hospital. The presence of other injuries must be assumed and treated accordingly, e.g. cervical spine injury.

Specific treatment for an inhalation injury in the pre-hospital setting is to assume its presence, to administer high concentration oxygen, and to ensure early transfer to an appropriate Accident and Emergency Department.

Accident and Emergency Department

The priorities here are exactly the same as for any other major trauma:

- Primary survey to find and treat immediately life-threatening injuries
- Analgesia titrated to response

- Secondary survey to find and treat other injuries
- Referral to appropriate definitive care

If all of the above are performed, then the patient with a cutaneous burn and an inhalation injury will receive optimal emergency care.

Specific investigations and treatment for the inhalation injury should follow the standard model of history, examination, investigation and treatment (see Table 7.1).

History

The most consistent findings in the histories of patients with inhalation injury are a history of entrapment in a smoke-filled environment, the occurrence of explosions and an impaired level of consciousness at the time of rescue. Disorientation or altered conscious level may indicate brain injury or effects of inhalation injury and should not be assumed to be due to alcohol or other drugs. For symptoms and signs of carbon monoxide toxicity, see Table 7.2. Other indicators in the history are related to respiratory symptoms, which should be actively sought. The patient may complain of sore throat, retrosternal burning, chest tightness and difficulty breathing. Patients may complain of voice change or the

Table 7.1 Indicators of inhalation injury

History	Entrapment in smoke-filled, enclosed space
	Explosions at fire scene
	Altered level of consciousness at time of rescue
	Change in voice or cry
	Retrosternal burning
	Dyspnoea
Examination	Altered level of consciousness
	Tachypnoea
	Perioral or perinasal burns
	Singed nasal hair
	Hoarseness
	Stridor
	Soot in oropharynx
	Erythema or oedema of tongue or uvula
	Wheeze
Investigation	Carboxyhaemoglobin >15% at time of rescue
	Low PaO_2 or increased $(A-a)O_2$ gradient
	Soot or erythema of bronchial mucosa on bronchoscopy
	CXR changes

Table 7.2 Symptoms and signs of carbon monoxide toxicity

% COHb	Symptoms and signs
0–10	None, levels found in smokers and drivers
10–20	Headache, mild confusion
20–40	Nausea, fatigue, disorientation, dizziness, muscle tremor
40–60	Hallucinations, ataxia, syncope, convulsions, coma
>60	Death

parents of an injured child may state that the child's cry sounds abnormal. These vocal changes may represent early indicators of laryngeal oedema.

Examination

Tachypnoea may be present and may be the only initial finding. Further examination may reveal the presence of perioral and perinasal burns, evidence of burns to the inside of the nose or mouth (singing of nasal hair, erythema or oedema of the tongue or uvula), soot in the oropharynx, the presence of hoarseness or other, later, indicators of laryngeal oedema, e.g. stridor. Chest examination can initially be normal or may show signs of bronchospasm. In severe cases, clinical signs of pulmonary oedema may be present. In the presence of strong historical indicators of possible inhalation injury, the absence of findings on the initial examination does not exclude injury. The patient must be monitored and reassessed carefully.

Investigation

Arterial blood gas (ABG) analysis should be performed (noting the inspired oxygen concentration at the time of measurement). Low arterial partial pressure of oxygen (PaO_2) relative to the inspired concentration, an $(A-a)O_2$ gradient, is highly suggestive of an inhalation injury. Blood gas analysers measure the plasma partial pressure of oxygen and they assume the presence of normal haemoglobin in order to calculate the oxygen saturation of haemoglobin. This can lead to two potential pitfalls in interpretation of results. Firstly, the partial pressure of oxygen in a sample can be normal or even raised despite significant levels of COHb. Secondly, the calculated oxygen saturation will be falsely high. Similarly, pulse oximeters cannot differentiate between COHb and normal oxygenated haemoglobin and may give falsely high readings.

Carboxyhaemoglobin (COHb) must be measured using a co-oximeter. Some analysers now perform this analysis routinely, but it may need to be requested in addition to standard ABG analysis. For treatment of carbon monoxide poisoning, see below.

Chest radiography (CXR) will have been performed in the primary survey and may be helpful but can, initially, be normal.

Fibre-optic bronchoscopy is unlikely to be available in the Accident and Emergency department but can be useful in diagnosis (see below).

Treatment

The mainstays of treatment of inhalation injury in the Accident and Emergency department are airway protection, oxygenation and treatment of bronchospasm.

The finding of any evidence of upper airway oedema is an indication for urgent tracheal intubation in order to prevent total upper airway obstruction as the oedema increases. Other indications for tracheal intubation include reduced conscious level and severe respiratory distress.

If it is decided that intubation is not required, the decision must be reviewed frequently following equally frequent reassessment of the patient. If the patient is to be transported within or between hospitals then further consideration should be given to protecting the airway. **If in doubt, intubate!**

Induction of anaesthesia and tracheal intubation should be performed by a senior anaesthetist with skilled assistance, as there may be considerable difficulty due to oedema. The tracheal tube should be cut to a longer length than normal to allow for the subsequent formation of facial oedema. This will reduce the risk of accidental tracheal extubation and the potential inability to reintubate.

Oxygen therapy should be given at the highest available concentration until it can be guided by the results of ABG and COHb analysis.

Bronchospasm should be treated aggressively with standard bronchodilators including steroids in severe cases if necessary (usually patients with a history of severe asthma).

Carbon monoxide

Treatment of carbon monoxide poisoning is based upon the competitive way in which CO and oxygen bind to haemoglobin (Hb). As previously stated, CO binds to Hb 250 times more readily than oxygen. At normal atmospheric pressure and in the presence of 21% inhaled oxygen, the half-life of COHb is approximately 250 minutes. If the inspired concentration of oxygen is raised, the half-life decreases. With 100% inspired oxygen, the half-life of COHb is reduced to approximately 50 minutes. If 100% inspired oxygen is given at 2.5 times normal atmospheric pressure (hyperbaric oxygen therapy) then the half-life is reduced to approximately 20–25 minutes. Unfortunately, the complex treatment needs of a patient with both a cutaneous burn and an inhalation injury, the tiny size of the majority of the hyperbaric treatment chambers and the geographical distances to the treatment centres makes hyperbaric oxygen therapy inappropriate in most cases.

Inspired oxygen concentration can be raised to 50–60% if high airflow oxygen equipment (HAFOE or 'Venturi' masks) is used. The use of a mask with a non-rebreathing reservoir bag can increase this to 80%. Tracheal intubation allows the administration of 100% oxygen and may be indicated in the patient with reduced conscious level.

Levels of COHb above 10% should be treated by high concentration inspired oxygen until they fall to normal. Such levels usually indicate that much higher levels were present at the time of rescue. Because of the predictable half-life of COHb, the blood level at the time of rescue can be calculated using a standard nomogram (Clark, Campbell and Reid, 1981) and this may be a useful prognostic indicator for any subsequent deterioration in lung function.

Intravenous fluid therapy

Intravenous fluid therapy for the cutaneous burn will be guided by the assessment of burn size calculated in the secondary survey. The type of fluid used (crystalloid or colloid) is less important than that it is administered in the appropriate volumes. Adjustment of therapy should be guided by urine output in the initial phase with a urine output of 0.5–1ml/kg/hour being adequate. It is just as important to reduce fluid therapy in the presence of excess urine production as it is to increase it in the presence of inadequate urine volumes because excessive fluids will lead to increased oedema formation and possible deterioration of the burn wound and lung function.

Communication

Early communication with the receiving Burn Unit is essential both for advice and to check the availability of a bed of the appropriate dependency level.

Burns Unit/ITU

Treatment already commenced should continue and a full reassessment of the patient's history and examination should be performed, specifically looking for any alteration. Analgesia and nutritional support should be given early and are discussed in other chapters.

ABG analysis should be repeated as regularly as clinically indicated. If COHb levels were raised initially, they should be repeated until they return to normal. Presence of a persistent metabolic acidosis despite apparently adequate oxygenation and fluid resuscitation should raise the suspicion of cyanide toxicity.

Significant cyanide toxicity in smoke inhalation is rare. Cyanide levels cannot be measured in time to be clinically useful in most hospitals but there is a correlation between initial levels of COHb above 15% and significant levels of cyanide. Most cyanide toxicity can be treated by supportive measures alone but specific therapy may be indicated in severe cases. The specific antidote therapies themselves carry a significant risk and many hospitals have their own policies on diagnosis and treatment. Therefore, full discussion of the treatment of cyanide toxicity is beyond the remit of this chapter but is well covered elsewhere (Langford and Armstrong, 1989).

Repeat CXR at 48 hours may be of more diagnostic significance than the initial film but should only be performed if clinically indicated.

Fibre-optic bronchoscopy may be used to assess airway damage. Some units advocate early inspection of the larynx as part of the assessment of upper airway injury. Bronchoscopy is extremely easy to perform when the trachea has been intubated and can be both diagnostic (the presence of soot and erythema in the lower airway) and therapeutic (to guide removal of casts and mucus plugs). Scrupulous attention to asepsis is required as the injured lung is very prone to infection.

The level of monitoring required by patients will vary with their condition. The absolute minimum is for the patient to be continuously observed by the nursing and medical staff.

Pulse oximetry is a very useful, non-invasive, continuous and simple guide to oxygenation. However, it should be remembered that it is a poor monitor of adequacy of ventilation.

Continuous ECG monitoring may be helpful but can be difficult in the presence of extensive burns.

The insertion of an arterial line for direct arterial pressure monitoring is useful, as non-invasive measurement may be made difficult or inaccurate by the presence of bandages. They also allow painless repeat blood sampling.

Urinary catheter and hourly measurement are mandatory in order to monitor ongoing fluid resuscitation.

Opinion on the benefit of other invasive monitoring has changed markedly in recent years. The use of central venous pressure (CVP) monitoring and measurement of cardiac output studies with pulmonary artery (PA) catheters can guide use of fluids, inotropes and vasoconstrictors to optimise cardiac performance. The presence of an inhalation injury in addition to a cutaneous injury increases the volume of intravenous fluid required for resuscitation by an unpredictable amount. Patients with this combination of injury require very careful monitoring of their resuscitation in order to avoid both under perfusion and fluid overload, as both cause deterioration in the cutaneous burn and the lung injury. Appropriate use of CVP and PA monitoring can avoid these complications. The risks of infection from the catheters were previously thought to outweigh the advantages but, as experience in interpretation and use of the information they provide has increased, it is now felt that the benefits outweigh the risks if they are used judiciously.

After the initial resuscitation phase, oxygen therapy should be guided by the results of ABG analysis. Humidification is needed, as the normal humidification function of the upper respiratory tract will have been impaired by the injury. Chest physiotherapy should be commenced as soon as it is practical. Physiotherapy aims to maintain small airway patency and prevent atelectasis, clear mucus secretions and casts, maintain and improve gas exchange (Keilty, 1993). All of these contribute to reducing risk of infection.

In addition, increasing failure of gas exchange may occur and the patient may require ventilatory support. Respiratory support is based around positive end expiratory pressure (PEEP) in mechanical ventilation and continuous positive airway pressure (CPAP) in spontaneous ventilation. The aim is to prevent airway collapse and thus improve gas exchange and reduce infection risk.

Older literature suggests that tracheostomy is contra-indicated in patients with burns. This is no longer felt to be the case (Barrett, Desai and Herndon, 2000). Tracheostomy should not be performed through burned skin (unless in an emergency for airway obstruction) as these have a very high incidence of infection and mediastinitis. Early tracheal intubation by the oral route should avoid the need for emergency tracheostomy for airway obstruction. However, when performed through unburned or healed skin, tracheostomy holds no increased risk above that for patients with other types of injury or illness.

Many treatments have come and gone without success in improving outcome from inhalation injury. Review of the current literature clarifies some areas while others areas remain unclear. Some of the most relevant are discussed here.

- There is no place for prophylactic antibiotic therapy for inhalation injury. Clinical indications and available culture results should guide antibiotic therapy.
- The use of high dose steroids does not appear to be of any value and may increase the incidence of infection.
- Hyperbaric oxygen therapy has been discussed earlier. Extracorporeal membrane oxygenation (ECMO) and intravenocaval oxygenation (IVOX) are still highly experimental in the situation of a cutaneous burn and an inhalation injury but may have a place in the treatment of lung injury alone.
- One very encouraging treatment is bicarbonate lavage. There is an increasing amount of evidence from work in children, that hourly bronchial lavage with isotonic sodium bicarbonate (5ml in infants, 10ml in larger children) reduces the incidence of late deterioration in lung function (Lord, 1997). This is thought to work by neutralising the acidic component of soot and by speeding the clearance of that soot. There are presently trials ongoing in both children and adults (Lord, personal communication).
- Timing of surgery should be as early as possible since early wound closure limits one very significant source of infection.

Summary

There are no specific physical or pharmacological interventions that will 'cure' lung damage from inhalation injury. Treatment is purely supportive, avoiding further lung injury and allowing healing to occur. Management of the patient with an inhalation injury in addition to a cutaneous burn can best be summarized as follows:

- high index of suspicion
- airway protection
- oxygenation
- optimal resuscitation and post-resuscitation care
- early burn wound closure

References

Barret JP, Desai MH, Herndon DN (2000) Effects of tracheostomies on infection and airway
    complications in pediatric burn patients. Burns 26: 190–93.
Clark CJ, Campbell D, Reid WH (1981) Blood carboxyhaemoglobin and cyanide levels in fire
    survivors. Lancet i: 1332–35.
Keilty SEJ (1993) Inhalation burn injured patients and physiotherapy management.
    Physiotherapy 79: 87–90.
Langford RM, Armstrong RF (1989) Algorithm for managing injury from smoke inhalation.
    British Medical Journal 299: 902–5.
Lord WD (1997) Burns management in children. Clinical Anaesthesiology 11: 407–26.

Further Reading

Haponik EF, Munster AM (1990) Respiratory Injury, Smoke Inhalation and Burns. New
    York: McGraw Hill.
Herndon DN (1996) Total Burn Care. London: WB Saunders.
Kinsella J (1997) Burns. Clinical Anaesthesiology 11(3).
Settle JAD (1996) Principles and Practice of Burns Management. London: Churchill
    Livingstone.

CHAPTER 8

Management of Pain for an Individual following Burn Trauma

OWEN JONES

The aim of this chapter is to highlight the importance of pain management in the burns patient. Pre-injury psychological sequelae, the traumatic nature of the injury, and the fear of pain result in burns pain being a very complex matter to manage. The intense pain and anxiety suffered both at the time of injury and throughout the healing phase is described as the tormenting consequence of a burn injury by Jonsson et al. (1998). This pain presents itself in three forms, background pain, breakthrough pain and procedural pain (Ulmer, 1998). The management of pain in the burns patient is recognized as the most important aspect of nursing care requiring extensive research (Gordon et al., 1998). The complexity of the pain experienced by the patient sets burns apart from all other injuries.

Pain cannot be quantified as there is no physiological measure of intensity of pain or a common language that objectively describes the suffering of the patient. Successful pain management depends on the effectiveness of the intervention initiated by the Burns team. The success of this intervention is directly related to the knowledge of the health professionals, the use of a structured approach to pain management and the priority placed on pain management by the Burns team. The provision of effective mechanisms for pain relief is an indicator of the quality care given (Audit Commission, 1993). To achieve effective pain control nurses must be able to understand the physiological and psychological aspects of pain. Appropriate use of assessment tools will aid effective communication between the patient, their family and the carers, which will facilitate effective pain management. A collection of pain assessment tools that have a direct relevance to clinical practice have been reproduced in *Prevention and control of pain in children* (Royal College of Paediatrics and Child Health, 1997).

The degree of pain experienced by people who have sustained burn injuries varies greatly. It is as dependent on the severity of tissue damage as it is to the individual's response to pain. No two patients will suffer the same degree of discomfort and pain from the same injury. Although it is impossible to quantify the severity of pain associated with a particular injury it is reasonable to predict that they will have some pain. For moral, humanitarian, ethical and physiological reasons pain should be anticipated and active intervention commenced (Fisher and Morton, 1998). Laterjet and Choinere (1995) suggested that inadequate pain relief was a major contributing factor to the psychological morbidity in burns patients.

The need for analgesia during the initial treatment is variable. The direct correlation between anxiety and pain makes it obligatory to consider the use of sedatives in conjunction with analgesics. Loss of skin integrity will expose nerve endings that will be sensitive to both the atmosphere and the application of any form of wound dressing. In the initial period of treatment the application of a layer of plasticized polyvinyl chloride (cling-film) over the wounds to exclude the air and reduce the loss of moisture can reduce the level of discomfort (Thomas, 1989). This form of covering will enable the wound to be assessed without the need to remove conventional dressings, which are painful to remove and time-consuming to apply, and may damage some healthy tissue when frequently applied and removed during the assessment stage. Cling-film is an ideal covering during both the assessment and transit stages and can remain in situ until an appropriate dressing is applied (Wilson and French, 1987).

Burn injuries are rarely uniform and different levels of damage to the skin will be present resulting in varying levels of pain. Pain is often exacerbated by the involvement of health professionals undertaking active treatment such as wound management or physiotherapy.

What is Pain?

In order to take appropriate action, the nurse must understand what pain is and what the word pain means to the individual. Pain is a complex, distressing experience, involving sensory, emotional and cognitive components. The word 'pain' is derived from the Greek word 'poire' meaning punishment. The International Association for the Study of Pain (1986) produced the following definition:

> Pain is an unpleasant sensory and emotional experience with actual or potential tissue damage. Each individual learns the application of the word through experiences related to injury in early years.

Almost every patient who has sustained a burn injury experiences pain. Although patients who have sustained a severe burn injury present with many problems, pain is often their most significant complaint. Therefore, the assessment, prescription and administration of effective analgesia are of paramount importance. Burns nurses are in an ideal position to assess and evaluate the management of pain because of the amount of time they spend in direct contact with the patient.

Studies of orthopaedic patients have shown that prolonged pain can increase hospital inpatient stay and prevents patients from attaining their full potential, because they are unwilling or unable to fully participate in the rehabilitation phase of their recovery (Crocker, 1986). By promoting communication between all members of the multidisciplinary team, in order to coordinate painful procedures and to give effective analgesia in advance, the intensity and frequency of pain can be reduced to a minimum. To do this effectively, the patient's day must be planned and the level of discomfort assessed over a 24-hour period. The level of discomfort over a period of time can be assessed using a pain diary, discussion or the use of observations of physiological measures and pain assessment charts. In this manner patient cooperation is increased and the level of discomfort is reduced.

Nurses' perceptions of pain can become dulled because of their frequent exposure to suffering. There is also a tendency to associate particular levels of discomfort or pain with different procedures or degrees of trauma. However, there appears to be little or no correlation between the severity of the injuries sustained and the pain experienced, and this demonstrates that pain and discomfort are very much individual experiences.

It is necessary therefore to adopt an operational definition of pain and have a clear understanding of our aims when managing individuals in pain. Consider McCaffery's (1979) statement: 'Pain is whatever the experiencing person says it is, existing whenever he says it does.' This can be adapted to create a nursing aim, which becomes the functional definition of our actions associated with pain management. This aim has three elements:

- to observe and listen to the patient
- to recognize the level of physical and emotional pain
- to initiate an effective plan of management to reduce this pain to a minimum

This aim takes into consideration the many factors that affect the level of discomfort that an individual experiences. However, it also emphasizes that the nurse should be forming a partnership with the patient, using his or her knowledge, understanding and expertise to reduce the pain.

Factors that Influence Pain

The benefits of reducing any pain to a minimum include increased patient satisfaction, reduced morbidity and mortality. However, although each individual will feel and display discomfort in different ways, there are many common factors that can affect the severity of pain which must be considered when planning patient care (Table 8.1).

Table 8.1 Factors that influence the severity of pain

The depth of the burn	The manner of the initial management
The percentage of body surface area burnt	The psychological response to injury
Other injuries	Fear and anxiety
Analgesia already administered	Previous painful experiences

The effectiveness of any particular form of therapy is variable: the Burns team, therefore, must be prepared to use a variety of methods to manage the pain. The amount of psychological support and analgesia required will never be the same for two patients. Factors such as age, gender and the cultural background of the patient will affect the pain experienced by an individual. It is sometimes difficult for people to express their feelings and fears with someone of another gender or from a different cultural background (Helman, 1990), and this can be exacerbated if communication is difficult because of language or speech problems. This can be overcome by the use of an interpreter. The use of a picture board with symbols that demonstrate discomfort, the severity of the pain, and the need for analgesia can help promote effective communication. The patient indicates his or her feelings and wishes by pointing to the relevant symbol; this can also be used with patients who have endotracheal tubes in situ.

The Rationale for Addressing the Problem of Pain Management

If adequate pain relief is not achieved, the patient begins to anticipate pain every time a member of the Burns team attempts to carry out a procedure, whether or not it is potentially painful. This can result in poor patient cooperation and an increasing tendency towards dependence, because the patient is afraid to move for fear of experiencing pain. The problem of pain management must be addressed as soon as the patient arrives in hospital. Pain itself can act as a barrier between the patient and members of staff, because a patient in pain is unlikely to communicate freely with carers if in pain. Staff members can actively work towards reducing this barrier by effectively reducing the level of discomfort and keeping the patient fully informed about their care. Hayward (1979) demonstrated that information given to the patient actively decreases anxiety levels, and therefore reduces the amount of pain.

In order for us to be able to assess and manage pain effectively, we must have an understanding of the factors that affect the perception of pain in the individual. We must also be aware of the different types of pain and how this 'pain' is transmitted and interpreted by the body (the mechanism of pain).

The pain experienced by an individual post-burn injury will change through the phases of recovery. Initially, there may be acute pain that has had a rapid onset giving individuals no time to prepare themselves; there will also be a time during this phase when they will have had no analgesia. The individual may also have been denied emotional or psychological support if the injuries were sustained in an isolated area.

Admission to hospital is the start of treatment and rehabilitation; they will have to undergo many painful procedures, often resulting in unpredictable levels of discomfort. The type of pain felt during the different stages of treatment will vary and can present the team with different management problems. Some of the activities that will increase the level of pain felt by the patient can be anticipated (see Table 8.2) and should become part of the planned programme of pain management.

It is this planned discomfort that can be reduced to a minimum. By looking at the factors that influence pain and establishing which ones are variable, staff can work with the patient to reduce the level of pain as much as possible. Hayward (1979) demonstrated that information and active patient participation reduces anxiety levels and thus reduces the level of post-operative pain. Health professionals must be honest with

Table 8.2 Activities that increase the level of pain experienced by the patient

Clinical examinations	Physiotherapy
Clinical procedures, e.g. the insertion of intravenous lines, venepuncture and catheterization.	Mobilization
Dressings/wound management.	Daily activities of living, e.g. eating, dressing and washing.
Surgery – graft and donor sites.	

patients and actively work to keep them as informed about future treatments and their possible side effects, such as pain or discomfort. Alternative methods of pain control can be discussed, and the patient can take an active part in their own care.

The Way the Body Reacts to Pain

To achieve pain-free therapy, one must have a greater understanding of the way in which the body reacts to pain. Everybody has a different pain threshold, but each individual's pain threshold is affected by the same factors, which may lower or raise the threshold. Some of these factors are included in Table 8.3.

Table 8.3 Factors affecting the pain threshold

Threshold lowered	Threshold raised
Discomfort	Relief of symptoms
Insomnia	Sleep and rest
Fatigue	Sympathy
Fear and anxiety	Understanding and companionship
Mistrust	Trust
Anger, sadness and depression	Diversional activities
Boredom and introversion	Reduction in anxiety
Mental isolation	Elevation in mood
Social abandonment	Analgesics and antidepressants

The Anatomy and Physiology of Pain

To manage pain effectively it is essential to have a good understanding of the mechanisms and theories of pain. The theories of pain are just that –'theories' – and although such theories are commonly used to explain the process of pain and pain management it is worth noting that many are unproven hypotheses (McCaffery and Beebe, 1994).

The Pain Mechanism

The structures that enable us to feel pain are the receptors (nociceptors), which are sensitive to painful stimuli. The impulse pathways (routes) carry the impulses to the interpreting centres in the brain that decode and act on these impulses. There is also an analgesic system that modulates and controls pain.

Pain receptors

The concentration of pain receptors (nociceptors) varies greatly within the body, but they are found in nearly all tissue types. The nerve fibres are small and non-myelinated. Simulation of the nerve endings results in the release of kinins. The rate of release is increased in the presence of prostaglandins, which themselves are released by damaged cells as part of the inflammatory process.

Pain stimuli

A variety of agents either physical or chemical can become stimuli, and the degree of stimulation felt is directly proportional to the intensity of the agent applied. Thus for heat, the higher the temperature, the greater the stimulus.

Pain impulse pathways

These are the paths or routes along which the impulses travel to reach the spinal cord or brain stem. They are made up of small (non-myelinated) and large (myelinated) nerve fibres, myelin being a fatty insulating sheath. When impulses travel along both types of fibres, we are aware of pain, but the sensation produced is different. Impulses travelling along the non-myelinated fibres travel slowly, producing the throbbing, dull, burning type of pain, whereas when impulses travel along the myelinated fibres, they travel at speed, creating the sharp, stabbing, localized pain often linked to an initial burns injury.

There are many theories that have been written to try to explain the physiology of pain, the two most common being the Specificity Theory and the Gate Theory. Using both theories together can explain most methods of pain control.

Theories of Pain

The Specificity Theory

This theory proposes that specific structures, namely nerve fibres, central nervous system pathways and neurones, are responsible for the passage of information to the brain. The areas that are covered by similar systems are pain, temperature, light touch and pressure.

Impulses travel from the site of injury or stimulus via specific sensory nerve fibres to the spinal cord (first-order neurones), the route of entry to the spinal cord being via the posterior root ganglia and into the horn of grey matter. Many interconnections occur here, but most impulses travel to the brain via the spinothalamic tract (second-order neurones).

These impulses travel through the brain stem to the thalamus (Figure 8.1a and 8.1b). The fibres associated with pain and temperature terminate in the ventral posterior lateral nucleus of the thalamus where conscious recognition of pain and temperature occurs.

From this point, the impulses are carried to the somesthetic area of the cerebral cortex by third-order neurones. This is where the pain is localized and, through past experience, the source of the pain identified. Pain is experienced when impulses reach the thalamus and brain stem, but interpretation of that pain is carried out in the cortex.

The theory of specificity can be used to explain the benefits of the physical aspects of pain management, such as surgery, which can be used to sever or interrupt the pathway, thus stopping the passage of impulses.

Adjacent to the spinothalamic tract lies the anterior (ventral) spinothalamic pathway, which transmits nerve impulses relating to light touch or pressure. The touch fibres (mechanoreceptors) are located in the same areas of the skin as the pain receptors. It is these large, myelinated fibres that, when stimulated, close the pain gate and prevent pain impulses travelling up the spinothalamic tract. This is achieved by bombarding the first synapse with impulses, which explains why rubbing a painful area or applying transcutaneous nerve stimulation (TENS) is an effective method of managing pain.

However, not all impulses take this route: some are passed to the motor neurones at this first junction in the spinal cord. This process facilitates the instinctive or reflex-type reaction, e.g. removing the hand from a hot object.

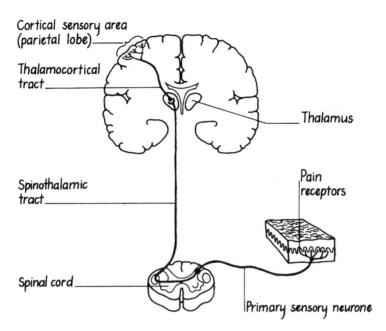

Figure 8.1 (a) Pathway of pain impulses.

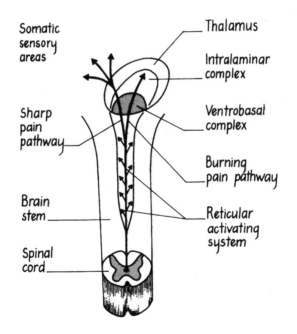

Figure 8.1 (b) Pain pathway.

The Gate Theory

The Gate Theory, initially proposed by Melzack and Wall (1965), suggests that there is an analgesic system within the brain and spinal cord that actively works to diminish the passage of pain impulses and thus reduce the level of discomfort experienced. The impulses carried to the spinal cord by the nerve fibres are blocked at their synapses in the posterior horns in the spinal cord. It is thought that this blocking is brought about by the action of a group of specialized neurones (the substantia gelatinosa) located close to each posterior column of grey matter.

The action of rubbing or the application of heat – or, specifically in the case of burn injuries, the cooling of the affected area – will produce increased activity in the large fibres. This increased activity 'closes the gate', but when the predominant nerve activity is along small fibres the gate opens and allows the impulses to pass to the posterior horn cells and on to the higher centres of the brain. This suggests that the position of the gate and the ability for impulses to pass through the system is related to the intensity of nerve activity in either the large or small nerve fibres.

The Chemical Control of Pain

The pain control system is also susceptible to the effect of a variety of chemicals, some of which are produced naturally by the body and some of which are introduced into the body specifically to control the sensation of pain. These substances primarily work by suppressing or enhancing the passage of nerve impulses.

Endogenous chemicals (Table 8.4) form the basis of the body's analgesic system. When the body is under stress, it produces its own opiates, which can be generated by exercise, fear, excitement or a combination of all three.

The previous mentioned theories of pain can be used to rationalize the use of the following methods of pain management:

- distraction, relaxation, hypnosis or guided imagery (very effective with children: Langley, 1999)
- local application of hot or cold substances
- reduction in anxiety or fear
- electrical stimulation (TENS)
- acupuncture
- analgesics (chemicals)

Table 8.4 Endogenous chemicals affecting the sensation of pain

Name	Location	Function
Encephalins	Thalamus, hypothalamus, spinal cord pathways	Limit production of substance P
Endorphins	Pituitary gland	Limit production of substance P
Substance P	Sensory nerves, spinal cord pathways, areas of the brain involved with pain	Stimulates perception of pain
Serotonin	Brain stem	Alters sensory perception and mood

The passage of most pain impulses can be inhibited chemically at the synapses by analgesics. Most forms of pain will respond to a combination of chemical and other therapies. The dynamic process of pain means that it is essential to review the effectiveness of the pain management to establish the most effective form of therapy.

The Assessment of Pain

In selecting the most appropriate method of pain control it is necessary to understand as much as possible about the pain itself. This is a difficult task, because pain is a subjective experience. It is impossible to measure it in purely physiological terms, because of the psychological factors that influence the severity of pain or its importance to the individual. Therefore the nurse must look beyond such factors as blood pressure, pulse and respiration rates. In the acute stages of burn trauma management, it is helpful to look for ways of assessing and managing both the current and future physical and psychological pain. In this way, it is possible to plan pain relief to correspond with projected levels of pain.

When assessing a patient for the most effective methods of pain control, consideration must be given to the needs and goals of the patient and members of the Burns team. This should include an assessment over a period of 24 hours and take into account the level of pain felt during physical therapy and also the pain endured at night. Pain is always difficult to measure, because it is only the person experiencing the pain who knows its nature, intensity and location. There are many guides that can be employed as an aid to pain assessment but most rely on a certain level of cognitive and communication ability. This makes them unsuitable for young children, or people with a learning disability or a communication problem (Stevens, Hunsberger and Browne, 1987). These may take the form of a checklist, or they can include the use of tools to measure pain (McCaffery and Beebe, 1989). The use of assessment tools will promote a systematic approach to pain management and help to remove the subjective aspect. Appropriate tools are provided for the patients themselves to assess their pain, and this information should then be used in building up a complete picture, rather than being taken as a definitive value of pain. There is no one tool that is totally satisfactory for all patients, so an element of flexibility is required at all times (McGrath, 1989).

One of the most frequently used tools is the Visual Analogue Scale (VAS) or linear scale (Huskisson, 1983). These scales are normally in the form of a ten-centimetre line with the words 'No Pain' at one end, and 'Unbearable Pain' at the other. The user then describes the severity of the pain by pointing to the corresponding part of the line or stating the equivalent numerical value (Figure 8.2a). A variation of this commonly used with children is the 'Pain thermometer', in which the range extends vertically from 0 (No Pain) to 4 (Unbearable Pain). Another system commonly used with children is a series of six pictures depicting a child in various degrees of discomfort (Figure 8.2c)

Any such tools can prove helpful when looking at the intensity of pain, but it is necessary to be consistent once one has been chosen in order to prevent any misunderstanding. VAS forms a small but essential part of the construction of pain assessment charts. Completion of pain assessment should be an integral part of the nursing observation process. To facilitate this observation charts should incorporate routine observations of temperature, pulse, blood pressure, respiration rate, and pain and nausea scores.

Gordon et al. (1998) found that the preferred methods for reviewing pain in burns nursing were the Adjective Pain Rating Scale (APRS) or Faces Pain Rating Scale (FPRS) shown in Figure 8.2b and c.

Pain assessment charts such as The London Hospital Pain Chart (Sharpe, 1986) can be adapted, especially for Burns patients, to gain a better all-round picture of the pain. The overall objective is to establish a pain profile over a 24-hour period so that analgesia requirements and pain management techniques can be matched with activities.

To illustrate this thought process consider the following example. A young man is six days post-injury: he has sustained 22% burns to hands, feet, face and left lower leg (Figure 8.3). He has not required any surgery but he has been experiencing a considerable amount of pain, particularly

(a) **Visual Analogue Scales (VAS)**

0	1	2	3	4	5	6	7	8	9	10

No Pain   Unbearable
                                                                            Pain

(b) **Adjective pain Rating Scale (APRS)**

0.   No Pain

1.   Slight Pain

2.   Mild Pain

3.   Moderate Pain

4.   Severe Pain

5.   Unbearable Pain

(c) **Faces Pain Rating Scale (FPRS)**

0	1	2	3	4	5

No Pain   Unbearable Pain

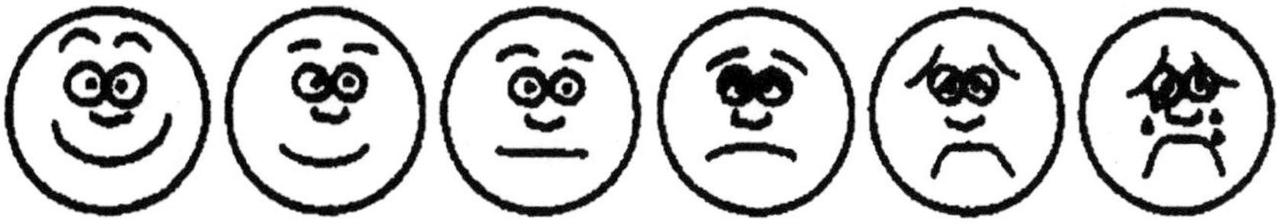

Figure 8.2 Examples of pain scales.

during dressing changes and physiotherapy. He has been on his present medication regimen for 48 hours. The mainstay of his analgesia is 30mg of controlled release morphine tablets (MST Continus) twice daily. It is found that he requires additional analgesia for breakthrough pain: for this, dextromoramide (Palfium) is used, in conjunction with 50% nitrous oxide/50% oxygen (entonox) as required.

Using the chart, it is possible to plot a 24-hour profile of this patient's pain (Figure 8.4): the resulting pain profile or graph can then be used to adjust the type, dose of timing of any analgesia that is being administered. The profile can also be used to coordinate painful procedures so that events such as dressing changes and physiotherapy coincide with the

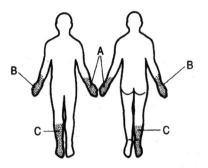

Date 15/4/94

Name Anon Anon

Age 21 years

Diagnosis 22% Burns

Linear scale for the assessment of pain

0　1　2　3　4　5　6　7　8　9　10

No pain　　　　　　　　　　　Unbearable pain

Time	Pain score				Analgesia		Activity/comments
					Type	Dose	
	A	B	C	Total			
0000	2	3	2	7			Watching television
0200	0	0	0	0			Asleep
0400	0	0	0	0			Asleep
0600	4	6	5	15	MST	30 mg	Hands stiff/aching
0800	6	6	3	15			Washing/eating Dressing change
1000	8	8	6	22	Palfium Entonox	20 mg 15 mins	Physiotherapy
1200	3	4	2	9			Eating
1400	1	2	0	3			Visitors present, mind occupied
1600	7	7	0	14	Palfium Entonox	20 mg 15 mins	Visitors leave Physiotherapy
1800	4	3	1	8	MST	30 mg	Eating
2000	2	1	1	4			Watching TV
2200	3	2	2	7			Hands elevated in slings

24-hour pain profile

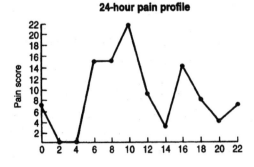

Plot total pain score/time to produce a 24-hour profile. This can then be used to assess the effectiveness of the action taken and assist in the planning of future management.

N.B. Compare 'peaks' of pain to activities carried out at any given time.

Figure 8.3 Pain assessment chart for burns.

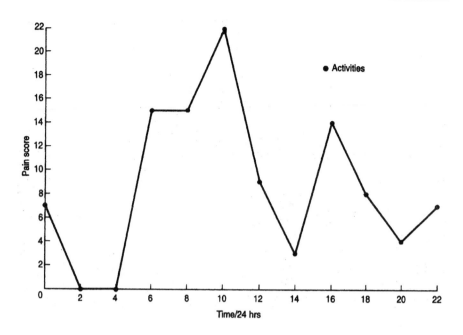

Figure 8.4 24 hour pain profile.

maximum effort to control the pain. The use of such charts can also be used to promote patients' involvement in managing their own pain. This is achieved by establishing what the optimum level of pain control is for the individual. When the profile is plotted, the patient can draw the optimal and maximum level of pain as horizontal lines on the graph. This then forms part of the plan to control pain. By observing the peaks and troughs of pain over a period of days, the analgesia regimen can be adjusted to achieve the optimum level of pain relief.

However, the importance of a thorough physical examination, an accurate history and a good understanding of the effects of pain on the patient cannot be over-emphasized.

The following is a checklist of points to note when assessing a patient for pain:

- Physical examination, to establish the source or cause of the pain.
- Characteristics of the pain:
- Type: crampy, sharp, stabbing, dull, throbbing, burning, etc.
- Intensity: mild or severe, on a scale of 0–10
- Frequency
- Duration

- Changes in the site: tenderness, swelling and colour
- Associated symptoms:
- Nausea and vomiting
- Altered level of alertness
- Confusion or disorientation
- The patient's priorities and aims.

Achieving Successful Pain Control

The assessment of a patient in pain may take only seconds, perhaps on arrival in the Accident and Emergency department. However, this is likely to be the beginning of a continuous period of assessment and the trial of a variety of methods until the goal of optimum pain relief is achieved.

The most widely recognized approach to pain management involves the use of a 'step-up' or 'ladder system' but because of the acutely painful nature of the burn injury, a 'step-down' policy for analgesia is usually indicated. Most burn injuries will require intravenous opiates to achieve effective analgesia. Intramuscular injections are inappropriate in the initial management as the absorption may be greatly delayed in the shock phase of the injury. Good analgesia is not only humane but it will gain patient and family trust and allow for adequate assessment of the burn wound.

Intravenous opiates are the method of choice for the initial period of care following a significant burn injury. They should be titrated in small increments every two to five minutes until an adequate level of analgesia is obtained. Only when an adequate loading dose has been given should an infusion be commenced otherwise a delay will occur before good analgesia is achieved.

Analgesic Drugs in Common Use

Opioids

The term 'opioids' refers to any drug acting on the body's opioid receptors, e.g. morphine, diamorphine, codeine and dextromoramide. Opioid drugs are used to relieve moderate to severe pain. Morphine and diamorphine have proved to be the most effective method of controlling pain in the initial stages of treating the burns patient. However, they need to be administered as a continuous infusion, preferably via a syringe driver. Side effects such as a reduced respiratory rate should not inhibit the use of this category of drug. However, patients receiving an opioid infusion should be monitored as frequently as their condition dictates. It is also necessary to assess the patient frequently with regards to the danger of constipation. The risk of dependence should not be taken into consideration when trying to control severe pain. Patient-controlled analgesia delivery systems (PCAs) are a valuable tool for the delivery of opiates such as morphine, diamorphine or alfentanil. PCAs have been shown to be useful in children as young as three years old (Hodges, 1998).

Oral morphine can be used in small doses at two to four hour intervals as required. If frequent doses are required, then consideration should be given to an intravenous infusion or the regular use of slow release morphine tablets (MST). Converting from intravenous infusions of opiates to oral doses is imprecise but a rough guide is to take the previous 24-hour intravenous requirement of diamorphine and treble or quadruple it for the daily dose of MST, which should be given in two divided doses for the next 24 hours. To convert from intravenous morphine, the previous 24 hours' requirements should be doubled for the oral daily dose, again given in two divided doses.

Response to opiates by any route shows enormous variability. Many patients with burns will require larger doses while small children and frail adults may need less. The most appropriate dose for dressings changes can be best judged according to observed response to previous opiates given. Dextromoramide is very effective for breakthrough pain while an adequate MST dose is being sought. It has a rapid onset of effect and is only effective for two to three hours. It can be used for short painful procedures such as a small dressing change or transfer from bed to chair or trolley.

Non-opiates

In this group are drugs such as paracetamol, as well as the non-steroidal anti-inflammatory drugs, e.g. ibuprofen and aspirin. These drugs are usually found to be most effective on mild to moderate pain that originates in the musculoskeletal system. Paracetamol is effective when prescribed on a regular basis for background pain (Howell, 1999). Non-steroidal anti-inflammatory drugs (NSAIDs) should be used with caution in patients with a history of peptic ulceration and renal impairment. Care should be taken during treatment to elicit onset of new symptoms such as indigestion. NSAIDs are best avoided until good urine output is established in the resuscitation phase.

Patients with asthma should be asked if they have taken any of the NSAIDs without incident, as a small group of asthmatics are made worse by these drugs. Paracetamol and NSAIDs can be prescribed concurrently and be an affective analgesic regime (Morton, 1993). Only one drug from the NSAID group should be prescribed at any one time.

Local Anaesthetics

Local anaesthetics may be administered by injection or by the application of a cream or other agent directly onto the skin. A topical cream such as EMLA (Lignocaine 2.5% and Prilocaine 2.5%: Maunuksela and Korpela, 1986) or AMETOP (Amethocaine Gel: Woolfson, McCafferty and Boston, 1990) is frequently used to site intravenous lines or for venepuncture on children. EMLA is not licensed for use in children less than one year of age but AMETOP can be used for children over one month old. Other forms of local anaesthetic include local filtration, regional nerve blocks and epidural analgesia.

Table 8.5 lists types of analgesics and their form of administration for different levels of pain. Frequently, more than one form of analgesic agent is required, and the use of a sedative in conjunction with an analgesic has been shown to be effective. This is of particular relevance when undertaking painful procedures such as dressing changes. It may also be necessary for some patients to undergo repeated general anaesthesia for procedures such as dressing changes in order to minimize their pain and discomfort.

Summary

Effective pain management is every health professional's responsibility. All patients regardless of age, creed or gender deserve our utmost efforts to control their fear, anxiety and pain. Liebeskind and Melzack (1989) said: 'The young and the elderly have the most to fear from pain as they are the most defenceless against it.' The management of pain in children has been widely researched and the failing of health professionals to adequately treat preterm infants or non-verbalising children was in an overview of the literature by Schechter (1989). Much of the proposals for good practice associated with the care of children apply equally to other age groups. Honari et al. (1997) found that elderly patients with burn injuries received less opiates than other age groups and commented that they were unsure if this was mismanagement or clinically appropriate.

Table 8.5 Analgesics used for different degrees of pain

Drug	Form
Mild Pain	
Ibuprofen	Tablet, liquid
Paracetamol	Tablet (soluble), liquid, suppository
Aspirin	Tablet (Dispersible), suppository
Moderate Pain	
Coproxamol	Tablet
Codydramol	Tablet
Dihydrocodeine	Tablet, liquid, injection
Codeine phosphate	Tablet, liquid
Diclofenac	Tablet, suppository, injection
Entonox	Gas (50% nitrous oxide/50% oxygen)
Severe Pain	
Pethidine	Tablet, liquid, injection
Morphine	Tablet, liquid, suppository, injection
Diamorphine	Liquid, injection
MST Continus	Tablet
Dextromoramide (breakthrough pain)	Tablet (oral/sublingual), suppository, injection

Further research is needed to fully understand the metabolism of opiates in those patients at either end of the age spectrum.

In order to improve the management of pain in the burns patient, it is essential to be proactive in the field of pain management. Often the pain cannot be prevented but much can be done to reduce its intensity and severity. It is this that presents the greatest challenge to those involved in burns care. This single aspect of care will have a lasting effect on the patient and their family so it is worthy of the greatest commitment on the behalf of the health professional to achieve maximum effect.

The following points should be considered when reviewing pain management of an individual following burns trauma:

- Prevention is better than cure.
- Understand the importance of pain control.
- Be aware of the physiology of pain.
- Be aware of the various factors that affect the process of pain.
- Do not rely on drugs alone.
- Assess the patient for pain in an objective manner at regular intervals.
- Promote patient involvement in the management of pain.

- Encourage communication and cooperation between members of the multidisciplinary team.
- Be prepared to investigate the effectiveness of the wide variety of pain control methods that are available.

Pain is a complex phenomenon involving physical, psychological and social elements: it demands ,therefore, a holistic approach to its management. The best approach to pain management is a team approach, and expertise from outside the Burns team should be sought early on. With effective pain management it is possible to care for burns patients so that their discomfort and suffering is reduced to a minimum. This will optimize both the physical and psychological recovery from the burn injury.

References

Audit Commission (1993) Children first – a study of hospital services. London: HMSO.

Crocker CG (1986) Acute postoperative pain: cause and control. Orthopedic Nursing 5(2): 11–16.

Fisher S, Morton NS (1998) Pain prevention and management in children. In Morton NS, (Ed) Acute Paediatric Pain Management. London: Saunders. pp 1–11.

Gordon M, Greenfield E, Marvin J et al. (1998) Use of pain assessment tools: is there a preference? Journal of Burn Care Rehabilitation 19: 451–54.

Hayward J (1979) Information: a Prescription Against Pain. London: Royal College of Nursing.

Helman C (1990) Culture Health and Illness. 2nd edn. London: Wright.

Honari S, Patterson D, Gibbons J et al. (1997) Comparison of pain control medication in three age groups of elderly patients. Journal of Burn Care Rehabilitation 18: 500–4.

Howell T (1999) Paracetamol use in children. Care of the Critically Ill 15(6): 208–13.

Huskisson EE (1983) Visual analogue scales. In Melzack R, (Ed) Pain Measurement and Assessment. New York: Raven Press. pp 33–37.

International Association for the Study of Pain (1986) Classification of chronic pain. Descriptions of chronic pain syndromes and definitions of pain terms. Pain (supp. 3).

Jonsson CE, Holmssten A, Dahlstrom L et al. (1998) Background pain in burn patients: routine measurement and recording of pain intensity in a Burns Unit. Burns 24(5): 448–54.

Langley P (1999) Guided imagery: a review of effectiveness in the care of children. Paediatric Nursing 11(3): 18–21.

Laterjet J, Choinere M (1995) Pain in burn patients. Burns 21(5): 344–48.

Maunuksela EL, Korpela R (1986) Double blind evaluation of lignocaine-prilocaine cream (EMLA) in children. British Journal of Anaesthesia 58: 1242–45.

McCaffery M (1979) Nursing the Patient in Pain. Lippincott Nursing Series. (Adapted for the UK by Sofaer B) London: Harper and Row.

McCaffery M, Beebe SA (1989) Pain: Clinical Manual for Nursing Practice. St. Louis: Mosby.

McCaffery M, Beebe SA (1994) Pain: Clinical Manual for Nursing Practice. UK edn. London: Mosby.

McGrath PA (1989) Evaluating a child's pain. Journal of Pain and Symptom Management 4(4): 189–214.

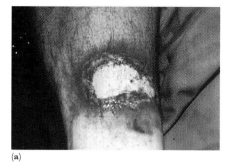

(a)

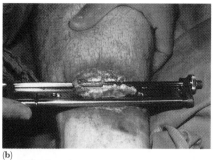

(b)

Plate 1(a).
Deep burn of calf.

Plate 1(b).
Tangential excision
(shaving) of deep
burn of calf.

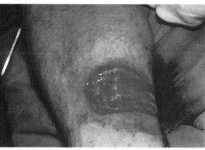

(c)

Plate 1(c).
Bleeding dermis in
the wound base.

Plate 2.
Minimal blood loss
during skin
harvesting.

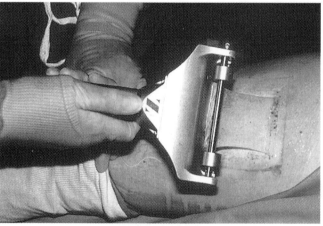

Plate 3.
Meshed skin applied
to a shaved burn on
the foot, secured with
Superglue.

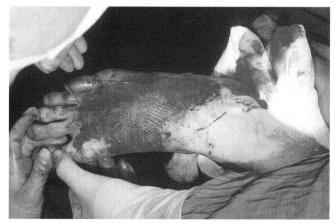

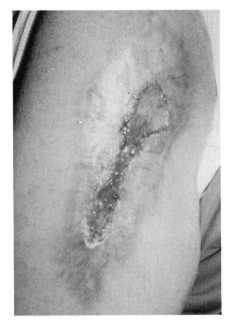

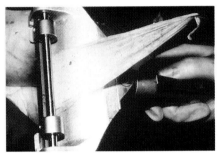

Plate 4.
Hypertrophic scar developing in a burn of a right shoulder, not fully healed.

Plate 5.
The dermatome actually cutting a split thickness skin graft which may be taken of different thickness.

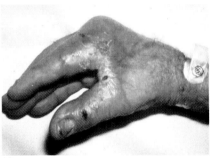

(a)

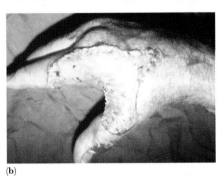

(b)

Plate 6(a).
Contracture of 1st web space of right hand

Plate 6(b).
Contracture released with insertion of thick skin graft

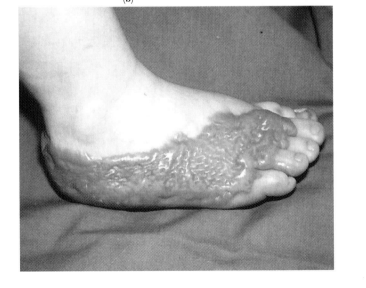

Plate 7.
Active hypertrophic scarring.

Melzack R, Wall PD (1965) Pain mechanisms: a new theory. Science 150: 971.

Morton N (1993) Balanced analgesia for children. Nursing Standard 7(21): 8–10.

Royal College of Paediatrics and Child Health (1997) Prevention and Control of Pain in Children. London: BMJ Publishing Group.

Sharpe S (1986) The use of the London Hospital Pain Chart. Nursing 11: 415–23.

Schechter NL (1989) The under-treatment of pain in children: an overview. Pediatric Clinic of North America 36: 781–94.

Stevens B, Hunsberger M, Browne G (1987) Pain in children: theoretical, research and practice dilemmas. Journal of Paediatric Nursing 2(3): 154–66.

Thomas S (1989) Pain and wound management. Community Outlook 15: 11–13.

Ulmer JF (1998) Burn pain management: a guideline-based approach. Journal of Burn Care and Rehabilitation: 19(2): 151–59.

Wilson GR, French G (1987) Plasticised Polyvinylchloride as a temporary dressing for burns. British Medical Journal 294: 556–7.

Woolfson AD, McCafferty DF, Boston V (1990) Clinical experience with a novel percutaneous amethocaine preparation: prevention of pain due to venepuncture in children. British Journal of Clinical Pharmacology 4: 273–79.

Further Reading

Carroll D, Browser D (1993) Pain Management and Nursing Care. Oxford: Butterworth-Heinemann.

Morton NS (1998) Acute Paediatric Pain Management: a Practical Guide. London: Saunders.

CHAPTER 9

Early Wound Excision and Grafting

FIONA BAILIE AND DAVID WILSON

It is now acknowledged that early excision and grafting of the burn wound allows rapid wound healing, with a significant decrease in the incidence of wound infection, compared with a more conservative approach. However, experience is needed in selecting cases and the type of surgical excision.

The General Principles of Early Excision

Indications

Early burn wound excision is indicated in situations in which the wound will be slow to heal, i.e. taking longer than 2–3 weeks, which applies to deep partial thickness and full thickness burns. The procedure is used for larger wounds and also small deep burns in significant sites, such as the fingers.

Only superficial burns with bright pink wounds, demonstrating that a dermal circulation is present, and displaying wound sensation are obviously suitable for conservative treatment.

There are also other advantages of early surgery. Excision of the dead skin removes bacteria potentially harmful to the patient (Jackson and Stone, 1972), and early wound closure allows quicker recovery for the patient, with less pain, a reduced hospital stay (Muller and Herndon, 1994) and, hopefully, less scarring in the long term (Jackson and Stone, 1972).

Previously, a more conservative approach allowed the eschar (dead skin) to lift off gradually as a result of underlying bacterial action. This involved many dressings, pain and the need to graft on to granulation tissue after approximately 2–3 weeks, with an increased chance of developing hypertrophic (thickened) scarring (Clarke, 1992a).

Early excision therefore helps to:

- heal wounds more quickly
- minimize infection
- reduce the degree of scarring

Timing

Early excision, also called tangential excision ('shaving'), was first introduced by Janzekovic in 1969. Timing of surgery was between 3–5 days, when the burn wound had demarcated ('declared itself'). This is because progressive vascular changes are taking place in the first few days after the burn (Janzekovic, 1970). In the authors' Burns Unit, we routinely check burn wounds at 48 hours post-injury and plan surgery, if needed, at that time. If it is obvious at the outset that the burn is largely full thickness earlier surgery may be performed.

Blood Loss

One of the acknowledged disadvantages of tangential excision is the increased blood loss during surgery (Jackson and Stone, 1972; Heimbach and Engrav, 1984). This is anticipated, however, and there are many ways to limit the blood loss, as well as limiting the amount of burn surface area treated. With major burns, although it may be desirable to remove all the eschar at one operation, it may be advisable to do this over several procedures to limit the resultant blood loss.

Infection

Burns are, by their nature, enough to sterilize the skin immediately following a thermal injury. Bacteria take some time to recolonize the area, and it is common for wound swabs to show no growth for the first 3–5 days after the injury. Most organisms will hopefully be removed, if present, at the time of surgery, but we routinely repeat wound swabs just prior to operating to determine the current wound flora. Immediate skin cover then protects the excised wound.

Antibiotic cover is given routinely, according to a set protocol, for 24 hours from induction of anaesthesia, to cover a possible bacteraemia (bacteria entering the blood stream) or septicaemia (growth of bacteria in the blood stream).

Healing

All skin grafts heal within 5 days, having initially survived for the first 3 days by diffusion of nutrients from the underlying bed. During this time new capillaries grow in to the graft – a process known as 'inosculation' (Jankauskas et al., 1991) producing a true capillary circulation by 5 days. At this time the graft should be pink, with a dermal circulation, and be adherent to the wound bed, but will lack a nerve supply. (Skin grafts are not innervated tissue, although they may pick up some cutaneous nerve supply from adjacent nerves in due course.)

Scarring

Early grafting can produce very acceptable results despite the need to mesh the skin grafts (Clarke, 1992a). The best results are obtained where the burn wound is deep dermal as opposed to full thickness. Shaving the burn wound during tangential excision attempts to preserve as much viable dermis as possible whilst removing the dead eschar. The more dermis that can be preserved, the better the scar and the more the elasticity of the skin is maintained. Where the burn extends down to the level of the fat and all the dermis is destroyed, it is more likely that the grafts will contract significantly, and that the resultant scars will be hypertrophic. Pressure therapy is vitally important in helping to overcome this problem and also in the treatment of existing hypertrophic scars (see Chapter 13 and Plates 4 and 7).

The Process of Surgical Excision

Types of Surgical Excision

Tangential excision

Tangential excision is also called 'shaving'. This implies that a surgical knife (with a guard) is preset at a given thickness, to allow dead skin to be removed (as in planing wood) until bleeding dermis is reached in the wound base (Plate 1a, b, c).

Fascial excision

Fascial excision is carried out where the burns are deep, down to fat, with no chance of any viable dermis remaining. All the skin and fat are therefore removed down to the fascial level, usually overlying muscle, which has a better blood supply than fat and will therefore support a skin graft

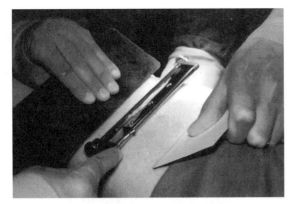

Figure 9.1(a) Harvesting of skin using an Watson hand knife.

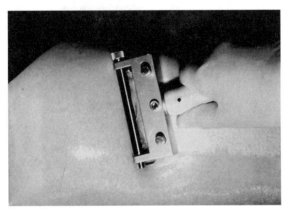

Figure 9.1(b) Harvesting of skin using an electric dermatome.

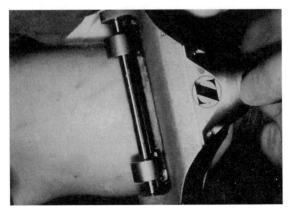

Figure 9.1(c) Harvesting of skin using an air driven dermatome.

better. The procedure results in less blood loss than tangential excision and may be a faster procedure, both of which may be important in a frail or unstable patient. However, there is a distinct disadvantage in that the contour is altered, resulting in a 'dip' or a 'wasted' appearance on a limb (Heimbach and Engrav, 1984). This technique may, however, be the best means of providing rapid debridement (removal) of burnt tissue and wound healing, particularly in major burns, with enhanced survival as a result.

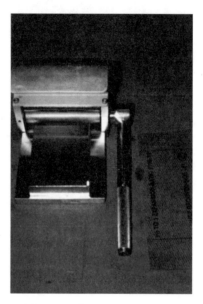

Figure 9.2(a) Skin mesher and dermacarrier.

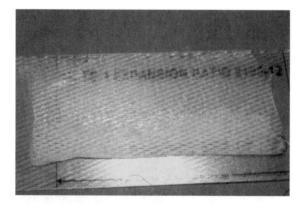

Figure 9.2(b) Meshed skin spread on dermacarrier, meshed 1.5:1 (lower margin doubled over to obtain maximum benefit).

Blood Loss

Blood loss in burns surgery can be quite dramatic!

In order to be prepared for this, most patients need to have blood cross-matched before surgery: for example, as much as 10 units may be the starting point for a major burn, and other blood products such as platelets and clotting factors may be needed as well. Surgeons should try to minimize blood loss by as many means as possible. A number of procedures can be used to accomplish this.

- Tourniquet on limbs – This makes surgery slightly more difficult as viable dermis cannot be assessed by its bleeding. Experience is needed to ensure all the burned tissue has been removed, without taking off a layer of healthy tissue. Usually pink or red dermis and thrombosed vessels need to be removed – healthy dermis is pale white/yellow.
- Simple elevation of limbs using ceiling-mounted suspension hooks or an assistant will also help.
- Diathermy – cutting tissue with this technique during fascial excision will reduce blood loss. Also, the use of coagulation diathermy (monopolar or bipolar) can be used for cut vessels rather than capillary 'ooze'.
- Subcutaneous infiltration of Epinephrine (Adrenalin)/Hyalase solution (1mg of Epinephrine and 1500iu Hyalase in 500ml normal saline). This solution can be infiltrated under pressure under both the burn wound and the donor site to reduce blood loss. Blanching of the skin at the donor site will be seen, and again experience is needed to gauge the correct depth of excision. Slow capillary bleeding is considered the best guide (see below) along with a healthy appearance to the dermis. This technique is particularly helpful in reducing blood loss from the donor site (Plate 9.2) even in non-burn patients. Kahalley et al. (1991) report a similar experience using a subcutaneous injection of a saline/vasopressor solution under donor sites and debrided areas with no problems in the healing of either.
- Topical agents – Epinephrine soaks may be used directly on to the wound to control capillary 'ooze' (Heimbach and Engrav, 1984). Alternatively 5 vol-strength hydrogen peroxide may be used similarly (Cort and Herbert, 1971): this helps because of its exothermic reaction, which coagulates the capillaries. More recently, clotting factors such as Thrombin and Fibrin have been marketed as topical agents to reduce blood loss from wounds and have been used in burns surgery.

Certain dressings such as calcium alginate have haemostatic properties and are widely used on donor sites and may be applied temporarily to
the excised burn wound (NHS Surgical Dressings Information, 1988).

- Skin – It should not be forgotten that skin contains tissue thrombo-
  plastin which initiates the 'clotting cascade' (Tortora and Anagnostakos, 1990). Hence, ready-prepared skin grafts are really one of the
  best means of controlling capillary bleeding, either autograft (patient's
  own skin) or allograft (donor skin).

All swabs are weighed during surgery to provide an accurate and up to
date account of the blood loss during the procedure.

Skin Cover

Prior to tangential or fascial excision, the first step should be harvesting
(taking) skin grafts as this is the cleaner of the two procedures. Also, as
mentioned above, application of skin grafts speedily stops oozing from the
shaved wounds.

Skin can be meshed (best avoided on cosmetically sensitive areas such
as the face and hands) to allow drainage, easier contouring and to allow
the available skin to cover a larger area. Various mesh ratios are used
depending on need.

Where area is not a problem but prevention of haematoma (a collection of blood under the graft) is the main priority a ratio of 1:1.5 is
commonly used (Plate 3). The small splits in the graft heal in 48 hours in
a moist environment (James, 1992).

Where large areas require cover, ratios from 1:3 up to 1:9 may be used
and the mesh spread widely. In this case the holes in the mesh will take
longer to heal and leave a significant scar pattern. With widely spread
mesh grafts it is advisable to cover with a layer of allograft to maintain the
viability of the exposed dermis in the mesh holes and to allow the autograft to heal in an ideal environment.

Cosmesis

Although meshed grafts (even minimally meshed 1.5:1) are not ideal,
they can be fairly unobtrusive at 1–2 years and acceptable to patients.
Some surgeons prefer non-meshed sheet grafts, even with tangential excision, but there is a greater risk of haematoma formation.

Hypertrophic Scarring

This is a frequent finding in burns scarring following more severe injuries (Plates 4 and 7). It is due in part to:

- The depth of the burn – deeper burns with loss of dermis and down to the fat are more likely to develop thickened scars.
- The site of the burn wound – it is more likely to occur on the chest, shoulders and neck areas.
- Racial factors – for example, those of Afro-Caribbean descent may develop the worst form of hypertrophic scarring, known as keloid scars (Hugo, 1991).
- Possible genetic causes – hypertrophic scarring in Caucasians is more common in certain individuals e.g. those with red hair and adolescents.

Skin Grafting

Split Skin Grafts

Thiersch grafts

Karl Thiersch (1822–1895) was a German Army surgeon in the Franco-Prussian War of 1870, who described the use of split-thickness skin grafts. The grafts are taken from a predetermined part of the body, using a skin knife (dermatome), electric or air driven dermatome (Figure 9.1 and Plate 5). Different thicknesses may be taken, depending on the need and donor area.

Meshed grafts

Split skin is laid on a dermacarrier (mesher board) and fed through a skin mesher which produces a series of splits in the graft, like a string vest (Plate 9.2). The main purpose is to allow drainage and prevent haematoma formation under the graft, and to allow the graft to conform to the bed better. When there is a shortage of skin, however, the meshed skin can be spread wider opening up the holes (expanded), enabling a larger area to be covered.

Expansion ratios commonly used are 1.5:1, 3:1, 6:1 and 9:1, although there may be other combinations with different meshers which are adjustable and some do not require carrier boards for the graft. If the mesh is very wide, it is preferable to cover the skin with a biological dressing (e.g. specially prepared porcine skin or cadaver skin) to protect the interstices whilst they heal.

Any surplus skin grafts, either meshed or unmeshed, can be stored (clearly labelled) at 4°C in the refrigerator on the Burns Unit for up to three weeks and used for further grafting if necessary. Skin may be stored for longer periods if kept in tissue culture fluid, frozen or treated with preservatives such as glycerol to prolong its shelf life. These latter procedures are used mostly for the storage of cadaver skin (Allograft) in skin banks (Achauer, 1987).

Securing the skin graft

There are numerous methods used to secure grafts which may be applicable in different situations. Remember the letter 'S':

- Superglue or fibrin glue
- Staples, usually stainless steel but may be absorbable
- Stitches, absorbable or non-absorbable
- Steristrips, or strips of other adhesive tape
- Simple vaseline gauze
- Splints
- Secure dressings

Remember also that skin grafts that lose their blood supply will **S**lough off, so do not apply the dressing with excess pressure.

Wolfe grafts

Julius Wolfe (1836–1902) was an Austrian ophthalmologist who later settled in Glasgow. In 1873, he described the repair of an eyelid using a full thickness postauricular skin graft (skin from behind the ear).

The term 'Wolfe graft' has now come to be applied to most full thickness skin grafts. There is little place for them in the acute management of burns as they do not heal well in adverse conditions, i.e. possible wound infection and a potentially poor wound base. Also, donor sites are limited due to the area of skin that can be harvested without resorting to a split thickness skin graft to close the donor site. In general, split-skin grafts are more appropriate in the acute wound.

However, deep burns exposing tendon or bone require flap cover with a vascularized piece of skin containing fat and its own blood supply. A Wolfe graft may be used in this situation for the donor site, e.g. if a cross-finger flap is used for a burn on the hand (Smith, 1990). Burns of this sort, where avascular tissue such as tendon or bone is exposed, will not heal with a simple skin graft.

Hand burns benefit from moderately thick skin grafts to try to prevent the subsequent development of tight scarring. Also, some surgeons prefer sheet grafts to meshed grafts in this area: however, as stated earlier, the risk of haematoma formation is higher as a result, and great care is needed at surgery.

Full thickness grafts find greater use in the secondary and reconstructive surgery following burns, and occasionally large grafts will be used to resurface areas such as the face (Parkhouse, 1999).

Contracture Formation

The thinner the skin graft and the less dermis present, the more it may contract. However, if the underlying dermis is partly present, this can prevent contraction, and a reasonable scar can result.

Where the dermis is virtually or totally lost, the skin graft is liable to become thickened (compare an elastic band allowed to relax having been stretched). This is especially likely to occur over fat.

Longitudinal bands of scarring may develop underneath, resulting in formal contracture bands (Plate 6a, b) needing release at a later date. This is necessary to prevent restriction in joint movement and limitation in range of motion.

Cultured Skin

Cultured epidermal autografts (grown from the patient) have lost their initial popularity to a certain extent, due to the need for laboratory facilities, high production costs, high failure rate and the quality of graft survival (Muller and Herndon, 1994). They are still used in major burns where donor sites are scarce and can aid survival as a result. In recent years the time taken to culture skin has reduced although there is still no dermal element to the grafts. However, combining cultured epidermal autograft with some of the dermal skin substitutes is a method of overcoming this problem.

Biological Dressings

If skin graft donor sites are lacking in patients with major burns, temporary cover with allografts – either live donor or cadaver – may be used. The donor skin may be fresh or fresh frozen and therefore viable, or preserved by a variety of techniques (such as Glycerol) and non-viable. In either case, the donors should be appropriately screened to exclude viral transmission, but prion-transmitted diseases such as BSE remain a worry, as with all human products. Another, less ideal, alternative is porcine skin (xenograft) which is preserved, non-viable and lasts for a relatively short period of time.

Skin Substitutes

Various skin substitutes are now being marketed and many are used in the treatment of burns. These may be entirely artificial, such as Integra (Integra LifeScience Corporation, USA), or composed partly or entirely of human skin elements treated to make them inert and free from the risk of infection transmission. At present, most simply replace the dermal layer and require covering with epidermal autograft at some point. Integra is a bilaminar membrane composed of a dermal layer of collagen and glycosaminoglycan (CAG), with an epidermal layer of silicone rubber. The dermal layer is incorporated into the wound bed providing a template for the ingrowth of the patient's cells and collagen. Once incorporated, the silicone layer is removed (at 2–3 weeks) and a thin split-skin graft or cultured autograft is applied.

Other substitutes include treated human dermis, which again provides a template for the patient's own healing process and requires an epidermal layer to be applied. Some substitutes are also treated with neonatal cells which secrete growth factors into the dermal element and thus improve healing.

To date, a complete ideal substitute skin has not been produced but this is an area of intense research and development.

The Procedure for Obtaining a Skin Graft from Donor Sites

Donor Sites

Split-skin grafts can be taken from virtually anywhere on the body. However, places to avoid if possible are the face, neck, hands, feet, perineum and breasts. This leaves the commonly used sites of:

- limbs
- buttocks
- back
- chest
- abdomen
- scalp

However, in large burns where donor sites are at a premium, any site may be used and, if necessary, used again once it has healed.

For small grafts in children, the buttocks are a good site: they heal well, despite concerns to the contrary, and the result is cosmetically acceptable in the long term. In adults, the inner thigh is a suitable site, although it may be more awkward than the upper arm, but this site may heal slowly and cause an obvious cosmetic defect.

Skin thickness varies in different parts of the body (Tortora and Anagnostakos, 1990). The areas of thickest skin lie on the back and soles of the feet. The outer thigh skin is thicker than the inner thigh, an important point when looking for donor sites in the elderly, who have generally thinner skin. Care needs to be taken when harvesting skin in these patients: too thick a graft could result in a donor site not healing for many months, or even requiring a skin graft itself.

Lubrication

Friction is produced between the skin and the knife when harvesting skin which may make the process more difficult. Liquid paraffin wiped over the skin lubricates it satisfactorily, and some surgeons also like to lubricate the knife.

Equipment for Harvesting Skin Grafts

- Liquid paraffin – to lubricate the skin
- Dermatome (powered or hand held) – to cut the skin graft
- Skin boards – to steady and tense the donor site
- Skin mesher – to mesh the graft if required
- Dermacarriers – for the mesher
- Storage jar or tin – to store any excess graft at 4°C for up to three weeks in a refrigerator

Blood Loss

Bleeding occurs from shaving or excision of the burn wound as well as from the donor sites.

A recent paper estimated the total blood loss following surgery to be 2.6% for adults, and 3.4% for children, of their total blood volume for each percent of burn excised or donor site harvested (Budny et al., 1993). The use of the various techniques described earlier to reduce operative blood loss, including epinephrine infusion, can be very helpful and may avoid the need for a blood transfusion and its attendant risks.

Reharvesting

It is possible to take skin from the same donor site, once it has healed, a number of times in order to provide adequate skin cover (Cort and Herbert, 1971; Clarke, 1992b). Techniques to improve donor site healing times such as types of dressing, application of tissue growth factors and the use of growth hormone (Herndon, 1995) have all been used to allow more rapid repeat harvesting. However, each time the site is harvested there is a degree of permanent thinning of the dermis.

Dressings

There are many dressings on the market (NHS Surgical Dressings Information, 1993) for donor sites and new wound dressings are being developed on a regular basis. Different Burns Units may have individual preferences, as do individual surgeons. Some of the currently popular dressings are given below, but the list is not exhaustive:

- Non-/low-adherent dressings, e.g. NA, N/A Ultra, Mepitel
- Calcium alginates, e.g. Kaltostat, Sorbsan
- Foam type dressings, e.g. Lyofoam, Allevyn
- Hydropolymers, e.g. Tielle
- Hydrocolloids, e.g. Granuflex, Duoderm
- Film dressings, e.g. Opsite, Tegaderm
- Semi-occlusive, e.g. Flexipore
- Synthetic collagen based, e.g. Omniderm, Biobrane

Healing Time

Children's donor sites tend to heal slightly faster than adults', at around 10 days as opposed to 14 days. However, the general health and nutrition of the patient will also have a significant effect as may the dressing applied. Wounds certainly heal quicker in a moist environment and many of the newer wound dressings claim to give improved healing times. Certainly calcium alginate has been shown to be more effective than paraffin gauze. Other methods of increasing healing time have also been tried, such as the use of growth hormone as mentioned earlier. Healing times as low as 5–7 days have been reported.

If possible, we avoid donor sites on the upper arms which have been shown to have poor healing rates (Cort and Herbert, 1971). If thick skin needs to be taken, it is possible to graft that donor site with a thinner graft from elsewhere, allowing both sites to heal reasonably quickly (Press, 1991).

Cosmesis

Most donor sites heal very well with minimal scarring, and sensation is unaffected. The thinner the graft that was taken, the better the donor site will heal. Quite often the only evidence of injury is exaggeration of the hair follicles or less hair growth. The area may be a little paler than the surrounding normal skin and this may be exaggerated if the area is tanned. Very occasionally, hypertrophic scars develop but these are usually associated with delayed healing.

Post-operative Care of the Wounds

Dressings

If paraffin gauze is used, it needs to be very well padded, to prevent 'strike-through' (leakage of blood or serum through the dressing). This must be treated quickly to prevent bacteria entering the wound through the wet dressing; applying additional dry dressings may be all that is required. Otherwise, all wet dressings down to the paraffin gauze may need to be removed and replaced.

However, calcium alginates need fewer dressings due to their haemostatic properties, and some of the newer dressings combine a layer of alginate with a padded outer layer as a single dressing.

Exposure of the applied skin grafts may be carried out, if appropriate, on awkward areas in older children and cooperative adults, e.g. the buttocks, as this ensures a greater chance of graft survival. The grafts are checked frequently, any slippage corrected, haematomas expressed and any other problems treated as they arise.

Splintage is often necessary to prevent grafts from moving or shearing on the underlying bed, particularly if near or over a joint. This is usually achieved with plaster of Paris back-slabs or abduction splints. Custommade thermoplastic splints may also be used particularly if the splint may be needed for more than a few days. Preformed splints such as the Richards splint for the knee or abduction splint for the shoulder may also be used.

Removal of Dressings

Dressings should be left undisturbed, unless infection occurs. This is identified by pain, odour, seepage through the dressing or a raised temperature. The dressing should then be removed and the wound or skin graft inspected. If feasible, the patient is bathed or showered, and if the wounds or donor sites are heavily infected a topical treatment with, for example, silver sulphadiazine cream may be necessary, as may systemic antibiotics if the patient is generally unwell.

Prevention of Deep Vein Thrombosis

All patients receive subcutaneous Heparin (Drugs And Therapeutics Bulletin, 1993) if they are on bed rest as a result of their burn injury or following surgery. Heparin is given twice or three times daily (if the patient is at increased risk), until they are fully mobile. Where practicable, anti-embolism stockings are also worn. Deep vein thrombosis can occur in burn patients despite the use of Heparin, and early detection is essential to prevent more catastrophic complications.

Aftercare

Once the dressings are removed, the skin grafts and donor sites are very dry, owing to the lack of sebum, which is normally produced by the sebaceous glands in the area (Janzekovic, 1970). Moisturizing with a bland aqueous cream up to five times daily is advised to keep these areas supple. It may also help to reduce itching, a common complaint once the grafts and donor sites are healed, although the use of antihistamines is often helpful. Creaming may especially help where the scars have become hypertrophic. The frequency can be reduced with time as the skin's own ability to secrete sebum returns, although this will never be complete in the grafted areas.

Sun Avoidance

Scars react badly following exposure to strong sun, which exacerbates symptoms of irritation, redness and heat intolerance. It can also exaggerate areas of pigment change.

All burn patients need to avoid the sun or use total sunblock creams (applied regularly) for at least the first few years following injury. Ideally, overseas holidays are better avoided the first summer after a significant burn injury, and as a general rule grafts and donor sites should be treated as a baby of the same age. Holidays should, hopefully, be trouble free, although may only become so for the burn patient several years after the injury.

References

Achauer BM (1987) Management of the Burned Patient. University of California: Appleton and Lange. Ch. 6.

Budny PG, Regan PJ, Roberts AHN (1993) The estimation of blood loss during burns surgery. Burns 19(2): 134–37.

Clarke JA (1992a) Late management of burns surgery, Plastic Surgery10(5): 117–19.

Clarke JA (1992b) A Colour Atlas of Burn Injuries. Roehampton: Chapman and Hall. Ch 5.

Cort DF, Herbert DC (1971) Practical aspects of skin grafting. British Journal of Hospital Medicine (Apr): 462–71.

Drugs and Therapeutics Bulletin (1993) Preventing and treating deep vein thrombosis. 30(3): 9–12.

Heimbach DM, Engrav LH (1984) Surgical Management of the Burned Wound. University of Washington: Raven Press. Chs 1, 2, 4.

Herndon DN et al. (1995) Characterisation of growth hormone enhanced donor site healing in patients with large cutaneous burns. Annals of Surgery 221(6): 649–59.

Hugo NE (1991) Hypertrophic scars and keloids. In Smith JW, Aston SJ, (Eds) Grabb and Smith's Plastic Surgery. 4th edn. New York: Little, Brown. p 851.

Jackson DM, Stone PA (1972) Tangential excision and grafting of burns. British Journal of Plastic Surgery 25: 416–26.

James MI (1992) The effect of synthetic dressings on wound contraction. MD thesis, University of Edinburgh.

Jankauskas S, Cohen K, Grabb WC (1991) Basic techniques of plastic surgery. In Smith JW, Aston SJ (Eds) Grabb and Smith's Plastic Surgery. 4th edn. New York: Little, Brown. p 28.

Janzekovic Z (1970) A new concept in the early excision and immediate grafting of burns. Journal of Trauma 10(12): 1103–8.

Kahalley L, Dimick AR, Gillespie RW (1991) Methods to diminish intraoperative blood loss. Journal of Burn Care and Rehabilitation 12(2): 160–61.

Muller MJ, Herndon DN (1994) The challenge of burns. Lancet 343: 216–20.

National Health Service (1988) Welsh Common Services Authority Surgical Dressings Information. Pontypridd: Welsh Centre for the Quality Control of Surgical Dressings.

Parkhouse N (2000) Reconstruction of the burned face. Presented at British Burn Association Annual Meeting, Durham.

Press B (1991) Thermal and electrical injuries. In Smith JW, Aston SJ, (Eds) Grabb and Smith's Plastic Surgery. 4th edn. New York: Little, Brown. pp 706, 709.

Smith PJ (1990) Skin loss and scar contractures. In Burke FD, McGrouther DA, Smith PJ (Eds) Principles of Hand Surgery. Derby/London: Churchill Livingstone. p 57.

Tortora GJ, Anagnostakos NP (1990) Principles of Anatomy and Physiology. 6th edn. New York: Harper and Row. Chs 5, 10.

CHAPTER 10

Nutritional Care for an Individual following Burn Trauma

LISA NORMAN, DAVID ANDERTON AND SARAH HUBBARD

A burn injury places unique metabolic demands upon the body. Approximately 36–48 hours post-burn injury, following successful resuscitation from the shock ('ebb') phase, a severe catabolic state develops. This is associated with significant weight loss, which can prove fatal. Nutritional support is vital to restrict weight loss and preserve lean body mass, thereby ensuring donor site and graft healing.

Nutritional support consists of three closely linked components: assessment of nutrient requirements, planning and implementation of dietary regimens, and monitoring the adequacy of the nutrients provided. This chapter discusses the theory behind current nutritional rationale and describes how this can be applied in practice.

Burn injuries occur more commonly in certain groups of the population than others. Those groups most at risk include young children, the elderly and people who abuse alcohol or drugs. Risk factors within these groups include poor economic and social circumstances, confusion, mental health problems, learning difficulties and physical disabilities. These population groups tend to be at greater risk of being malnourished prior to the burn injury. It is important that these patients are assessed by a dietitian to determine their nutritional status, however minor the burn.

Minor Burn Injuries

Burn injuries of less than 15% body surface area burned (BSAB) in adults and less than 10% BSAB in children are classified as minor. Intravenous fluid resuscitation therapy is generally not required. The increase in basal metabolic rate (BMR) is related to the size of burn injury (BSAB).

The BMR is the amount of energy required to maintain physiological equilibrium while at rest in the fasted state. It represents a person's minimal daily energy requirement. Patients with minor burn injuries show a small increase in BMR, so that their nutritional requirements are similar to those estimated for the general population (Department of Health, 1991). Body weight can usually be maintained through eating and drinking amounts similar to the patient's normal intake.

Both weight (kg) and height (m) measurements are necessary if the dietitian is to determine whether a patient is over, under, or adequately nourished. Weight should be taken before wound dressings are applied.

These measurements should be calculated differently for adults and children. For children, growth charts should be used. When the measurements for weight and height fall on the same centile, this represents a child who is the ideal weight for his height. Where children's weights are more than a centile below that for their heights this suggests that they are underweight. Extra attention should also be given to those children whose measurements fall on or below the third centile for both weight and height. The hospital admission may be a valuable time for the dietitian to assess the adequacy of the diet in such children and to identify any problems, which should be addressed at a later stage.

In adults, a formula called the Body Mass Index (BMI) is used (Figure 10.1). Particular attention should be paid to the dietary intake of patients with a BMI of less than 20. Use of oral nutritional supplements is likely to be necessary. Food intake should not be restricted in overweight patients while wound healing is being promoted.

$$BMI = \frac{Weight\ (kg)}{Height\ (m^2)}$$

(measured in indoor clothing and without shoes)
Grades of obesity are defined as follows:

	BMI
Grade 0	20–24.9
Grade 1	25–29.9
Grade 2	30–39.9
Grade 3	>40

Grade 0 indicates a desirable weight range
A BMI of much less than 20 is suggestive of malnutrition
Grade 3 indicates severe obesity

Figure 10.1. Body Mass Index.

Major Burn Injuries

The flow phase is characterized by an increased production of catabolic hormones (adrenaline, noradrenaline, glucagon, and corticosteroids). These hormones cause a state of hypermetabolism, characterised by accelerated protein and fat breakdown, negative nitrogen balance and altered carbohydrate metabolism (De Bandt and Cynober, 1996). The abnormalities of carbohydrate metabolism include elevated blood glucose levels, increased gluconeogenesis (glucose production from amino acids), altered insulin levels and insulin resistance. If a patient also becomes septicaemic, this will further accentuate insulin resistance. Additional insulin should be given to treat hyperglycaemia. A reduction in carbohydrate and other nutrients is not appropriate and would be detrimental to the patient.

The hypermetabolic response is minimized by a thermoneutral environment, early excision and closure of burn wounds, prevention of wound sepsis and good pain control. Larger burn injuries produce a greater rise in BMR and it may become impossible for a patient to meet their nutritional requirements by eating normal amounts of food.

Nutritional Assessment

Nutritional assessment should be carried out as soon as possible for all patients who may be at nutritional risk (Figure 10.2).

It is important to obtain a pre-burn weight in patients with major burns, as true weight will become distorted through oedema, resuscitation fluid and bulky wound dressings. If this is not possible, the admission

---

Intensive nutritional support is indicated if:

1. Burn   > 30% total body surface area in adults
           > 25% total body surface area in children
           > 20% total body surface area in infants
   The range of values is due to differences in the surface area:volume ratio that exists between the different age groups.

2. The clinical course is likely to involve multiple operations; ventilatory support or compromised mental status.

3. For minor burns, the pre-nutritional status as assessed by growth charts or BMI and dietary/social history, is poor.

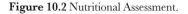

Figure 10.2 Nutritional Assessment.

weight minus that of the resuscitation fluid administered will be representative of the most accurate weight available. Inaccurate weights may result in poor fluid resuscitation and nutritional management. The dietitian will also carry out a nutritional assessment based on energy and protein intake prior to injury, food allergies, recent weight changes, cultural/religious restrictions, food preferences and any past medical history which is likely to affect nutritional status – such as gastritis or IBS. Weight loss is expected in all patients. Dietitians aim to prevent a loss of more than 10% ideal body weight in adults. However a loss of 10% ideal body weight in children is far more significant, as it represents deviation in weight from the normal growth curve.

Nutritional Requirements

Fluid requirements

All fluid requirements in the first 48 hours are met through the standard fluid resuscitation procedure. Hence, any nutrition provided will be in addition to this. Following this period, requirements should be based on the recommended fluid intake (Department of Health, 1991; Elwyn, 1980) plus losses through evaporation. Evaporation losses are high in patients with larger burns, owing to loss of the water-impermeable barrier. Wilmore and McDougal (1977) estimate fluid loss to be:

$$(25 + \%\mathrm{BSAB}) \times \text{body surface area } (\mathrm{m}^2) = \text{ml water lost/hour}$$

This loss will reduce as the burn wounds heal.

Energy requirements

Energy requirements are based on estimated energy expenditure. Total energy expenditure represents the sum of a number of factors including:

- Basal metabolic rate
- Resting energy expenditure (REE)
- Diet-induced thermogenesis (DIT)
- Physical activity

DIT represents the energy expended during digestion and absorption of food.

Energy requirements can be determined by direct or indirect calorimetry, or from a formula. Direct calorimetry involves measuring the heat produced by a subject placed in a sealed chamber. This is impractical in the clinical setting.

Indirect calorimetry is becoming more widely used. A metabolic monitor may be situated at the patient's bedside and a canopy placed over the patient's head for between 20 and 30 minutes. This measures the amount of oxygen uptake and carbon dioxide produced. It provides a measure of the patient's resting energy expenditure (REE), i.e. the energy requirements at rest in the fasted state. Although this is the best method available for determining energy requirements, as it accounts for individual variability, it is expensive, complicated, time-consuming and labour-intensive.

The most widely used methods of calculating an individual's energy requirements use formulae that are simple and incur no cost.

The most frequently used formulae in the UK for adults are represented in Table 10.1. Although many formulae over-estimate requirements, the calculated intake is rarely achieved, owing to frequent interruptions related to nursing and surgical procedures. There is

Table 10.1 Equations for estimating energy requirements in adults

Estimation of BMR (Schofield, 1985) + determination of energy requirements (Elia, 1982, 1990).

Age (years)	Male	Female
15–18	BMR* = $17.6 \times wt^\dagger + 656$	BMR = $13.3 \times wt + 690$
18–30	BMR = $15.0 \times wt + 690$	BMR = $14.8 \times wt + 485$
30–60	BMR = $11.4 \times wt + 870$	BMR = $8.1 \times wt + 842$
Over 60	BMR = $11.7 \times wt + 585$	BMR = $9.0 \times wt + 656$

*BMR is kcal/24 hrs. †Weight = wt (kg). The dietitian will adjust the BMR to account for stress, energy expenditure, DIT and pyrexia.

Elwyn (1980) provides some useful starting points for adults:

Change in BMR (%)	Nitrogen (g/kg)	Energy (kcal/kg)	Fluid (ml/kg)	Sodium (mmol/kg)	Potassium (mmol/g N)
0–25	0.16	30	30–35	1.0	5.0
25–50	0.2–0.3	35–40	30–35	1.0	5.0
50–100	0.3–0.5	40–60	30–35	1.0	7.0

Energy requirements should not exceed twice the BMR.

substantial agreement that energy requirements plateau for burns of 50% BSAB and above, and energy expenditure rarely exceeds twice the predicted normal REE.

In children it is suggested that although they also have a hypermetabolic response, because of a large reduction in physical activity their overall energy requirements are not greatly increased. This is because physical activity contributes a greater proportion of their normal total energy requirements than in sedentary adults. However, it is important to remember that young infants and toddlers need to grow, so are particularly vulnerable to the effects of an inadequate diet. It is thought that post trauma, growth stops temporarily. The energy normally used for growth can then be utilized in the healing process. Currently in the UK, children's energy requirements are assessed using the DRV (Department of Health, 1991). These are recommended intakes for energy and nutrients derived by an expert committee. In larger burns, formulae developed specifically to estimate energy requirements in burned infants and children can be used (Table 10.2).

Protein requirements

Severe burn trauma is known to increase protein requirements, due to increased protein turnover and protein losses through open wounds. It is not possible to prevent loss of body protein. However in adults, the provision of protein at 1.3–1.8g/kg body weight/day (Elia, 1990), representing approximately 20% of the total energy intake, is sufficient to promote wound healing. Cunningham et al. (1990) concluded that in infants and young children a protein intake of 2.5–3.0g/kg body weight/day achieves the best utilization for recovery.

Protein cannot be used without an adequate supply of energy. Therefore, nutritional requirements are often expressed as non-protein

Table 10.2 Equations of estimating energy requirements in infants and children

---

1. Infants under 1 year (Hildreth et al., 1993)
   2100 kcal/m^2 total body surface area + 1000 kcal/m^2 body surface area burned*
2. Children under 12 years (Hildreth et al., 1990)
   1800 kcal/m^2 total body surface area + 1300 kcal/m^2 body surface area burned**
3. Adolescents (Hildreth et al., 1990)
   1500 kcal/m^2 total body surface area + 1500 kcal/m^2 body surface area burned**

---

* Equation devised to maintain weight where BSAB > 25%
** Equations devised to maintain weight where BSAB > 30%

energy:nitrogen (N) ratio. In adult burn patients, this ratio is relatively low, owing to the large amount of protein required. It is suggested that a ratio (kcal/gN) in the range of 100:1 to 150:1 be provided.

Research has focused on the manipulation of specific amino acids to improve clinical outcome. Two of interest are discussed below (Paxton and Williamson, 1991).

Glutamine is an amino acid that serves as a major fuel source for rapidly dividing cells, especially intestinal mucosal cells and lymphocytes. It is suggested that the addition of glutamine to feeds improves mucosal cell integrity and prevents bacterial translocation (see 'Early Feeding' below). Glutamine is unstable in aqueous solutions, and enteral feeds containing the free amino acid are in powder form, which has to be reconstituted with sterile water. Unfortunately, this increases the risk of contamination. More recently, however, ready-to-use enteral feeds have been enriched with glutamine by combining it with other amino acids.

Arginine is an amino acid that is thought to stimulate the immune system by improving delayed hypersensitivity responses and clearance of bacteria. It also enhances wound collagen synthesis and decreases nitrogen loss. Arginine-enriched enteral feeds are also available.

Carbohydrate and fat requirements

Carbohydrate and fat are both used to meet the non-protein energy requirements. Carbohydrate is a fuel for all cells and has a protein-sparing action by inhibiting gluconeogenesis. However the amount of carbohydrate that can be provided is limited by the body's capacity to oxidize glucose. The maximum glucose oxidation rate for an individual is calculated as 4–7mg glucose/kg body weight/minute/day. If excessive carbohydrate is given, fat deposition in the liver is increased and over a prolonged period will lead to hepatic steatosis (fatty liver). Carbon dioxide production will also increase. In order to remove excess carbon dioxide from the blood, and so prevent acidosis, the respiratory effort will increase and this is of particular importance in ventilated patients. Carbohydrate usually comprises 50–60% of the total energy intake.

Carbohydrate is provided as dextrose solutions (glucose source) for parenteral (intravenous) feeding, and as glucose polymers or maltodextrins in nutritionally complete enteral feeds and high calorie/high protein sip feeds.

Fibre (non-starch polysaccharides) is suggested to have an additional role in the treatment of critically ill patients, and is added to some nutritionally complete enteral tube and sip feeds. Soluble fibre is fermented to short-chain fatty acids by the action of bacteria in the colon and may influence the integrity of the gut, thereby reducing the risk of bacterial translocation. Short-chain fatty acids also stimulate sodium and water absorption and may therefore be useful as an antidiarrhoeal agent (Paxton and Williamson, 1991). More recently attention has been paid to fructo-oligosaccharides (FOS). These are also fermented to short-chain fatty acids in the colon, and are in addition thought to act as a prebiotic by stimulating the growth of bifidobacteria in the colon, thus helping to maintain the correct balance between beneficial bacteria and potentially harmful pathogens. Enteral feeds containing FOS are now available.

As energy requirements are high and cannot be met through carbohydrate alone, fat is also used. This is a useful energy source and should provide approximately 20–30% of the total energy intake. Linoleic acid is an essential fatty acid and should be present in the feed to prevent essential fatty acid deficiency. Some of the total fat intake can be provided by medium-chain triglycerides (MCTs), which are readily absorbed as an energy source (Paxton and Williamson, 1991).

Long-chain triglycerides fall into two categories depending on whether they contain ω-6 or ω-3 fatty acids. The former are suggested to compromise the immune system in large quantities, whereas ω-3 fatty acids, which are found in high concentrations in fish oils, may improve immunity. They have a possible role in the reduction of REE and catabolism (breakdown of body protein), improving protein synthesis and nitrogen balance, and better maintenance of overall patient weight.

Vitamin, mineral and trace element requirements

Specific vitamin, mineral and trace element requirements for patients with burns have not been established. A dietitian should make recommendations on an individual basis, taking into account pre-burn nutritional status and amounts that will be supplied via sip and tube feeds. Care should be taken as it is possible to overdose the patient.

It can be assumed that the requirements for certain vitamins, minerals and trace elements will be increased owing to their roles in either energy and/or protein metabolism, or as antioxidants or in the immune system. Losses in urine and burn exudate will also affect their requirements. The requirements of B group vitamins will increase in proportion to energy requirement. The levels of most other vitamins should meet, but not exceed twice their DRVs (Department of Health, 1991). Vitamin C can be supplemented by up to 10 times the DRV, owing to its role in wound healing. Additional iron should be provided if the patient is anaemic.

Table 10.3 shows some of these vitamin, mineral and trace element requirements and suggested supplements, which exceeds the DRV as detailed above. Commonly, Ketovite (Paines and Byrne) tablets and liquid plus ascorbic acid tablets are given to adults. Children may also receive Ketovite or alternatively Abidec (Warner Lambert Ltd). If anaemia is present, iron is given as iron sulphate tablets in adults or as Sytron (Parke-Davis Medical) in children.

Research shows that the trace elements Zinc, Copper and Selenium are lost in large amounts in the burn exudate (Berger et al., 1992; Gosling et al., 1995). It is recommended that patients with burn injuries over 20% should have their serum levels monitored and be supplemented if necessary (Berger et al., 1994).

Implementing Dietary Therapy

Calculated nutritional requirements are delivered via the enteral or parenteral route.

Enteral feeding

Enteral nutrition consists of oral diets (plus nutritional supplements), nasogastric or nasojejunal feeding or feeding via a gastrostomy or jejunostomy. The latter two routes are rarely used in burn patients. The

Table 10.3 Vitamin, mineral and trace element requirements.

Vitamin, mineral or trace element	UK DRV (adults)	Suggested supplement
Vitamin A	600–700µg	5ml Ketovite® liquid or 0.6ml Abidec®
Vitamin B complex	B_1: 0.4mg/1000 kcal B_2: 1.1–1.3mg B_6: 15µg/g protein	3 × Ketovite® tablets or 0.6ml Abidec®
Folate	200µg	3 × Ketovite® tablets
Vitamin C	40mg	200mg ascorbic acid or 0.6ml Abidec®
Iron	9–15mg	200mg $FeSO_4$ tablets bd or 2.5ml bd – 5ml tds Sytron®
Zinc	15–20mg	220mg $ZnSO_4$ tablet or 5ml $ZnSO_4$ mixture
Copper	1.2 mg	2mg Copper Citrate
Selenium	60–75µg	100µg Seleno–L-methionine

Supplements only apply if enteral or parenteral feeding is not being used. The suggested supplements are of a common dosage, prophylactic in some cases, therapeutic in others, which aim to meet or exceed the DRV.

enteral route is preferable for feed administration: it is simple, economical, safe and usually well tolerated. Enteral delivery is associated with preservation of intestinal integrity, including increased intestinal blood flow, reduced bowel oedema, improved gut motility and reduced rates of bacterial translocation.

It is now widely accepted that enteral feeding should be started within 6–12 hours post burn to minimize weight loss. Commencing enteral feeding this early is of great benefit, owing to reduction in the hypermetabolic response.

The dietitian will see and assess all patients identified as being at risk (see 'Nutritional Assessment' above). Likes, dislikes, food intolerances and any other specific dietary requirements are identified. A dietary care plan is devised, comprising problems identified and aims and objectives of treatment. The nurse plays an important role in encouraging patient choice over food, ensuring that patients have ample time to eat and digest their meals. Treatments, procedures and other interruptions should be avoided during meals. Many patients will require assistance in eating. The nurse and dietitian will determine whether a normal diet is sufficient and, if not, dietary supplements are offered in the form of high-calorie/high-protein sip feeds and/or the addition of a glucose polymer to fluids (Table 10.4). If nutritional requirements are not met orally within 2–3 days of commencing the diet, some form of tube feeding should be used. Patients with major burns should automatically have a tube sited during the initial resuscitation period when the majority of invasive treatment is carried out.

Nasogastric (NG) feeding is still the most common form of tube feeding in the UK, although there is a risk of aspiration in patients who require supine immobilization. The type of NG tube used depends upon the patient, body size and projected duration of feeding. Commonly, a wide-bore tube, for example, a Ryles tube of 12 French gauge (FG) or more, is used in the Intensive Care Unit, as it facilitates gastric aspiration. However, a wide-bore tube is uncomfortable for the patient, as it is large and made from PVC, a fairly inflexible plastic, which may inhibit a patient from taking fluids orally. Therefore, a fine-bore tube, preferably of 5–8FG (1–2mm internal diameter), made of polyurethane or silicone, should replace it at the earliest possible moment. PVC tubes should be changed every seven to ten days, whereas tubes made of polyurethane/silicone can remain in situ for up to six months, although they are usually changed after one month.

Approximately 50cm NG tubes are usually used for children, and 70–100cm for adults. Longer tubes are available for nasojejunal (NJ)

Table 10.4 Oral supplements

Product	Description	Energy kcal/100ml	NPC:N*	Protein (g/100ml)
0 years–adult				
Maxijul® (SHS)	Glucose			
Polycal® (Nutricia)	Polymer	100**	–	–
Polycose® (Ross Products)	Powders			
Duocal® powder (SHS)	Glucose + Fat	100**	–	–
1–6 years				
Fortisip® (Nutricia)	Complete	150	167:1	5.0
Frebini® (Fresenius Kabi)	Complete	100	225:1	2.5
Peadiasure® (Ross Products)	Complete	101	200:1	2.8
7 years–adult				
Build Up® (Nestle)	Made up with Whole milk	120	82:1	7.0
Ensure Plus® (Ross Products)	Complete	150	125:1	6.3
Entera® (Fresenius Kabi)	Complete	150	140:1	5.6
Fortisip® (Nutricia)	Complete	150	167:1	5.0

*Non-protein calorie:nitrogen ratio (kcal/gN)
**A 1kcal/ml solution is usually derived from:
10g (2 scoops) glucose polymer/100ml whole milk or formula
8g (2 scoops) Duocal)/100ml whole milk or formula
25g (5 scoops) glucose polymer/100ml water or squash.
NB this is a selection of products available. Others not mentioned here may be used on some units.

feeding. NJ feeding involves placing the tube by endoscopy beyond the pylorus so those patients with a gastric ileus can be fed safely, although siting of these tubes places high demand upon the endoscopy team. There is increasing use of NJ feeding as it allows the patient to be fed up to the point of anaesthesia and can be restarted immediately post surgery, thus reducing the period of starvation (Bengmark, 1998). It may even be possible to continue feeding certain patients throughout theatre (Jenkins et al., 1994).

Early feeding

Early enteral feeding, i.e. within the first few hours after a burn injury, is thought to be advantageous to the severely burned patient, even if only a small volume of feed is administered (MacDonald et al., 1991). Without enteral feeding, changes in the gastrointestinal mucosal lining may facilitate the entrance of intestinal endotoxin and bacteria into the lymphatic circulation (bacterial translocation). This in turn stimulates the release of catabolic hormones responsible for the hypermetabolic state. Early enteral feeding maintains intestinal integrity, thereby reducing bacterial translocation. It is also thought to prevent paralytic ileus. The benefits are not seen, however, if feeding is not instigated within the first 24 hours post-burn. Figure 10.3 represents an example of a flow chart suitable for the early feeding of patients with major burns.

By the end of the fluid resuscitation period (36 hours post burn) early feeding should have been established. The dietitian will then prescribe the most appropriate enteral feed for each individual and outline the method of administration in terms of the pump rate and time span. Feed can be administered via gravity, but it is recommended to use a pump to ensure accuracy of delivery. Table 10.5 illustrates some commonly used feeds for burn patients and for which age group they are most appropriate. For infants with minor burns, continuing with their existing infant

---

Admission
↓
Age and % burn

Infant/toddler	(0–3 years)	BSAB > 15%
Child/adolescent	(4–14 years)	BSAB > 15%
Adolescent/adult	(>15 years)	BSAB > 20%

or if ventilated
↓
Pass a nasogastric tube
↓
Resuscitation period, administer:

Age	Enteral feed	Administration rate
0–1 years:	Infatrini	5ml/hr
1–3 years:	Nutrini	10ml/hr
4–6 years:	Nutrini	15ml/hr
7–10years:	Nutrison Standard	25ml/hr
11years–adult	Nutrison Standard	30ml/hr

Feed to be administered continuously via enteral feeding pump for first 36 hours post burn injury. Gastric contents to be aspirated every 4 hours to check tolerance.

Figure 10.3 Suggested guidelines for early feeding of critically ill burns patients (first 36 hours post burn) – based on the Nottingham City Hospital protocol.

formula is recommended. For infants with larger burns a 1kcal/ml formula should be used (see Table 10.5). Normal paediatric feeds are suitable for children between 1 and 6 years of age, although high energy feeds of 1.5kcal/ml are also available which are useful when fluid restrictions apply. Normal adult feeds are suitable for children aged 7–12 years, and high protein feeds for adults and adolescents over 14 years of age.

The feed is usually introduced at full concentration but using small volumes, governed by a low pump flow rate, usually 50ml/hour over 24 hours in adults. This rate is gradually increased over the next 1–2 days, usually by 25–50ml increments over 4–6 hour periods. A slower rate and smaller increments will be used in young children. Interruptions of feeding due to nursing and surgical procedures, however, may delay this process. Once established, tube feeding continues until the patient can consume sufficient nutrition orally. Usually, 24-hour feeding changes to overnight feeding in an attempt to stimulate the patient's appetite during the day.

Table 10.5 Appropriate enteral feeds for burns

Product	Energy		Protein
	kcal/100ml	NPC:N*	(g/100ml)
0–1 years			
Infatrini® (Nutricia)	101	221:1	2.6
1–6 years			
Frebini® (Fresenius Kabi)	100	225:1	2.5
Nutrini® (Nutricia)	100	202:1	2.8
Paediasure® (Ross Products)	101	200:1	2.8
Nutrini Extra® (Nutricia)	150	252:1	3.4
Paediasure Plus® (Ross Products)	151	200:1	4.2
7–14 years			
Fresubin® (Fresenius Kabi)	100	141:1	3.8
Nutrison Standard® (Nutricia)	100	133:1	4.0
Osmolite® (Ross Products)	100	134:1	4.0
15 years–adult			
Fresubin 750 MCT® (Fresenius Kabi)	150	100:1	7.5
Stresson® (Nutricia)	125	79:1	7.5
TwoCal HN® (Ross Products)	200	125:1	8.4

*Non-protein calorie:nitrogen ratio (kcal/gN)
NB this is a selection of products available. Others not mentioned here may be used on some units.

Poor tolerance of enteral feeding is indicated by vomiting, severe abdominal cramps and/or abdominal distension, worsening diarrhoea, or if the aspirated gastric content is greater than 50% of the volume administered during the previous 4-hour feeding period. The most frequent gastrointestinal complication is that of diarrhoea. This may be as a result of antibiotic therapy, infective organisms, sorbitol in drug preparations, feed hypertonicity or a too rapid administration rate (Edes et al., 1990; Heimburger, 1990). There should be an attempt to diagnose the cause of the diarrhoea: stool samples should be sent for microbiological testing and antibiotic and other drug therapy reviewed. Antidiarrhoeal drugs should be prescribed if appropriate. If these causes are eliminated, the feed rate should be reduced, and then increased more gradually. It is important to ensure the patient still receives adequate fluid and electrolytes.

Blockage of enteral feeding tubes is one of the most common mechanical complications. This can be caused by adherence of feed residue to tube walls or impactation of medications. Therefore it is important to flush tubes with 20–50ml sterile water, using a 50ml syringe, before and after administering drugs and feed.

Parenteral feeding

Parenteral nutrition (PN) is the aseptic delivery of nutritional substrates directly into the circulatory system, usually via a central venous catheter. It should involve a dedicated feeding line to reduce the risk of sepsis, and be administered via a volumetric pump to ensure accurate delivery. PN carries a significant risk of sepsis, metabolic complications (metabolic acidosis and hepatic steatosis) and is the most expensive form of feeding.

PN should only be considered when the gut is inaccessible or none functional, after NG and NJ feeding have failed.

If no central venous access is available, the use of a peripheral vein may be considered: this is known as peripheral parenteral nutrition (PPN). However PPN is not appropriate as the sole source of nutrition in patients with major burns because concentrated parenteral feeds, necessary to meet the high nutritional requirements, would cause phlebitis and occlusion of the peripheral veins. It can be a useful adjunct to enteral feeding for those patients who are unable to achieve full nutrition via the enteral route alone as it carries lower risk of sepsis than does centrally administered PN and is easier to instigate.

The dietitian liaising with the medical team should determine the PN prescription. The volume of PN required is determined by the patient's

calculated fluid requirements. There are two nutritional components of
PN: the water-soluble mixture, which is continually infused, and the lipid
solution. The water-soluble mixture comprises carbohydrate, protein,
electrolytes, minerals and water-soluble vitamins.

Carbohydrate is provided in the form of hypertonic glucose solution,
usually dextrose of 10%, 20% or 50% concentration. The amount of
dextrose that can be administered parenterally is limited by the body's
ability to oxidise glucose (see 'Carbohydrate and Fat Requirements'
above). Occasionally, hyperglycaemia occurs. Insulin can be used to
increase the clearance of glucose, but this is associated with increased fat
deposition in the liver. Therefore, prior to administering insulin, a reduction in dextrose concentration without reducing the parenteral nutrition
infusion will decrease the glucose load without compromising amino acid
delivery. The lipid component can be increased accordingly to prevent a
reduction in energy. If hyperglycaemia persists, however, insulin will be
necessary. Protein is provided as amino acids. These can be obtained in
differing concentrations, although in adult burn patients the more
concentrated amino acid solutions (for example 18 or 24g Nitrogen/l) are
most commonly used because of the high protein requirements.

Electrolytes are added initially to meet normal requirements and then
adjusted daily, depending on serum electrolyte levels. Vitamins and minerals are added to the mixture at standard recommended levels for PN.
These are slightly lower than for oral requirements, as the gut is one of the
regulatory organs that protect against trace element toxicity. However, in
burns of over 30% BSAB where exudate losses are high during the acute
phase, higher levels of supplementation may be necessary.

As discussed above, fat (lipid) is also a useful energy source and forms
the second component of PN. Emulsions of various concentrations, 10%,
20% and 30% lipid, are available. Lipid usually provides approximately
40% of the non-protein energy provided in PN. This should not exceed
more than 60% of the total non-protein energy in adults, 4g/kg of lipid in
infants or 2.5g of lipid in adolescents.

The lipid solution, together with fat-soluble vitamins, is commonly
added to the water-soluble compartment to form a 'big bag' solution. These
are mixed in pharmacy production units under strict aseptic conditions.

PN in infants may be made up daily by the pharmacy department.
The water-soluble component should be given separately from the fat
compartment. The latter, often only being a small amount, can be delivered via a syringe pump over 18 hours. This allows 6 hours for the lipid to

clear from the blood prior to blood sampling, to ensure accurate results and check that the fat is being cleared from the blood. The concentration of divalent cations, for example Ca^{2+} and Mg^{2+}, is often too high in the young infant to allow mixing in one bag. Separate regimens allow for greater flexibility if alterations need to be made according to results from monitoring procedures.

Full concentration PN can be introduced in adults immediately. A flow rate of 1.5–1.6 ml/kg per hour is a good guide, depending on total fluid requirements. In infants and children, introduction is more cautious. The concentration of the regimen is usually increased over a few days, along with a gradual increase in the flow rate. The PN flow rate is normally increased by the same amount as the intravenous solution used to prevent dehydration is reduced. Full nutritional requirements are therefore not met for the first few days on PN.

Monitoring

Monitoring is crucial to ensure that nutritional goals are being met. There is no single parameter that indicates nutritional adequacy. A combination of measurements, such as nutrient intake, body weight, nitrogen balances and laboratory analyses, should be used and interpreted in the light of the clinical situation.

The nurse is responsible for administering the diet and monitoring the outcome. Oral intake (food and fluids, including nutritional supplements) is usually estimated by visual assessment and should be charted by nurses on a feeding form for all patients described as being nutritionally at risk. It is important to provide enough detail of the amounts of each individual food, drink and supplements taken (Table 10.6). The dietitian can use this information, plus amounts of intravenous or enteral feed delivered, to calculate the patient's actual energy and nutrient intake and express it as a percentage of estimated requirements.

Body weight should be monitored weekly without wound dressings. Serial measurements can be compared to the pre-burn weight to calculate percentage weight loss. Weight loss should be no greater than 10% for adult patients with large burns, and preferably less in children.

Nitrogen balance is used as a measure of catabolism and helps to assess the adequacy of protein intake. It requires a complete 24-hour urine collection and accurate determination of protein intake. Nitrogen balance should be measured at least weekly. A simplified nitrogen balance calculation adapted from Lee and Hartley (1975) is commonly used by dietitians:

Nitrogen balance = Nitrogen input (g) – Nitrogen output (g)
Nitrogen output (g) = Urinary urea (mmol/24 hours) x 0.033 + obligatory losses
(hair, skin, faeces) of 2–4g Nitrogen
+ extra renal losses:
pyrexia 0.6gN/1°C
burn exudate 0.2gN/% BSAB

The amount of burn exudate decreases as healing progresses. This occurs rapidly if the burn is of partial thickness. In full-thickness burns, exudate losses continue at 0.2gN/% BSAB until the wound is grafted or the tissue has granulated. At each dressing change nursing or medical staff should reassess the burned surface area, and the nurse should inform the dietitian of any changes. As the burn heals, nutritional requirements will alter. Metabolic rate and nitrogen losses peak at 5–12 days post burn, but may continue to be raised for at least the first month post injury (Elia, 1991).

Table 10.6 Format for completing food record charts

Time	Food Offered	Amount eaten
8 a.m.	2 rashers streaky bacon	1 rasher
	2 large sausages	All
	1 grilled tomato	All
	2 slices thick white bread with butter (thickly spread)	1 slice
	Tea with 30ml full cream milk + 1 tsp sugar	1 cup
10 a.m.	2 digestive biscuits	All
	Full-cream milk 200ml	All
Noon	Fried fish in batter	Half eaten
	Chips – medium portion	All
	2 tbsp peas	1 tbsp
	100ml custard	80ml
	200ml orange squash	All
etc.		

Laboratory analyses for enteral feeding should include serum urea and electrolytes and C-Reactive Protein 2–3 times a week for the first 2 weeks, and then weekly. Blood glucose levels should be measured daily for the first 2 weeks. Liver function tests, full blood count and serum calcium, phosphate and magnesium levels are required at least on a weekly basis. Weekly transferrin, albumin, mineral and trace element levels are also valuable. However the plasma proteins are poor predicators of nutritional status in the short term, owing to injury-induced changes. Although transferrin has a shorter half-life (8 days) than albumin (20 days), and is therefore a more sensitive measure, it is affected by falls in haemoglobin which are often seen in the burns patient. The trend in serial measurements of plasma proteins plays a more useful role.

Biochemical monitoring needs to be more aggressive when feeding parenterally, owing to the increased risk of complications. Laboratory analyses of urea and electrolytes, glucose and haemoglobin are required on a daily basis. And calcium, phosphate, albumin and transferrin levels and liver function tests should be recorded three times a week until the patient appears to be clinically stable. The frequency can then be reduced to comply with the standard monitoring procedure for enterally fed patients. When introducing lipid parenterally as a separate component, lipidaemia should be tested for daily until the full dose of lipid is achieved. This cannot be done if a single-bag mixture is being used as the lipid has to be withdrawn prior to testing.

The Multidisciplinary Team

Good communication is essential if nutritional therapy of the burned patient is to be effective. The medical team is responsible for biochemical monitoring and decisions on the stages of treatment. Nurses are involved in the important role of assessing, feeding and monitoring their patients. It is obviously important to have good liaison with the catering department if a patient's needs are to be met within the constraints of the hospital environment. Pharmacists help in formulating PN regimens and determining the most appropriate vitamin, mineral and trace element supplements. Occupational therapists help in ensuring that feeding is made possible though the use of specialized equipment. Play therapists can help young children by making eating fun, and psychologists can be invaluable through use of relaxation techniques and reducing patients' fears. Ward rounds provide a great opportunity to disseminate information from each of the professionals involved.

On discharge, patients who are of appropriate weight for height and who have been receiving a high level of nutritional support should be given advice on reducing their intake to normal. However if the quality of the diet prior to admission appears to be poor, advice should be given on how to improve the nutritional balance within the context of patients' food preferences. Where concerns exist, follow-up by the GP, health visitor or dietitian may be recommended. It has been shown that some children who sustain burn injuries will fail to maintain normal growth centiles (Hubbard, unpublished data). Particular attention should be given to children who are not eating on discharge.

The use of any method of nutritional support requires careful administration and scheduled monitoring to ensure its safety and efficacy. Nurses have an integral role to play in ensuring the appropriate nursing care and monitoring measures are performed.

References

Bengmark S (1998) Progress in perioperative enteral tube feeding. Clinical Nutrition 17: 145–52.

Berger MM, Cavadini C, Bart A et al. (1992) Cutaneous copper and zinc losses in burns. Burns 18(5): 373–80.

Berger MM, Cavadini C, Chiolero R et al. (1994) Influence of large intakes of trace elements on recovery after burns. Nutrition 10(4): 327–34.

Cunningham JJ, Lydon MK, Russell WE (1990) Calorie and protein provision for recovery from severe burns in infants and young children. American Journal of Clinical Nutrition 51: 553–57.

De Bandt JP, Cynober L (1996) Metabolic response and nutritional management in burns patients. British Journal of Intensive Care 6(3): 93–102.

Department of Health (1991) Dietary Reference Values for Food, Energy and Nutrients for the United Kingdom. Report on Health and Social Subjects No. 41. London: HMSO.

Edes TF, Walk BE, Austin JL (1990) Diarrhoea in tube-fed patients: feeding formula not necessarily the cause. American Journal of Medicine 88: 91–93.

Elia M (1982) The effect of nitrogen and energy intake on the metabolism of normal, depleted and injured men. Clinical Nutrition 1: 173–92.

Elia M (1990) Artificial nutritional support. Medicine International 82(Oct): 3392–96.

Elwyn DH (1980) Nutritional requirements of adult surgical patients. Critical Care Medicine 8: 9–20.

Gosling P, Rothe HM, Sheehan TMT et al. (1995) Serum copper and zinc concentrations in patients with burns in relation to burn surface area. Journal of Burns Care and Rehabilitation 16: 481–86.

Heimburger DC (1990) Diarrhoea with enteral feeding: will the real cause please stand up. American Journal of Medicine 88: 89–90.

Hildreth MA, Herndon DN, Desai MH et al. (1990) Current treatment reduces calories required to maintain weight in paediatric patients with burns. Journal of Burn Care and Rehabilitation 11: 405–9.

Hildreth MA, Herndon DN, Desai MH et al. (1993) Caloric requirements of patients with burns under one year of age. Journal of Burn Care and Rehabilitation 14: 108–12.

Jenkins ME, Gottschlich MM, Warden GD (1994) Enteral feeding during operative procedures in thermal injuries. Journal of Burn Care and Rehabilitation 15: 199–205.

Lee HA, Hartley TF (1975) A method for determining daily nitrogen requirements. Post Graduate Medical Journal 51: 441–45.

MacDonald WS, Sharp CW, Deitch EA (1991) Immediate enteral feeding in burn patients is safe and effective. Annals of Surgery 213: 177–83.

Paxton J, Williamson J (1991) Nutrient substrates – making choices in the 1990s. Journal of Burn Care and Rehabilitation 12(2): 198–202.

Schofield WN (1985) Predicting basal metabolic rate, new standards and review of previous work. Human Nutrition, Clinical Nutrition 39C, suppl 1(5): 41.

Wilmore DW, McDougal WS (1977) Nutrition in burns. In Richards JR, Kinney JM (Eds) Nutritional Aspects of Care in the Critically Ill. Edinburgh: Churchill Livingstone. pp 583–94.

CHAPTER 11

Rehabilitation

NICOLE GLASSEY

The role of the physiotherapist is vital to the rehabilitation of the burn-injured patient. However, a team approach is essential and the roles of the individual members of the multidisciplinary team often overlap (Biggs et al., 1998). The nursing staff, physiotherapists and occupational therapists need to work together closely with good communication to ensure that everyone works towards agreed goals (Biggs et al., 1998). The ultimate objective of rehabilitation is for the patient to return to full independence, managing their former occupation and hobbies wherever possible (Harden and Luster, 1991). To achieve this everyone, including the patient, must have a clear understanding of the aims of physiotherapy (Clarke, 1997).

The aims of physiotherapy treatment are to:

- Maintain clear airways
- Prevent joint contracture
- Aid functional independence
- Provide psychological support

Maintenance of Clear Airways

Smoke Inhalation

A smoke inhalation injury is diagnosed if the patient has been trapped in a smoke-filled room and has facial burns, singed nasal hairs, soot in the airways, impaired voice and signs of respiratory distress (Mathur, 1986). Smoke consists of heat, gases and particulate matter (Kinsella, 1988). Its main gaseous content is oxygen, carbon dioxide, carbon monoxide and hydrogen cyanide. The concentration of oxygen is reduced as it is consumed in the process of combustion. Inhalation of carbon monoxide further reduces oxygen availability as it binds preferentially to haemoglobin forming carboxy-haemoglobin. Any remaining oxygen is more tightly bound, reducing delivery to the tissues. The result is that the patient rapidly becomes hypoxic making carbon monoxide poisoning a major cause of death in fire victims (Keilty, 1993). Cyanide poisons mitochondria and affects cellular metabolism, aggravating the metabolic acidosis caused by hypoxia (Kinsella, 1988).

Smoke particles irritate the airways and the heat produces thermal damage to the mucosa. This results in bronchospasm, pulmonary oedema and the production of carbonaceous sputum. Therefore, there is potential for the development of respiratory complications, e.g. pneumonia and adult respiratory distress syndrome (Darling et al., 1996). The requirement of large volumes of fluid during resuscitation can further aggravate the pulmonary injury by overloading the lungs with fluid (Darling et al., 1996). As airway oedema resolves the damaged mucosa begins to slough, mucus production is increased and cilial action is reduced. Sputum retention is inevitable and if not treated effectively atelectasis and infection will follow.

Patients with an inhalation injury often have accompanying facial burns. The head and neck become grossly swollen and the patient's vision may be occluded. It is therefore particularly important that the physiotherapist gives clear explanations of all procedures. To allow gravity to assist drainage of facial oedema patients are nursed in an upright position. However, repositioning is often necessary during physiotherapy treatment to aid drainage of sputum.

Hough (1996) divided physiotherapy respiratory treatment techniques into three categories, according to their aims:

- to increase lung volume
- to decrease the work of breathing
- to clear secretions

Increasing lung volume

An increase in lung volume reduces airway resistance and improves ventilation (Menkes and Britt, 1980). The patient should mobilize as soon as possible, as this is the best method of increasing lung volume (Dean, 1994). If mobility is not possible high sitting or transferring from bed to chair is sufficient. Jenkins (1988) demonstrated that functional residual capacity increases sequentially when a patient progresses from lying through sitting to standing. Gas exchange can also be modified by altering a patient's position to achieve a better ventilation/perfusion (V/Q) match (Mackenzie et al., 1989). Deep breathing exercises combined with end inspiratory holds and sniffs utilize collateral ventilation to distribute air between lung segments, and abdominal breathing encourages air into dependent areas of the lung (Hough, 1996). Once inflated, alveoli will remain patent for an hour (Bartlett et al., 1973). Continuous positive airways pressure (CPAP) and intermittent positive pressure breathing (IPPB) will also increase lung volume.

Decreasing the work of breathing

Burn-injured patients will tire very easily and the addition of a pulmonary complication, e.g. infection, could cause fatigue and even respiratory failure. Medical management includes bronchodilation and provision of oxygen. Sleep disturbance can cause a deterioration in respiratory status (Cooper and Phillips, 1982) and therefore physiotherapy treatment sessions should be short but frequent (Hough, 1996). Positioning the patient as described above will increase the lung volume and consequently decrease the respiratory effort required. Again CPAP and IPPB can also be used.

Clearing secretions

Clearance of sputum depends upon mucociliary transport and coughing. Mucociliary transport is depressed in a patient with an inhalation injury due to dehydration, hypoxia, thick carbonaceous secretions and damaged airways. Heated, nebulized humidification of inspired oxygen is used continuously with additional saline nebulizers as necessary (Keilty, 1993). This prevents dehydration of the airways and therefore maintains the mobility of the cilia (Clarke, 1989). Techniques that increase lung volume, i.e. mobility and breathing exercises, liberate secretions that are trapped distal to closed airways, and gravity assisted positioning aids drainage of sputum – although this is contra-indicated if there is excessive head and neck oedema.

Percussion and vibrations are used to loosen secretions from the airways (Gallon, 1992). Pryor et al. (1990) stated that they should be accompanied by deep breathing exercises to increase lung volume and prevent oxygen desaturation. However, Jones et al. (1992) demonstrated that percussion had no effect on oxygen saturation, and Dallimore et al.

(1998) showed a significant increase in saturation when percussion was performed with thoracic expansion exercises. If cutaneous chest burns are present, care is taken and vigorous manual techniques are contra-indicated over recently grafted areas.

If the patient is unable to expectorate secretions that are detrimental to his or her respiratory status the physiotherapist may consider nasopharyngeal suction. This may be complicated by the presence of cutaneous facial burns. Consideration is given to patient comfort and the risks of hypoxia, infection and atelectasis. The insertion of a nasal airway aids suction if it is required frequently. If suction is necessary, it is performed gently and minimally due to the already damaged mucosa (Hough, 1996). If repeated suction is necessary, a minitracheostomy could be indicated. If possible, however, any form of tracheostomy should be avoided in the burn-injured patient due to the risks of infection (Boardman, 1991).

In severe cases of smoke inhalation admission to an Intensive Care Unit is necessary for endotracheal intubation and ventilation to prevent occlusion of the airway by oedema (Mathur, 1986). Once ventilated, the patient cannot clear sputum independently and regular chest physiotherapy and endotracheal suction is necessary.

Other causes of retained secretions

- Pre-existing respiratory pathology, e.g. asthma, COPD
- Repeated general anaesthetics
- Enforced bed rest to allow skin grafts to heal
- Reduced thoracic expansion due to burns to the chest and back

Prevention of Joint Contracture

It is important to differentiate between a skin contracture and a joint contracture. Damaged or grafted skin contracts as it heals. If this skin covers a joint, the joint will be pulled into the direction of the contracture. If identified early enough, a release of the skin contracture will allow resumption of full joint range of motion. However, if the skin contracture is allowed to persist, the joint structures that are being held in a shortened position, e.g. ligament, capsule, volar plate, muscle, will also contract. Joint structures, and hence a joint contracture, are extremely difficult to release surgically and rehabilitation is lengthy. Joint contractures must be prevented (Boswick, 1983), and early physiotherapy intervention that aims to do this can delay or alleviate the need for later surgical reconstruction (Bahnof, 2000).

Exercise

There has been debate over whether to rest or mobilize injuries (Salter, 1996). Recently, early motion has been strongly advocated but it is important to recognize the stages of wound healing (see Chapter 6) and arrange a balance between rest and exercise accordingly. For example, over-aggressive manipulation of a joint during the inflammatory stage can prolong this phase and delay healing, but gentle stress during the fibroplastic phase assists the development of new collagen and therapeutic stretching realigns collagen during scar maturation.

Initially, burn-injured areas are heavily bandaged, precluding movement. The first occasion for the physiotherapist to assess and encourage joint movement is when dressings are removed 48 hours after injury, when the depth of burn is assessed by the medical staff (Gairns and Martin, 1990). The physiotherapist encourages the patient to move each affected joint through as full a range of movement as possible (Kealey and Jensen, 1988). If this cannot be achieved, the physiotherapist uses passive exercises (Grigsby de Linde and Miles, 1995). Another ideal time for the physiotherapist to encourage the patient to exercise is during bathing (Raeside, 1992). Dressings do not impede movement and it is often more comfortable for patients to move in relaxing warm water. Treatment sessions in this instance are kept brief to avoid patients getting cold or prolonged exposure of wounds. Pain control is essential (Raeside, 1992). The physiotherapist endeavours to time treatment with the administration of analgesia. If oral analgesia is not effective and circumstances permit the physiotherapist can administer Entonox during treatment.

Exercise is stopped for five to seven days after skin grafting to allow the grafts to heal (Carmudie, 1980; Clarke, 1997). Once the skin grafts are stable, exercise can be resumed. Initially this should be with the dressings off so that the physiotherapist can observe the grafts (Grigsby de Linde and Miles, 1995).

Exercise becomes a regular part of the patient's daily routine. The physiotherapist encourages, advises and progresses the exercise programme but the responsibility for exercise is gradually given to the patient. This responsibility for rehabilitation is the start of the progression towards independence. Initially, the aim of exercise is to maintain a full joint range of motion. Eventually, the physiotherapist alters the emphasis of the programme to regaining muscle strength, motor control, endurance and function.

Most young children do not require physiotherapy treatment as they do not lose joint range of motion as quickly as adults (Clarke, 1997). If exercise is necessary, the physiotherapist needs to use imagination in devising play activities to encourage movement at the required joints (Raeside, 1992). The assistance of the nursery nurse/play therapist can be of great benefit in these circumstances.

Positioning

The position the patient rests and sleeps in needs to be monitored to control oedema and prevent contractures (Boswick, 1983). As a general rule the position of contracture for most joints is flexion. The patient should not spend any length of time with a joint in a flexed position if there are overlying skin grafts. Hence patients should not have pillows under their knees if the flexor aspect of the knee has been grafted (Figure 11.1). No more than one flat pillow under the head is allowed if the anterior aspect of the neck has been grafted (Figure 11.2). Hand burns need to be elevated (Figure 11.3) and patients with axillary burns should rest with their shoulder supported in abduction (Figure 11.4). The patient also needs to sleep in this position and encouragement by the nursing staff as well as the physiotherapist reinforces this. A patient who has burns to the flexor aspect of the hip needs to spend part of each day in prone lying to help prevent a flexion contracture (Figure 11.5).

Splinting

Patients who are fully compliant with exercise or who have minor burn injuries do not require splintage (Richard et al., 1996). However, if exercise and positioning are not sufficient in maintaining correct alignment of a joint, a splint is required (Schnebly et al., 1989). Initially, splints are worn at all times, only being removed for change of dressings and twice daily by the physiotherapist so that full range of active or passive movements can be carried out. The physiotherapist or occupational therapist will usually make the splint from thermoplastic material which is heated in hot water to soften it (Carmudie, 1980). When sufficiently cool it is moulded over the patient's wound dressings to hold the joints in the corrected position. The splint material becomes virtually rigid once it is completely cool. The splint is secured by a bandage or Velcro straps (Figures 11.6, 11.7, 11.8 and 11.9). Eventually, splints may only need to be worn at night, leaving the patient free to use the injured part and exercise regularly during the day.

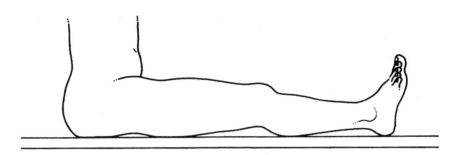

Figure 11.1 Resting position for leg burns.

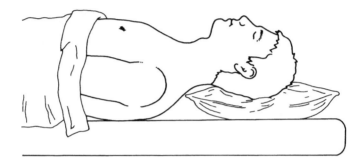

Figure 11.2 Resting position for anterior neck burns.

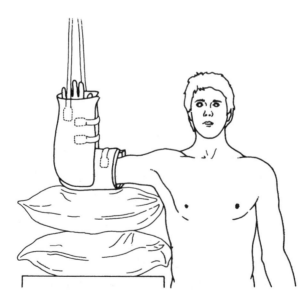

Figure 11.3 Resting position for hand burns, also illustrating a 'Bradford' sling.

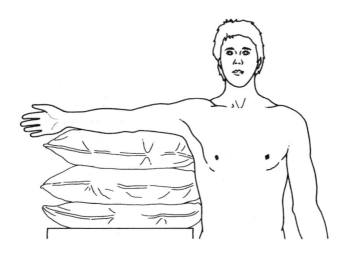

Figure 11.4 Resting position for burns to the axilla.

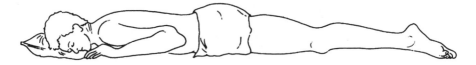

Figure 11.5 Position for a patient with burns to the flexor aspect of the hips.

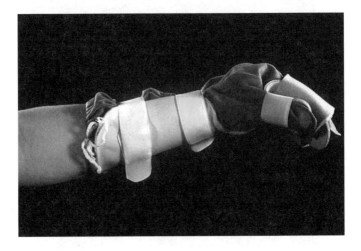

Figure 11.6 Hand resting splint.

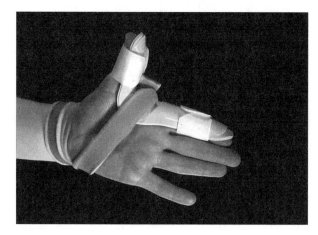

Figure 11.7 Thumb abduction splint for burns to thumb web.

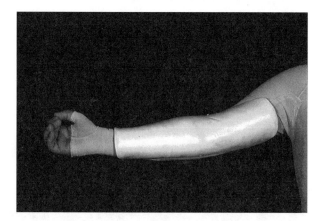

Figure 11.8 Elbow extension splint.

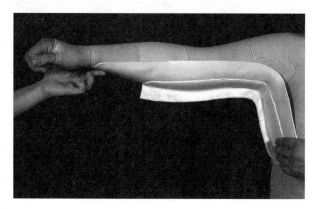

Figure 11.9 Arm abduction splint.

Hand Burns

Hand burns are worthy of a special mention and require physiotherapy from the earliest stage of wound management (Kealey and Jensen, 1988). Finger and thumb joints are very sensitive and the range of motion can be lost quickly. The burned hand becomes grossly oedematous. Uncontrolled oedema collects on the dorsum of the hand where the tissues are loose. This causes the metacarpophalangeal joints to hyperextend, stretching the long flexor tendons of the hand so that the interphalangeal joints are pulled into flexion: the result is a clawed hand. In this situation, the joint structures are in their shortened position and will contract, rendering the hand useless. It is therefore imperative that the hand is kept elevated in a Bradford sling at all times to allow the oedema to drain (Figure 11.3). Burns to the dorsum of the hand can easily expose the extensor tendons, particularly the central slip of the extensor digitorum tendon, over the proximal interphalangeal joint. Rupture of the central slip results in a Boutonnière deformity of the finger. Sheridan et al. (1995) identified that only 9% of patients who sustained damage to the extensor mechanism of their hand achieved normal function.

Dressings should be as light as possible so that the patient can exercise regularly both under the supervision of the physiotherapist and independently. The use of plastic or semi-permeable membrane bags are ideal as they allow free movement of the digits (Martin et al., 1990). Regular exercise of affected joints is encouraged as soon as possible after the patient is admitted. Exercise not only maintains joint range of motion but also aids oedema drainage by producing a muscle pump (Grigsby de Linde and Miles, 1995). Total active and passive ranges of motion are monitored and patients are taught exercises to obtain isolated tendon gliding and intrinsic muscle activity (Grigsby de Linde and Miles, 1995). The use of continuous passive motion machines in the rehabilitation of hand injuries is increasing (Adams and Thompson, 1996). Salter (1996) advocated their use and demonstrated a reduction in pain, maintenance of range of motion, reduction in complications and a shorter period of rehabilitation. However, Pope et al. (1997) investigated their use after surgery to the lower limb and demonstrated no significant improvement in function or range of motion. Of greater concern is the identification of increased blood loss and analgesic requirement (Pope et al., 1997). However, the application of repeated submaximal stress to scar tissue has been shown to be effective in achieving tissue lengthening (Kisner and Colby, 1990).

Splinting is particularly important for patients with hand burns who are ventilated and sedated and are therefore unable to cooperate with exercises. The hands are splinted in a position that will prevent joint contractures (Bach et al., 1984: Figure 11.6):

- Wrist: 15–30 degrees of extension
- Metacarpophalangeal (MCP) joints: 45–80 degrees of flexion
- Interphalangeal (IP) joints: full extension
- Thumb: abduction and 10–20 degrees of flexion at MCP and IP joints

Aiding Functional Independence

Ambulation

Patients with burns to the leg are encouraged to mobilize as soon as possible. Skin grafts to the lower limbs need to be supported by correctly sized, double-thickness tubigrip to control oedema and prevent venous stasis (Giuliani and Perry, 1985). The physiotherapist may need to provide suitable walking aids, e.g. a walking frame, crutches, a walking stick. The majority of Burns Units recommend that patients with skin grafts to their lower limbs remain on bed rest for a period of time post-operatively to ensure graft take and prevent shearing forces being applied to the grafts. However, Burnsworth et al. (1992) demonstrated that immediate ambulation did not impair graft take and decreased the average length of hospitalization. Close liaison with the nursing staff is essential so that the patient is encouraged to walk to the bathroom/toilet when the physiotherapist is not present. The physiotherapist also teaches the patient to negotiate stairs and ensures that they are safe and independent prior to discharge from hospital.

Exercise Tolerance and Muscle Power

Patients who have numerous operations resulting in lengthy periods of bed rest will become weak and debilitated (Giuliani and Perry, 1985). Muscle strength, exercise tolerance and endurance are developed by gradually increasing the frequency and intensity of exercise sessions (Hartigan et al., 1989). The patient is encouraged to make use of the facilities in the physiotherapy department gym. This removes the patient from the protected environment of the Burns Unit and begins the preparation for their return to society. If the patient is in isolation due to wound infection, equipment is kept in the patient's room, e.g. a static bicycle. Parrot et al. (1988) demonstrated that although a structured exercise circuit for burn-injured patients resulted in no change in the length of hospitalization, it did reduce the number of outpatient therapy visits required. St Pierre et al. (1998) demonstrated that patients with severe burns (>30% TBSA) remained weak for years after their trauma and suggested this was a result of either an inability to recover fully or insufficient rehabilitation.

Self Care and Independence

As a preparation for discharge home the patient is encouraged to be independent in all daily activities (Giuliani and Perry, 1985). Patients with injured hands should use them for functional activities as well as continuing with regular exercise. Patients need to be as independent as possible particularly if living alone. Prior to discharge from hospital the majority of patients need to be able to:

- Use hands for tasks, e.g. apply moisturizing cream to grafted areas
- Mobilize independently
- Transfer in and out of chair/toilet/bed independently
- Safely negotiate stairs

The physiotherapist needs to work closely with the patient and other members of staff to achieve these goals. It may be necessary for the physiotherapist to visit the patient's home to assess individual needs.

Psychological Support

Most burn-injured patients have difficulty in coming to terms with their injuries and go through various stages of anxiety, depression or even aggression (Giuliani and Perry, 1985). The physiotherapist has an ideal opportunity to establish a relationship with the patient during treatment sessions and is able to offer support and encouragement when necessary. Parents of a burn-injured child may need to supervise exercises or appropriate play activities when their child returns home (Raeside, 1992). The parents need help and support at this time particularly if the child is unwilling to cooperate. Patients often have many questions and anxieties about scarring, altered body image and how they will manage at home or work. These anxieties may be voiced to the physiotherapist during treatment sessions. When appropriate the physiotherapist will be able to offer reassurance and advice. Patients are encouraged to assume responsibility for their rehabilitation and Gripp et al. (1995) demonstrated that this gives patients a greater sense of motivation and accomplishment.

Outpatient Follow-up

After discharge from the Burns Unit the patient may need to continue with physiotherapy treatment as an outpatient (Raeside, 1992). The physiotherapist normally reviews the patient when they attend for a change of dressing, as this makes it easier to monitor joint movement. Hand burns in particular need monitoring for some time to ensure any graft tightness does not result in joint contracture. Younger patients who are keen to regain former fitness and strength may benefit from intensive physiotherapy and occupational therapy at a rehabilitation centre. This serves as an excellent preparation for the patient to return to work.

Conclusion

The patient's functional outcome is dependent on an integrated team approach at all stages of recovery (Clarke, 1997). The physiotherapist has an important and often demanding role in the rehabilitation of a burn-injured patient, requiring patience, adaptability and, often, a firm but caring approach. The ability to work with other members of the multidisciplinary team is essential and it is close teamwork that will help patients overcome their injuries. Each patient requires an individual assessment and reassessments; a prescriptive regime is inappropriate (Clarke, 1997) except during the initial management of mass casualty incidents (Barillo et al., 1997).

References

Adams KM, Thompson ST (1996) Continuous passive motion use in hand therapy. Hand Clinics 12(1): 109–27.

Bach J, Draslov B, Jorgensen B (1984) Positioning, splinting and pressure management of the burned hand. Scandinavian Journal of Plastic and Reconstructive Surgery 18: 145–47.

Bahnof R (2000) Intra-oral burns: rehabilitation of severe restriction of mouth opening. Physiotherapy 86(5): 263–66.

Barillo DJ, Harvey KD, Hobbs CL et al. (1997) Prospective outcome analysis of a protocol for the surgical and rehabilitative management of burns to the hands. Plastic and Reconstructive Surgery 100(6): 1442–51.

Bartlett RH, Gazzaniga AB, Gerachty TR (1973) Respiratory manoeuvres to prevent post-operative pulmonary complications. Journal of American Medical Association 224: 1017–21.

Biggs KS, de Linde L, Banaszewski M et al. (1998) Determining the current roles of physical and occupational therapists in burn care. Journal of Burn Care and Rehabilitation 19(5): 442–49.

Boardman S (1991) Treatment of respiratory problems. In Leveridge A, (Ed) Therapy for the Burn Injured Patient. London: Chapman and Hall. pp 29–33.

Boswick JA (1983) Rehabilitation after burn injury. Annals of the Academy of Medicine 12(3): 443–48 .

Burnsworth B, Krob MJ, Langer-Schnepp M (1992) Immediate ambulation of patients with lower-extremity grafts. Journal of Burn Care and Rehabilitation 13(1): 89–92.

Carmudie C (1980) Management of the burned hand. Australian Journal of Physiotherapy 26: 4.

Clarke J (1997) Burns to the hands – the perspective from Roehampton. British Journal of Hand Therapy 2(6): 9–10.

Clarke SW (1989) Rationale of airway clearance. European Respiratory Journal 2: 599–604.

Cooper KR, Phillips BA (1982) Effect of short term sleep loss on breathing. Journal of Applied Physiology 53: 355–58.

Dallimore K, Jenkins S, Tucker B (1998) Respiratory and cardiovascular responses to manual chest percussion in normal subjects. Australian Journal of Physiotherapy 44(4): 267–74.

Darling GE, Keresteci MA, Pugwash RA et al. (1996) Pulmonary complications in inhalation injuries with associated cutaneous burn. Journal of Trauma: Injury, Infection and Critical Care 40(1): 83–89.

Dean D (1994) Oxygen transport: a physiologically based conceptual framework for the practice of cardiopulmonary physiotherapy. Physiotherapy 80: 347–54.

Gairns CE, Martin DL (1990) The use of semi-permeable membrane bags as hand burn dressings. Physiotherapy 76(6): 351–52.

Gallon A (1992) The use of percussion. Physiotherapy 78(2): 85–89.

Giuliani CA, Perry GA (1985) Factors to consider in rehabilitation aspect of burn care. Physical Therapy 66(5): 619–23.

Grigsby de Linde L, Miles WK (1995) Remodelling of scar tissue in the burned hand. In Hunter JM, Mackin EJ, Callahan AD, (Eds) Rehabilitation of the Hand: Surgery and Therapy. London: Mosby.

Gripp CL, Salvaggio J, Fratianne RB (1995) Use of burn intensive care unit gymnasium as an adjunct to therapy. Journal of Burn Care and Rehabilitation 16: 160–61.

Harden NG, Luster SH (1991) Rehabilitation considerations in the care of the acute burn patient. Critical Care Nursing Clinics of North America 3(2): 245–53.

Hartigan C, Persing JA, Williamson SC et al. (1989) An overview of muscle strengthening. Journal of Burn Care and Rehabilitation 10(3): 251–57.

Hough A (1996) Physiotherapy in Respiratory Care: a Problem Solving Approach to Respiratory and Cardiac Management. 2nd edn. London: Chapman and Hall.

Jenkins SC (1988) The effect of posture on lung volumes in normal subjects and in patients pre and post coronary artery surgery. Physiotherapy 74: 492–96.

Jones AYM, Hutchinson RC, Oh TE, (1992) Effects of bagging and percussion on total static compliance of the respiratory system. Physiotherapy 78(9): 661–66.

Kealey GP, Jensen KT (1988) Aggressive approach to physical therapy management of the burned hand. Physical Therapy 68(5): 683–685.

Keilty SEJ (1993) Inhalation burn injured patients and physiotherapy management. Physiotherapy 79(2): 87–89.

Kinsella J (1988) Smoke inhalation. Burns 14(4): 269–79.

Kisner C, Colby LA (1990) Therapeutic Exercise, Foundation and Techniques. 2nd edn. Philadelphia: FA Davis.

Mackenzie CF, Imle PC, Ciesla N, (1989) Chest physiotherapy in the intensive care unit. 2nd edn. London: Williams and Wilkins.

Martin DL, French G, Theakstone J (1990) The use of semi-permeable membranes for wound management. British Journal of Plastic Surgery 43: 55–60.

Mathur NK (1986) Inhalation injury in major burns. Care of the Critically Ill 2(5): 195–96.

Menkes H, Britt J (1980) Rationale for physical therapy. American Review of Respiratory Disease 122: 127–32.

Parrot, M, Ryan R, Parks DH et al. (1988) Structured exercise circuit program for burn patients. Journal of Burn Care and Rehabilitation 9(6): 666–68.

Pope RO, Corcoran S, McCaul K et al. (1997) Continuous passive motion after primary total knee arthroplasty. Does it offer any benefits? Journal of Bone and Joint Surgery 79(6): 914–17.

Pryor JA, Webber BA, Hodson ME (1990) Effect of chest physiotherapy on oxygen saturation in patients with cystic fibrosis. Thorax 45: 77.

Raeside F (1992) Physiotherapy management of burned children: a pilot study. Physiotherapy 78(12): 891–95.

Richard R, Staley M, Miller S et al. (1996) To splint or not to splint – past philosophy and present practice: Part 1. Journal of Burn Care and Rehabilitation 17(5): 444–53.

Salter RB (1996) History of rest and motion and the scientific basis for early continuous passive motion. Hand Clinics 12(1): 1–11.

Schnebly WA, Ward RS, Warden GD et al. (1989) A non-splinting approach to the care of the thermally injured patient. Journal of Burn Care and Rehabilitation 10: 263–66.

Sheridan RL, Hurley J, Smith MA et al. (1995) The acutely burned hand: management and outcome based on a ten year experience with 1047 acute hand burns. Journal of Trauma 38(3): 406–11.

St Pierre DM, Choiniere M, Forget R et al. (1998) Muscle strength in individuals with healed burns. Archives of Physical Medicine and Rehabilitation 79(2): 155–61.

Further Reading

Chartered Society of Physiotherapy and College of Occupational Therapy (2000) Standards for Burns.

Hough A (1996) Physiotherapy in Respiratory Care: a Problem Solving Approach to Respiratory and Cardiac Management. 2nd edn. London: Chapman and Hall.

Leveridge A (1991) Therapy for the Burn Patient. London: Chapman and Hall.

CHAPTER 12

Social Reintegration for an Individual following Burn Trauma

JILL BLUNT

Introduction

In today's culture much seems to hinge on good looks, with great social significance attached to faces, which are described by Partridge (1990) as the outward canvas of our personality. The theory of stigma described by Goffman (1963) gives good insight into characteristic social responses to disfigurement. He claims that the stigmatized are treated as a discredited subgroup in society because assumptions are made about the cause of disfigurement, e.g. culpability for burns in terms of neglect, or scars resulting from fighting.

Disfigurement, which is a consequence of a physical condition as opposed to a condition itself, has also long been seen as a form of punishment. Throughout history, criminals were deliberately disfigured to mark them for all to see. The social impact of disfigurement is also often reinforced by negative images portrayed through the media and literature, e.g. Freddie Kruger in *Nightmare on Elm Street*, the Beast in the Walt Disney film of *Beauty and the Beast*, the Joker in *Batman*, and *The Phantom of the Opera*. Even the medical profession is guilty of making anything unusual scientifically interesting, e.g. *The Elephant Man*.

Body image is formed in a social as well as personal context, and alterations to it and the resulting reactions of others to it will be felt deeply. Social reintegration is a journey during which the patient gradually accepts the alteration to their body image and, through slowly regaining and re-establishing self-esteem and independence, they develop confidence in being accepted as a person with the disfigurement as part of their personality. It is a learning process that takes a long time, in some cases years. Members of the multidisciplinary team have important parts to play in helping patients and their families both to prepare for the losses that will occur and to cope with them as they arise in the future.

Issues of altered body image focus on two overlapping psychological consequences: bodily changes, or the way in which patients and others perceive their bodies; and changes of function, where patients will have to alter their activities and possibly roles. Often one is more affected than the other. Burns commonly cause both a loss of function and damage to body image, and in many instances pose a threat to life itself. Thus the effects of the burn injury impact not only on the injured person but everyone involved in their life. Although vast improvements to appearance can be made, patients will never regain the perfect smoothness of their skin following a significant burn injury. The skin will both feel and look different and, because burns often involve the unprotected face and hands, the resulting disfigurement may always be on show.

Bradbury (1996) notes that the loss of identity following an abrupt change to appearance is multifaceted, embracing various different kinds of loss: self identity (not recognizing the face in a mirror); family identity (no longer resembling siblings or parents); gender identity (feeling less feminine because of scarring, or less of a man because emasculated by hand injury); and racial identity (where burned tissue loses its dark pigment). Bradbury also maintains that this perception of loss of identity leads to anxiety/depression, isolation and a grieving response. All those with visible disfigurements face common problems that have their roots in psychological, social and historical processes. However, individuals differ in their ability to cope and reintegrate, and although the importance of rehabilitation is widely accepted, its profile in health care is heavily eclipsed by the acute services (Hurren, 1995).

Body image is categorized by Price (1990) into five modes of typical care intervention: preventative care; supportive care; patient education; patient counselling; and liaison with the social support networks. These categories are incorporated into the reintegration strategies that draw on the work of Watkins et al. (1996) and Morse and O'Brien (1995).

The Importance of Social Support Networks

The ability to reintegrate has been linked to a patient's pre-existing psychological state. Parkes (1975) suggests that those who had a long-standing tendency to anxiety or depression coped less well and suffered more than others. However Watkins et al. (1996) claim that more recent studies have identified and confirmed that the quality of family support is the single most important factor influencing a patient's post-burn adjustment. Despite this recognition of the importance of family support in the rehabilitation of patients, there is a paucity of studies into the needs of these families.

Price (1990) claims that body image is developed and sustained best within a supportive framework which includes family, friends and significant others. They provide the milieu in which a normal body image is first formed and an altered body image is reintegrated into society. Thus, patients with an active social support network are likely to make better progress. Burnside (1996) also identifies the presence of social support as a key element to successful reintegration, claiming that in the long term it is the patient's relatives and friends who fulfil the major support role. For this reason, interventions aimed at helping them are included in this text.

Stages of Adaptation

Watkins et al. (1996) describe family adaptation as a continuous process beginning at the time of the injury and proceeding at an individual pace to a conclusion and, although he identifies four common stages, they are separate points along this continuum. The emotional closeness/distance that a family member has with a patient to a large degree determines how many issues each member has to resolve. These issues need to be considered and assessed at each stage, although it is recognized that a family member may not need help at that time. It is important to recognize that the patient's adaptation will be out of synchrony with the family member's adaptation process. Whilst it is beyond the scope of this chapter to develop comprehensive rehabilitation programmes, one needs to be aware of the stages of adaptation in order to understand the behaviour exhibited by the family in order to select and implement interventions with them that can actually support the adjustment and reintegration programme. With the emphasis on early discharge, members of the multidisciplinary team will need to rapidly form sound relationships with the patient and family in order to achieve the best outcome for the patient.

Stage One – Vigilance and Crisis

The first stage of adapting to the effect of the trauma begins with the incident itself. Morse and O'Brien (1995) report that patients are acutely aware that their life is in peril and go to extraordinary lengths to preserve it. They display an immense increase in cognitive abilities and a heightening of senses, actually directing their own care if they feel that those assisting lack knowledge or appear incompetent. The focus is entirely on self.

If a family member (e.g. parent, sibling, spouse, partner – the list is not exhaustive) is present, he/she will be shocked and may display what Watkins et al. (1996) call behavioural disorganization. They believe that this calm, almost unconcerned behaviour, has survival value in that it allows the family member to function in a relatively normal manner so that further damage is limited, e.g. first aid can be performed. Once help is obtained, this 'emotional insulation' disappears and the focus is on their own feelings and needs as opposed to those of the patient. Watkins et al. (1996) describe the overwhelming intensity of feelings of confusion, fear, anxiety and guilt as an 'internal storm'.

At this initial stage, both the patient and his family focus on survival, pain relief, comfort, blame and guilt. Nursing care aimed at meeting the needs of both the patient and family in terms of these issues should be provided in a supportive, professional and respectful manner.

Immediate, effective analgesia for the patient is obviously vital. The family member should be allowed to express their feelings and practical assistance should be offered in terms of adequate facilities for meals and accommodation. This should then be followed with information on what is happening and why, explaining the patient's condition, treatment and needs, and should be given honestly, directly, compassionately and at a level appropriate to their understanding, thus forming the basis for a trusting relationship.

It is important to establish a relationship so that later one can move on to discuss problems and set aims. In burn trauma this is difficult as the early relationship takes place in an atmosphere of crisis. Giving information will undoubtedly provoke questions from the patient and involving the family members at the outset enables them to feel part of the patient's support team. From this foundation, nurses can begin to enlist their help.

Provision of information to the patient must be guided by their preferred coping style, described by Krohne et al. (1996) as either vigilant (where copious amounts of information should be given) or avoidant (small amounts of information given as too much increases anxiety). The patient will know, and confirm, their preference (Mitchell, 1997).

At an early stage, the family member will have to face the issue of the extent to which he or she is personally responsible for the injury and might have prevented it by doing something differently. Watkins et al. (1996) claim that the more devastating the injury, the more difficult it is for the family member to define and accept an appropriate level of responsibility.

Isolation increases all the stressors typically associated with hospitalization (Wong, 1997), with children feeling depersonalized from a decrease in interaction with the environment and people in it. Play is an enjoyable activity helping a child mature through various stages of childhood. One must aim to continue this natural development through play during hospitalization. A well-equipped playroom perceived as a safe environment by the child, where no medical or nursing interventions are undertaken, is essential but while they are too ill to use it appropriate toys should be provided at the bedside. Rodin (1983) concluded that children prepared for any intervention (including hospital admission) cope better than children who are not. Eiser (1984) supports this view and stresses that any attempt to improve communication with children and parents is to be welcomed.

There are comprehensive accounts in the literature on the short- and long-term distress caused by separating children from parents (Taylor et al., 1999). The three characteristics of a hospital experience quoted as affecting the risk of upset to children and parents are related to:

- The length of hospital stay
- Separation of child from parents
- The staff–parent relationship.

It is in the child's best interests that the hospital stay is not prolonged, with options for parents to have open access for visiting or, even better, encouraged to stay on the Burns Unit. The staff–parent relationship should be a trusting relationship in which the child's care can be planned and negotiated together so that the parents appreciate what is expected. It is also important to ensure that parents get adequate rest and regular meals as their needs are important too (Long, 1997; Palmer, 1993).

Morse and O'Brien (1995) found that although many patients do not voice their fears of scarring during the first stages of treatment, the thought is likely to be at the forefront of their minds. Swelling, particularly of the face, is very distressing to both the patient and their family. The temporary nature of this should be constantly reinforced, especially where vision is compromised, as this is both frightening and disorientating.

Nurses, along with other health care professionals, have competing pressures on their time, but critical physical care does not – and must not – negate the need for psychological care. Admission to the Burns Unit is a time of crisis not only for the patient but also for their family and friends. Failure to acknowledge and respond to their needs is to fail in the provision of holistic care.

Stage Two – Disruption and Control

During this stage Morse and O'Brien (1995) found that burn patients in particular suffered a loss of reality, with terrifying dreams or nightmares that rendered them unable to define reality in that the patients were unsure if they were alive or dead. Described as being 'in a fog', these dreams were in fact the reality of their predicament. This period of physiological instability was often spent in ITU or formed the initial period in the Burns Unit, where the priority was on preventing hypovolaemic shock.

Once the patient is stable, one needs to recognize the importance of assessing body image, guarding against marginalizing the psychological aspects of care because of the patient's physical needs. Concise, consistent information on the injuries and treatment remains a continuing priority to reorientate them. Talking to the patient about everyday activities including self-disclosure about interests, news, etc., can help to bring a sense of reality to the patient.

Price (1990) claims that even at this early stage patients will have an extended body image owing to intravenous infusion lines, nasogastric tubes, in-dwelling urinary catheters and a ventilator if one is utilized. Therefore, the temporary nature of these interventions should be stressed. Furthermore, he believes that pain itself can cause an alteration in body image in that patients may feel unable to 'trust' their body in the same way as before the burn injury. Effective pain relief attained through the use of Patient Controlled Analgesia (PCA) will not only provide the means for accurate pain assessment, but will also return a degree of control to the patient at a time when they are most overwhelmed.

Other strategies to aid the relief of pain include distraction therapy and allowing patients to help remove some of their wound dressings. Morse and O'Brien (1995) also found that patients at this stage distrusted their carers, frequently fearing the nurse was going to harm or even kill them. The patients wanted the continuous presence of someone they knew well, a relative or close friend who would help to provide reassurance and give a sense of reality. Thus there is a real need to promote open visiting and to encourage a close relative to stay, providing suitable accommodation or facilities at the patient's bedside.

At this stage, family members may now start to regain control of their own lives and routines of daily living, which is usually indicated by their focusing on practical details to support the family system. Watkins et al. (1996) found that they also try to determine responsibility for the injury but, instead of focusing on personal responsibility, they now focus on who or what outside the family system was to blame, e.g. faulty equipment, inadequate safety procedures, etc. The likely reason for this is that the family member needs to feel secure that there is no continuing threat, or simply that they are in control with regard to safety. They may therefore investigate the injury, seeking detailed information.

Strangely, family members rarely apportion blame to the patient, preferring to gloss over culpability for the injury even in cases where the individual was blatantly responsible. Watkins et al. (1996) claim it is a useful function linked to the resolution of other issues the family members face which overlap with those faced by the patient. During rehabilitation, the patient strives to regain self, the focus being on regaining autonomous functioning. His successes and failures cause him to accept his losses, accepting the long-term or permanent physical losses and the changes necessary in functioning to resume a meaningful life.

Likewise, the family member confronts the personal losses he/she suffers which affect his relationship and life. To acknowledge at this point that the patient was responsible for his own misfortune – and, consequently, for the losses of others – would force the family member to confront how little control he has over the patient and, ultimately, over the relationship. In essence, he would be confronting his emotional dependence on an untrustworthy person, a realization that is almost intolerable in the face of the helplessness and increased dependency of the injured.

The unpleasant behaviour exhibited by some family members is often related to unresolved issues of the extent of personal responsibility for the injuries. Watkins et al. (1996) note that some individuals can become demanding, disrespectful, arrogant, hostile and critical. They are essentially shifting intense self-blame or anger to those who now fulfil their usual role, finding it almost impossible to trust the care of the patient to anyone. The family member may in fact find relief from their guilt by ensuring the patient receives the best care – as a result of their constant vigilance!

To help them through this stage and to regain control of their lives, they need constant practical information about the patient's condition, progress, prognosis, and present and future needs. From this they will be able to determine the amount of help and support they will be able to provide within the framework of their daily life. Allowing and encouraging family members to participate in the care, praising their efforts and helping to develop the necessary skills will promote confidence in their ability to regain control in their lives.

The first time the patient views his injuries should be planned for in advance: this first glimpse, according to Partridge (1990), is critical, and can be devastating. The patient will need to have good outlets for talking to people following this, and there will remain a great need for open and frank conversations, allowing the patient to speak at length if he wishes.

This stage ends as the reality of the situation sets in. The patient may start to ask questions about the future.

Stage Three – Confronting and Regrouping

Patients can be dependent on the nurse for a long time, and during this period one should be gathering information on how their social networks function, and how past crises have been handled; this should help us to highlight how these coping strategies may help the patient adapt in the future. Family and friends provide a safe base from which patients begin to reintegrate into normal life and therefore represent one of the most important components in psychological recovery.

It has long been acknowledged that there is no relationship between the severity of burn and subsequent psychological adjustment but that the site of the burn and the degree of resulting disability are relevant factors. Burnside (1996) believes that the complicated relationship between burn injury and psychological adjustment is influenced by factors other than burn severity, such as: a premorbid personality; employment status; a lack of recreational activities; the coping style adopted; the visibility of burn scarring; the effect on mobility; the gender of the patient.

A number of reactions are usually observed by health care professionals in patients coming to terms with both the injury and its effect on their life. In this third stage, Morse and O'Brien (1995) found that although the physical suffering of patients was now largely controlled, the psychological suffering now became apparent as they recognized the meaning of the injuries and resulting losses. In order to make a positive adjustment to, and to accept, a new body image, patients need to develop or retain a sense of self-esteem despite the change in appearance. Salter (1997) claims that this adjustment follows the path of the grieving process described by Kubler-Ross (1969). The five phases she describes (denial, anger, bargaining, depression and acceptance) are experienced by both patient and family and, again, synchrony is unlikely.

The first three phases are usually experienced in hospital, and nurses need to probe gently to ascertain whether their patient has any concerns over their ability to cope when going home. Partridge (1993) found in his experience that nurses overlook their role as psychological support for the patient. It is imperative that time is allocated to sit with patients and utilize developed listening and communications skills. Likewise, Knowles (1993) identified nurses' inability to meet the psychological needs of patients, and he describes their lack of support as a downward spiral in which the patient feels depressed, requiring more support but in fact receiving less, and thus becomes more depressed. Anger and severe depression are natural reactions but should they become exaggerated or unmanageable, the help of a clinical psychologist may be appropriate.

Because body image is initially shaped by parents' attitudes to their children and then from significant others, it is important that relatives as well as health care professionals are encouraged to be positive and realistic about how the patient looks and how they will look upon completion of surgery. Health care professionals including Social Workers, psychologists, Occupational Therapists, etc., should be prepared in advance for the appearance of the patient so that they are greeted normally.

The aesthetic disability of disfigurement is frequently more severe then the physical disability. Partridge (1990) believes that disfigurement has two dimensions:

- Personal disfigurement: altered body image, your perception of yourself.
- Social disfigurement: how disfigurement is viewed in the eyes of others, how people to behave differently with you.

For example, Partridge felt his disfigurement when he noticed people in the pub staring or asking curious questions.

Feelings of inadequacy or inferiority must be challenged from the start for social reintegration to be real and effective, and the family needs to learn to develop skills to help the patient socialize and master encounters. Partridge's work around the SCARED acronym is a particularly useful tool to help patients challenge the reactions of people they meet. He claims these reactions are the first hurdles to overcome and the public need help to negotiate them (Partridge and Robinson, 1994). Fonagy et al. (1994) believe that factors helping individuals to cope with adversity include personal qualities such as intelligence, problem-solving skills, optimism, a sense of humour, acceptance by their parents and lack of early separations.

It is at this stage that patients are now moved from the confines and 'safety' of a single room to the open ward. They will need support during this change since it may well be their first encounter with strangers. Bradbury (1996) believes that a programme of controlled exposure to social encounters, or 'body presentation strategies' should begin with this first stage of moving the patient into the ward. Morse and O'Brien (1995) found that once patients orientated themselves, they were encouraged by the support the other patients gave them.

It can be useful to set clear objectives with defined parameters, and to guide the patient to anticipate the experience for himself/herself and others. A diary can be a useful tool for reviewing the experience, since evaluation is critical for turning the event into a positive learning experience – particularly if it was not a good experience. This diary, especially if supplemented with progressive photographs, becomes important in later weeks to demonstrate progress, and can also help family members to accommodate the alteration in body image. Partridge (1990), through his own experience, found that talking about the incident was a cathartic activity and he claims it enables people to let out all the emotion and feelings about the fire, cleansing them of the drama.

The helping process is rooted in:

* Facilitating patients to find ways of coping, as opposed to telling them how to cope.
* Promoting and aiming for normal social and family environments.
* Avoiding the dependence of patients on professionals.
* Empowering individuals by helping them to work through their problems, seeking solutions and constructively criticizing their individual skills.

Staff members need to build their confidence in their own ability to handle situations. It is also important to help patients bring about change: otherwise, warns Bradbury (1996), emotional support, whilst effective if it helps patients to cope, has no point if it maintains the status quo. Litt et al. (1995) clearly demonstrate the power of encouragement in helping patients to cope, and the need to offer support and voice words of encouragement.

Aims can be divided into short- and medium-term – e.g. moving the patient to the main ward, contacting school to obtain work, re-establishing relationships – and should be specific and focused. It is important to recognize that it may not initially be possible to set long-term aims and that, once set, they may not be achieved within the time span of our contact with the patient, but may eventually be achieved as a result of the help received. The patient must of course set the aims, but it is entirely appropriate to work with parents provided that conflicts between their needs and the wishes of the child are addressed. Bradbury (1996) points out the all too familiar situation where the child is untroubled by the disfigurement and consequently does not want further surgery, but the parents (perhaps through guilt) demand surgery.

The identification of problems can be made by helping the patient comprise a SWOT analysis (Bradbury, 1996):

- **Strengths**: Whom can he approach for support? What type of support can he expect? How can he get that support, e.g. telephone, writing, etc.?
- **Weaknesses**: What may work against him?
- **Opportunities**: What are the potential benefits from the situation?
- **Threats**: What are the potential problems? What are his fears about the future?

Partridge (1990) discusses the two interrelated emotions that people who knew the patient prior to the accident may experience as nostalgia and reparation. This special treatment they bestow, particularly on children, to try and compensate for the loss can be less than useful, as people's doubts about a patient's future can allow the patient to wallow in the past. Their attitude to themselves is very much influenced by the quality and quantity of support given by family and friends. Bradbury (1996) believes that there can be an element of self-stigmatization, since the power of stigma lies in its acceptance by those stigmatized.

Children have particular needs. There is much written about the benefits of play in hospital (e.g. Taylor et al., 1999). It provides diversion, a simple method of taking a child's mind off what is happening; it can be a way for the child to act out worries or problems; and it restores normal aspects of life. It also provides a way of understanding, allowing the child to become more aware of hospital and events and allows them to communicate fears.

A well-equipped playroom where no medical or nursing interventions are undertaken has already been described as a safe environment. This child-orientated atmosphere should have the presence of a trusted, permission-giving and responsive adult, who welcomes siblings. Education has similar functions to play, and hospital teachers will visit school-aged children, once well enough, to encourage them to begin school work. However, they cannot provide the social aspect of schooling normally experienced by a child and, for that reason, when children are well enough they are encouraged to go to the hospital schoolroom. Work sent in from the child's own school is also encouraged.

Regression

With illness, children always regress to the developmental level that allows them to deal with the stress (Wong, 1997). As their condition permits, children should be encouraged to do things they were capable of doing before. Allowing them to make decisions about the timing of their care and recreational activities provides a measure of control and makes them feel a worthwhile member of the team, gaining confidence and self-esteem.

Adolescents will have different needs, requiring a 'day-room' as opposed to a playroom. Their main needs are summarized by Taylor et al. (1999). Adolescence is a time of challenges and demands which can create feelings of inadequacy, pessimism, impatience and doubt.

At this time, family members must also resolve the issue of whether their altered relationship with the patient can be sustained through physical recovery and rehabilitation, since Watkins et al. (1996) claim that the alteration of the relationship is unavoidable. The patient's focus is primarily on his own needs, which appears to be a normal phenomenon and necessary for him to regain maximum function. However, a consequence is that he is unable to support anyone else.

The patient may not be able to perform all physical, emotional and social functions that were a feature of their previous relationship, with the increased dependence by the patient on the family member. The increased need for support from the family member and a decreased ability to provide for his family members' needs within the relationship is important. Watkins et al. (1996) believe that the family member has to decide, emotionally, whether or not to make the temporary, but prolonged, commitment to continuing the relationship with the patient in this altered form through recovery and rehabilitation.

Allowing the family member to gradually assume more responsibility for the patient's needs, perhaps through assisting with bathing, after-care and wound dressing, causes a gradual shift in control of the patient's care to the family members. Assisting with aftercare also demonstrates to both the patient and family members/friends that the healed burn wounds are not painful, and that it is acceptable to touch him. At this stage, the nurse would change from being the primary caregiver to a more collaborative role with the patient and his family, thus allowing family members to face the practicalities of their situation.

Nursing interventions in this stage include practical teaching and anticipatory guidance as well as providing physical and psychological comfort. The qualities of a skilled helper, quoted from the original work of Rogers (1959), are personal warmth, self-esteem, spontaneity, sincerity, unconditional positive regard, empathy, genuineness and non-defensiveness. Bradbury (1996) sees these qualities as being vital to the process of helping patients. One needs to be aware of the impact they have on individuals, developing them and using them to help bring about change.

The work of Lazurus (1966) is also useful, and describes four components of coping that can be utilized to help patients:

- Adjustment must be viewed as a process and not a single event. The process is interactive, during which patients should be encouraged to use their social resources (for example, friends and family to talk things through) and personal resources (problem-solving abilities).
- It is a dynamic process that needs to be managed rather than mastered. It is therefore a continuing learning process where experience of situations can be applied to other situations.
- It involves appraisal or evaluation, and patients should be helped to make subjective evaluations since a patient's behaviour is influenced by the sense that that person makes of it rather than the judgement of another.
- Coping requires mobilization of effort, both cognitive and behavioural – patients need to be encouraged to reflect on the experience and then implement changes to improve matters. Thinking alone is not enough as it cannot change the problems faced, and a purely behavioural change will not succeed if the patient does not understand what is happening.

Stage Four – Merging the Old and New Person

The patient is now regaining increasing independence. Reintegration into the community begins in hospital and continues well after discharge, with the nurse a source of information, advice and encouragement. A major difficulty is how to meet new people and make friends. The psychological care is perhaps the balancing of art with the scientific healing of the body.

Cronan (1993) believes that normalization is often neglected, and because exposure to everyday situations can be frightening, a gradual exposure should be encouraged. The first stages of reintegration began earlier, when the patient was first moved from the security of a single room into an open ward with other patients. This can then be built upon, with accompanied visits within the hospital, perhaps to Pharmacy to collect any prescriptions, etc., and then planned short shopping trips, followed by perhaps a visit to the cinema. One local strategy is to forge links with a local fast-food restaurant – a trip to the cinema followed by beefburger and chips is carefully planned as one of the first social visits outside the relative safe environment provided by the hospital.

Visits home

These include short visits for a few hours only, followed by an overnight/weekend stay and finally, if all is well, discharge home. This is an effective way of identifying needs that are not apparent in hospital and provide a 'safety net' for both the patient and carer.

Nearing discharge, individual coping mechanisms must be addressed. Burnside (1996) concludes in his extensive literature review that the adoption of coping mechanisms and higher levels of social engagement is associated with lower levels of stress in patients, and it is beneficial therefore to teach patients to confront issues and actively solve problems rather than avoid them. One needs to continue to emphasize desirable and attainable goals, reminding survivors that they have already demonstrated significant strength just by surviving a frightening and painful ordeal.

Paradoxically, the more an individual tries to do, the more they realize what they can no longer do. Morse and O'Brien (1995) note, however, that once the individual decides to move forward, it is then that they discover whether they are not able to go back to their former life and work. Learning one's limitations is regarded as an essential part of being able to reformulate the future. Patients may now reformulate expectations of self and of their future, seeking more information about their accident. This 'preserving' of self is thought by Morse and O'Brien (1995) to be crucial not only to survival but also the key to a successful rehabilitation.

Discharge Home

NHS hospitals are legally required to provide a discharge policy for all patients by the NHS and Community Care Act 1990 which came into force from 1 April 1993. As the average length of stay in hospital continues to be shorter, the necessity for effective discharge planning becomes essential. Many believe that planning for discharge should begin on admission (McBride, 1995; Salter, 1997; Elgie, 1998) and this is in fact demanded by some local health authorities whose policies take into account the Continuing Health Care guidance.

Discharge planning is part of an ongoing process that is, according to Armitage and Kavanagh (1996), part of the continuum of hospital care that is intended to prepare patients for their return to the community. It includes liaising with community services whilst providing the patient/families/carers with the skills and support they will need to manage the patient's health care. However, Partridge and Robinson (1994) found that after discharge many facially disfigured patients found a gap in resources. Their psychosocial needs were largely ignored with no preparation for life in the community and reintegration into society. Physical well-being alone is not a sufficient reason on which to base the discharge of a patient.

Nurses play a pivotal role in this multidisciplinary process as they probably have established a rapport with the patient better than any other member of the team. However, in the past they been accused of giving discharge planning a low priority (particularly in the acute care setting) where they have been found to under-rate the value of discharge preparation for the patient's welfare (Armitage and Kavanagh, 1996). Furthermore, McBride (1995) found that nearly half the patients in her study had their discharge arranged by more than one nurse, thus raising the importance of continuity of nursing actions and patient care.

After discharge there is a risk that patients will retreat into sheltered lives and never be fully reintegrated into society, suffering what Partridge (1998) claims a 'social death'. From his own experience, Partridge (1990) found that the feelings of isolation were strongest for the first few months after discharge. He likened the hospital support system to a wonderful cocoon, and he believes that there needs to be a system in place to gradually integrate and teach coping mechanisms. Like the American space shuttle, he claims people need an extra thick layer of protection for re-entry into their atmosphere, and that this extra-tough layer has to be capable of withstanding and deflecting the sometimes withering attention of other people. He stresses that this layer does not automatically appear but has to be constructed and with considerable help from others.

Partridge firmly believes that how you conduct yourself critically affects how others receive you, and that being honest will both allow people to express concern for you and in turn allow you to see that they acknowledge you as a whole and worthwhile person. Although patients need to toughen up for re-entry, Partridge stresses that it should not be in a defensive, armour-plated way. Rather, the armour comes from being willing to be open, deflecting curiosity or hostility and by trying to understand other peoples' initial reactions and then building on them, directing them to your own advantage. His registered charity 'Changing Faces' is renowned for its workshops for patients, healthcare members and carers, and is discussed more fully later in this chapter.

Partridge (1990) found that because fellow patients and staff do not relate to you with the awkwardness and hostility that you meet outside, there is great security to be derived from the Burns Unit where patients are totally accepted. Warden (1996) also found that the Burns Unit becomes a second home and it can be daunting to leave. Consequently, full emotional impact is often not felt until discharged from the protected environment of a hospital, when the reality of the emotional, physical and financial burden of the injury becomes apparent and has to be faced.

Telephone Support and Visits to the Patient at Home

A telephone call 36–48 hours after discharge to assess the ability to cope provides support in the same way that Mitchell (2000) found that a telephone conversation with a patient in the post-operative phase provided a positive therapeutic role.

Home visits and continued telephone support to the patient once discharged provide a valuable link and enables health care professionals to discuss and reflect on successful or negative encounters, and to refer the patient for professional help if it appears to be needed.

School Visits

Return to school is a critical milestone in the rehabilitation of children, and appropriate preparation is necessary to help teachers and children understand the situation. The child may have been away from school for some time and lost contact with friends and classmates, and they may return to school looking different. Teachers are helpful in maintaining the link between children with the burn injury and their peers to avoid estrangement. Bradbury (1996) suggests that a programme of re-entry should incorporate the teacher visiting hospital and bringing in school-work; friends should be encouraged to visit and, once home, they should be encouraged to call at the child's home.

A presentation, which gives them information on and the reasons for aftercare, with regard to scarring, creaming, splints and pressure garments, etc., will help them to be empathetic and supportive. Teenagers should be given the choice of having a school visit or not. Teachers may be concerned about allowing the child to resume sports, or even to play in the communal playground at breaks, and they may need basic first aid advice in case of further injury to the newly healed site.

The primary nurse plans and prepares objectives for the school visit, which should ideally be conducted before the child returns to school. Obviously, the child's family should be aware of the content of the presentation.

Some children, particularly teenagers, may be interested in preparing a video message to the class. This could be shown to the class by a nurse and followed up with an explanation of the treatment and how they can help the child to deal with it. This method allows the children time to get over the shock of the appearance of the injured child before he or she resumes school, and the teachers and children can ask questions that they may be reluctant to ask in front of the child. Teachers will then be able to work with the class before the child returns, guiding them towards a greater general understanding of people with disfigurement. The children could be encouraged to send cards and write to the patient, who should be aware of what is happening at school, and then encouraged to return even if only part-time initially.

This strategy for the future may also provide an opportunity to develop Outreach or Community Liaison Nurse posts, where nurses work in close contact with an outreach service that could include the Burns Unit psychologist, occupational therapist, physiotherapist, etc. The social worker is pivotal to dovetailing the resources of the hospital and community.

Returning to Work

Just as children can expect problems returning to school, so can adults experience problems returning to work, particularly if the accident occurred there. They may need structured counselling.

Issues faced by family members are related to determining the long-term consequences of the burn injury to that family member. Watkins et al. (1996) believe that there is an internal negotiation within a relationship about whether it has the potential to meet the emotional, social and economic needs of each member. In relatively less severe cases, they believe that a gradual return to the pre-burn relationship is the usual resolution, but in more severe injuries, this is much more complicated.

Amid agonizing guilt, some family members will choose to sever the relationship, unable to sustain the emotional commitment. This often happens when the pattern of the relationship and interaction since the injury has become entrenched and dysfunctional to the point where the family member cannot renegotiate a share of control within the relationship as the patient's functioning improves. They are faced with the choice of either meeting their own needs or continuing to meet those of the patient.

Watkins et al. (1996) found that it was rare for a spouse to divorce even the most severely injured patient during the first year after injury, but it became relatively common in the second and third years. Nursing interventions must focus on empathetic and non-judgemental listening. One needs to reassure the family member that it is legitimate for him to have personal needs that may be separate and quite distinct from those of the patient, and that it is fine to define them, assertively present those needs to others and ultimately take responsibility to meet them. This supportive interaction, which legitimizes their needs, corroborates the family member's feelings about the altered reality of his/her life.

Children

Some studies have revealed high maternal anxiety (see, for example, Kent et al., 2000; Zeitlin, 1997) suggesting that mothers may be at a higher risk than children for developing psychological sequelae. This has long-term implications for the child's outcome since it could affect treatment compliance, and it is important to identify mothers who could benefit from counselling. Sheldon (1997) claims that the successful psychological management of a sick child is influenced by the effectiveness of parents coping with illness.

In their study, LeDoux et al. (1996) discovered that children were aware of their resulting disabilities but seemed to have chosen to minimize their importance, presumably because these factors could not be changed. They did not deny their disabilities but rather denied the importance of the physical limitation to their overall success. The same children rated job competence, romantic appeal and scholastic appeal as most important – areas they can control and develop. Their value systems seem to reflect efforts to compensate in areas unaffected by the burn injury. It is useful therefore to develop such value systems as it offers a degree of hope for positive post-burn living. By emphasizing attainable/desirable goals it allows them to experience hope for achieving happiness and life satisfaction in spite of whatever impediments are imposed by the burn injuries. There is a need to communicate the belief that burned children can succeed both to the children and to the parents.

Counselling

Counselling should be viewed as a process through which one person helps another by talking in an understanding atmosphere, and is not advice giving. By establishing a helping relationship, patients and relatives are able to express their thoughts and feelings in a way that helps to clarify their own situation. Special counselling qualifications are not always needed but effective communication skills would seem to be essential.

Other family members may need help and although it is sometimes appropriate for the nurse to do this, other agencies may be required (see Chapters 13 and 14).

Support Groups

Self-help groups (for example, one Burns Unit has BUSH – the Burns Unit Self Help Group) allow people to meet others with similar problems, helping to legitimize them so that they appreciate that it is a problem of society and not unique to them. Hurren (1995) found that many self-help groups are combined with social skills training, with Price (1990) believing that group identity can enhance personal identity and provide a setting where the burn injury does not immediately intrude. It is useful to have members of the treatment team available if required to give advice and support, but the groups must remain patient-led.

Mothers and Young Children Groups

Riis et al. (1992) found that nearly all participating parents in her study expressed a wish to be in contact with parents who previously had a burned child. At one Burns Unit, a support group is run specifically for parents and young children in particular, responding to a particular need of that Unit. A nurse facilitates the group, which meets every 4–6 weeks and draws members from a wide section of the community – geographically and socially. They are able to discuss any issue of concern with parents who share a common experience.

Burn Camps

Burn Camps and holidays are of particular value to children. They are a relatively new concept in the UK but are rapidly becoming popular as a source of recreation and rehabilitation. The focus is to have fun but the principal goal is psychosocial adjustment through peer interaction and enhancement of self-esteem (Biggs et al., 1997). The children's lives were also thought to be enriched through providing new experiences, challenges and friends, giving fond memories for a lifetime. Verst (1996) also claims that in an atmosphere of openness and excitement, they were free to show their scars without embarrassment or shame, creating special bonds.

The merits of this type of intervention are reflected in the rapid development of similar camps/holidays and the high rate of repeat campers.

Changing Faces

This registered charity has school advisers, produces self-help guides and offers study days to professionals and workshops to patients and their families in order to learn strategies for coping and to raise awareness of the problems of disfigurement. The mix of activities (lectures, videotapes, slides, discussions) are intended to complement the work carried out by health care professionals, and acknowledges that health care professionals are often uncertain as to how to support patients (Clegg, 1998). The founder, James Partridge, suffered severe burns following a road traffic accident some years ago.

Let's Face It

This is another support group that helps patients to develop coping strategies through social skills training. Meetings are held at a number of venues and a newsletter is distributed. Although there is great emphasis in burns on facial disfigurement, to some people scarring on other visible parts of the body is also a problem.

Other helpful organizations include the British Red Cross Society which has an important role in the provision of camouflage make-up techniques. Advice should also be sought from appropriately trained people in the use of wigs, clothing styles, hairstyles and prostheses.

Conclusion

Society has always struggled to accept its members who do not conform to the accepted 'norm', deformity having been traditionally linked with evil or bad deeds. There is a need to equip patients with appropriate social skills that enable them to interact with others in a natural and uninhibited way, thereby helping those who appear to find it difficult to respond naturally when confronted with disability.

Many burn patients ask, 'When am I going to have the plastic surgery?', expecting to be returned to complete normality of appearance. This is an unrealistic expectation. Plastic surgery is a long-term process, usually performed on mature scars and has its limitations. Partridge (1990) warns of this quest for perfection actually deterring patients from making meaningful efforts to rebuild their lives, as surgical repair supersedes social rehabilitation.

There have been impressive advances in acute burn care during the last 25 years in terms of decreased mortality and decreased length of hospital stay (Warden, 1996), but these data on survival rates and length of hospital stay are not adequate measures of success for our specialty. As the ability to preserve life in burned patients improves, so too must concern for the quality of that life during reintegration into society. We need to equip staff with the skills to identify poor adapters so that appropriate help is obtained.

References

Armitage S, Kavanagh K (1996) Hospital nurses' perceptions of discharge planning for medical patients. Australian Journal of Advanced Nursing 14(2): 16–23.

Biggs KS, Heinrich JJ, Jekel JF et al. (1997) The Burn Camp experience: variables that influence the enhancement of self-esteem. Journal of Burn Care and Rehabilitation 18: 93–98.

Bradbury E (1996) Counselling People with Disfigurement. Leicester: BPS Books.

Burnside I (1996) Psychological aspects of burn injuries. In Settle JAD, (Ed) Principles and Practice of Burns Management. London: Churchill Livingstone. pp 443–51.

Clegg A (1998) Face value. Nursing Times 94(30): 30–32.

Cronan L (1993) Management of the patient with altered body image. British Journal of Nursing 2(5): 257–61.

Eiser C (1984) Communication with sick and hospitalised children. Journal of Child Psychology and Psychiatry 25: 181–89.

Elgie C (1998) Discharge planning. Nursing Management 4(8): 10–11.

Fonagy P, Steele M, Steele H et al. (1994) The Emanuel Miller Memorial Lecture 1992: The theory and practice of resilience. Journal of Child Psychology and Psychiatry 35(2): 231–57.

Goffman E (1963) Stigma: Notes on the Management of Spoiled Identity. Harmondsworth: Penguin Books.

Hurren JS (1995) Rehabilitation of the burned patient: James Laing Memorial Essay for 1993. Burns 21(2): 116–26.

Kent L, King H, Cochrane R (2000) Maternal and child psychological sequelae in paediatric burn injuries. Burns 26: 317–322.

Knowles HE (1993) The experience of infectious patients in isolation. Nursing Times 89(30): 53–56.

Krohne HW, Slangen K, Kleeman PP (1996) Coping variables as predictors of perioperative emotional states and adjustments. Psychology and Health 11(3): 315–30.

Kubler-Ross E (1969) On Death and Dying. New York: Macmillan.

LeDoux JM, Meyer WJ, Blakeney P et al. (1996) Positive self regard as a coping mechanism for pediatric burn survivors. Journal of Burn Care and Rehabilitation 17: 472–76.

Lazurus R (1966) Psychological Stress and the Coping Process. New York: McGraw Hill.

Litt MD et al. (1995) Preparation for oral surgery: evaluating elements of coping. Journal of Behavioural Medicine 18(5): 435–59.

Long S (1997) Being together as a family. Paediatric Nursing 9(6): 25–28.

McBride RC (1995) An audit of current discharge planning arrangements and their effectiveness on elderly care wards and community nursing services together with aspects of client satisfaction. Journal of Nursing Management 3: 19–24.

Mitchell MJ (2000) Nursing intervention for pre-operative anxiety. Nursing Standard 14(3): 40–43.

Mitchell MJ (1997) Patient's perceptions of pre-operative preparation for day surgery. Journal of Advanced Nursing 26(2): 356–63.

Morse JM, O'Brien B (1995) Preserving self: from victim, to patient to disabled person. Journal of Advanced Nursing 21: 886–96.

Palmer S (1993) Care of sick children by parents: a meaningful role. Journal of Advanced Nursing 18: 185–91.

Parkes CM (1975) Psycho-social transitions: comparison between reactions to loss of a limb and loss of a spouse. British Journal of Psychiatry 127: 204–10.

Partridge J (1998) Changing faces: taking up MacGregor's challenge. Journal of Burn Care and Rehabilitation 19: 174–80.

Partridge J (1993) The psychological effects of facial disfigurement. Journal of Wound Care 2(3): 168–71.

Partridge J (1990) Changing Faces. London: Penguin Books.

Partridge J, Robinson E (1994) Changing faces: two years on. Nursing Standard 8(34): 54–58.

Price B (1990) Body Image: Nursing Concepts and Care. Herts: Prentice Hall International (UK) Ltd.

Riis A, Anderson M, Pedersen MB et al. (1992) Long-term psychological adjustment in patients with severe burn injuries: a follow-up study. Burns 18(2): 121–26.

Rodin J (1983) Will This Hurt? London: RCN.

Rogers C (1959) A theory of therapy, personality and interpersonal relationships as developed in the client centred framework. In: Kock S (ed) Psychology: A study of a science Vol 3. Leicester: McGraw-Hill. pp 184–256.

Salter M (1997) Altered Body Image: The Nurse's Role. 2nd Edn. London: Baillière Tindall.

Sheldon L (1997) Hospitalising children: a review of the effects. Nursing Standard 12(1): 44–47.

Taylor J, Müller D, Wattley L et al. (1999) Nursing Children: Psychology, Research and Practice. 3rd edn. Cheltenham: Stanley Thornes (Publishers) Ltd.

Verst A (1996) Burn Camp: an unforgettable summer experience for children and teenagers. Plastic Surgical Nursing 16(4): 240–41.

Warden GD (1996) Functional Sequelae and Disability Assessment. In Herndon DN, (Ed) Total Burn Care. London: WB Saunders. pp 523–28.

Watkins PN, Cook EL, May SR et al. (1996) Postburn psychological adaptation of family members of patients with burns. Journal of Burn Care and Rehabilitation B17: 78–92.

Wong D (1997) Whaley and Wong's Essentials of Paediatric Nursing. 5th edn. Mosby-Year Book Inc USA.

Zeitlin REK (1997) Long-term psychological sequelae of paediatric burns. Burns 23(6): 467–72.

Further Reading

Bowlby J (1969) Attachment and Loss. London: Hogarth.

Dewing J (1989) Altered body image. Surgical Nurse 2(4): 7–20.

Doctor ME (1992) Helping the burned child to adapt. Burn Rehabilitation and Reconstruction 19(3): 607–14.

Leveridge A (1991) Therapy for the Burn Patient. London: Chapman and Hall.

MacGinley KJ (1993) Nursing care of the patient with altered body image. British Journal of Nursing 2(22): 1098–1102.

Parkes CM, Markus A (1998) Coping with Loss. London: BMJ Books.

Pruzinsky T (1998) Rehabilitation challenges for burn survivors with residual disfigurement: promising directions for interaction, research and collaboration. Journal of Burn Care and Rehabilitation 19: 169–73.

Rotter J (1966) Generalised expectations for internal vs external control of reinforcement. Psychological Monographs 80(1): 1–26.

Tarrier N (1995) Psychological morbidity in adult burns patients: prevalence and treatment. Journal of Mental Health 1: 51–62.

CHAPTER 13

Burns Aftercare and Scar Management

ROSEMARY GOLLOP

This chapter explores aspects of rehabilitation that concern the treatment of burn scarring, and the long-term consequences of scarring on the patient's recovery. The term 'patient' is used throughout for continuity, although facilitating the transition from patient to independent, functioning member of society is central to the occupational therapist's approach to rehabilitation.

The development of unsightly scarring is a common and distressing sequela to the healing of burned skin, and one which can pose major problems to the patient in the long process of rehabilitation. Although one of the purposes of skin grafting is to minimize scarring, scars do develop in grafted areas, as they do in burns that have been treated conservatively but have taken longer than 3–4 weeks to heal. Even donor sites may scar if the skin taken is anything other than extremely thin.

The scarring that occurs following burn injury is termed hypertrophic, which means literally 'overgrowth'. It is characterised by being raised, hard, red and pruritic (see Plate 7). Less commonly, keloid scars sometimes develop; these resemble particularly severe hypertrophic scars but are different in that they overgrow the margins of the original wound and can be quite resistant to treatment. A combination of both hypertrophic and keloid scars may occur concurrently in the same patient.

Aetiology

The causes of hypertrophic scarring are not yet fully understood, but several contributory factors have been identified, and may point to those patients who are at particular risk. These factors include:

- Depth of burn – damage to the dermal layers of the skin, particularly if the wound heals without grafting, is more likely to lead to hypertrophic scarring (Patino et al., 1998).
- Skin and hair colour – risk factors include very fair skin and red hair, and conversely, darkly pigmented skin.
- Age – more severe scarring is thought to be associated with youth and pregnancy (Baum and Busuito, 1998).
- Infection – the presence of infection delays healing and increases the chance of scar development (Lawrence, 1987).
- Type of graft – split skin grafts scar more than full thickness skin grafts.
- Personal and family history, i.e. genetic factors (Baum and Busuito, 1998).
- Wounds that heal under tension are thought to be more prone to scarring (Berman and Flores, 1998).

Pathophysiology of Scar Formation

The pathophysiology of wound healing and scar formation is complex, and for the patient it manifests itself in the change from healed flat graft to active, hypertrophic scar in a very short time. During healing, fibroblasts migrate into the wound and start to synthesize collagen. The normal process of collagen synthesis and lysis is unbalanced, and collagen is deposited at three times the normal rate, in lumpy whorls rather than the usual elongated fibres (Berman and Flores, 1998). Some of the fibroblasts become modified to form myofibroblasts, which possess the properties of smooth muscle cells and contribute to the contraction of scar tissue. During this stage, which can last several months, the scar is termed 'immature'. It is initially quite fragile, but rapidly becomes raised, thickened and hard (Plate 7). The colour may vary from deep red to purple. Itching may be severe and prolonged. Scar contraction can be particularly aggressive and, if the scar extends across a joint, unopposed contraction can lead to the development of deformity in a very short time. It can take up to 18 months, and occasionally longer, for the scar to become mature, at which time it will appear pale, contraction will have ceased and the itching will have subsided.

Treatment

At the present time, hypertrophic scarring cannot be prevented, but its effects can be minimized. Several treatment methods are available, and the therapist must make an early assessment of the healing wounds in order to plan the programme of treatment with the patient. Controlling the growth of scar tissue in its immature phase can produce a flatter, softer, more cosmetically acceptable scar. Controlling the contraction of scar tissue can prevent the development of disabling and unsightly deformities and the need for corrective surgery.

Non-surgical methods of management available to the therapist include pressure therapy, massage, the use of silicone gel sheets and elastomers, and splinting. These will be considered in some detail, as they constitute the mainstay of treatment in Burns Units throughout the UK.

Pressure Therapy

The use of pressure in the treatment of deforming scars and contractures was documented as long ago as the late-seventeenth century. Pressure has been used in a number of forms, including elastic bandages and adhesive plaster, with varying degrees of success throughout the centuries since then (Linares et al., 1993). Universal support of pressure therapy was only gained following the pioneering work of Duane Larson and his team at the Shriners Burns Institute in America in the late 1960s (Larson et al., 1971). Further research by Kischer and others (Kischer et al., 1971; Haq and Haq, 1990) confirmed pressure therapy as a widely accepted first-line treatment for hypertrophic scarring.

Although its mode of action is not yet proven, it has been postulated that a regimen of continuous pressure of at least capillary level (25mmHg) effects a realignment of the collagen bundles and, by producing a mild hypoxia of the cells, may control the overexuberant collagen synthesis (Figure 13.1). Leung and Ng (1980) also demonstrated a reduction in the discomfort of itching when pressure garments are worn.

However, one prospective randomized trial of burns treated with and without pressure therapy found no significant difference in scar maturation time (Chang et al., 1995). Further randomized controlled trials would be needed to determine whether pressure improves either the appearance or function of the burn scar, but since pressure therapy has become such an accepted treatment for scarring, withholding it in a clinical trial may raise ethical concerns.

Pressure can be achieved simply by using cotton elastic tubing, such as Tubigrip™, but made-to-measure garments of a Lycra® material are more commonly used and may afford more evenly distributed pressure. As soon as the grafts have healed, detailed measurements are taken and a

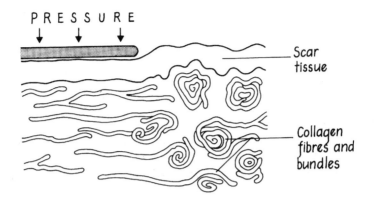

Figure 13.1 Hypertrophic scarring showing the effect of pressure.

decision as to the required style of garment is made. Although certain styles are commonly used, suppliers offer an individualized service so that particular deformities arising from contractures or amputations can be accommodated. It is sometimes helpful for the therapist to include extra measurements, drawings or photographs for an unusual request. There are several pressure garment manufacturers in the UK, and some occupational therapy departments make their own made-to-measure garments. Delivery times vary, but most patients can be fitted with their first garments within a week of measuring.

Care must be taken when the initial garments are applied, as newly healed grafts are fragile and may be easily damaged in the process of donning a garment. To avoid this problem, initial garments may be made with extra zips included, or may be manufactured with a lower pressure; some suppliers offer an 'interim' type of garment, made of a more yielding fabric. It is often best to order one set of garments for the initial fitting, as many patients request small changes, such as the positioning of zips, that can be made to subsequent garments without compromising their effectiveness. Patients should always have their first garments fitted by their therapist, to ensure accurate fit and provide an opportunity for a more detailed explanation of the need to check the condition of the skin, how to care for garments, when to remove them, etc. Written information regarding pressure therapy is usually given at the fitting appointment, to complement verbal advice. Subsequent orders can sometimes be posted directly to patients, in order to save an unnecessary hospital appointment, although arrangements for regular review and re-assessment are normally made at the time of first fitting.

In order to be of maximum benefit, pressure therapy must be applied for an average of 23 hours per day, the garments only being removed for washing, bathing and massage (Scott Ward, 1991). Since they are skin-tight, patients do not always find them easy to wear, especially during hot weather, and therapists need to be available to offer ongoing support and advice. Garments may be removed for swimming although some patients with very visible scars prefer to keep them on whilst in the water.

Scarring of the face poses particular problems to both patient and therapist in the choice of an acceptable pressure technique and material. Semi-rigid, transparent, plastic facemasks fabricated from high temperature thermoplastics are sometimes used. These can give excellent pressure, especially round the nose, where a fabric mask would not conform, but patients often find them hot and uncomfortable to wear over long periods (Rivers et al., 1979; Schons et al., 1981). Some practitioners contend that although no significant difference in pressure can be observed between the transparent and the fabric mask, the transparent mask is more socially acceptable and may be less likely to cause social withdrawal (Groce et al., 1999). Sensitivity and understanding are required in these situations, and the choice of treatment must rest with the patient. Compromise regarding wearing time may be required in the treatment of facial scarring since for some patients the treatment may cause more anxiety than the actual scars.

Inserts and conformers are sometimes used under garments to obtain pressure over areas of anatomical concavity, such as the palm of the hand, where pressure is difficult to obtain. Conformers can be made simply from high density sponge, or from low density thermoplastic splint materials or medical grade elastomers. Extra pressure may be required over areas such as web spaces, in order to prevent the development of 'web creep', where scarring forms tight bands between the digits and limits full spanning of the hand.

Pressure garments are discontinued when the scars are 'mature', normally 12 to 18 months post-burn. If no change in the scar is observed when the pressure garment is left off for 24 hours, the scar is deemed mature. At this stage it should be pale, soft and reasonably flat. Itching will normally have subsided. Occasionally scars remain active for longer periods of time, perhaps for three years or more.

Massage and Use of Emollient Creams

Sebaceous glands, which provide the sebum necessary for oiling normal skin, are destroyed in deep partial thickness and full thickness burns.

Since split skin grafts contain no sebaceous glands, the grafted skin is liable to be dry, inelastic and easily damaged. Massage with emollient creams is commonly recommended after healing, to improve the texture and comfort of the skin. It is also sometimes advocated as a way of improving the appearance of hypertrophic scarring, but empirical evidence for this is lacking. One study which compared the use of massage and pressure therapy with pressure therapy alone found no difference in the vascularity, pliability or height of scars, although some patients reported a decrease in itching (Patino et al., 1998). Creams containing vitamin E are sometimes recommended but also lack an evidence base to support their use. They can also be expensive and are not available on prescription.

In the clinical setting, patients often report that their scars feel more comfortable with regular massage, and that they obtain some temporary relief from itching. As soon as the graft is healed, patients are shown how to massage their burn scars. Initially, creams should be applied gently to prevent skin damage to the newly healed graft, but deeper massage can be started as the skin becomes stronger. The process is repeated at least three times a day during the stage of active scarring, as well as after bathing. Any non-perfumed, water based cream, such as E45, Aqueous cream or Nivea, may be used. Aromatherapy massage is being used in several Burns Units to reduce burn scar itching, although, as with other forms of massage, its effect on scar maturation is not proven. Overall, the benefits of massage may lie more in the psychological effect of therapeutic touch, with the patient benefiting from the implied acceptance of their appearance that the therapist's touch brings.

While regular showering or bathing is indicated to thoroughly cleanse grafted skin, the bathing process can be very drying, especially if the water is too hot, and the addition of a bath emollient such as BathE45 can help to prevent this.

Silicones

The use of topical silicone gels in the treatment of burn scars, originally described by Perkins and others in 1982, has become widespread as an adjunct or alternative to pressure. Research by Quinn (1987) in the UK, demonstrated a softening of hypertrophic scars with silicone gel but the mode of action was not identified. Further studies (Ahn et al., 1989, 1991) showed the gel to be efficacious in the prevention and treatment of scars, and that the effect did not appear to depend on pressure. Later research demonstrated that occlusion and hydration are the principal modes of action, rather than any particular properties relating to silicone itself (Sawada and Sone, 1990, 1992; Bieley and Berman, 1996). In fact comparable results have been achieved with a glycerin based sheeting, a less expensive alternative (Baum and Busuito, 1998).

The market for silicone products is expanding and they are now available in a number of formulations, including a liquid form, and a skin-tone self-adhesive sheeting. In the clinical situation, silicone gel is sometimes used in conjunction with pressure garments, particularly if there are areas of particularly resistant scar, but it is also useful in treating small, isolated scars, where pressure therapy would be inappropriate. It is applied directly to healed, dry skin and removed daily for skin inspection and cleansing. Early silicone products required a 'build up' time to prevent skin sensitivity, but some of the newer formulations permit immediate all-day use and possess improved adhesive properties. The glycerin-based sheeting may be used on open wounds to facilitate early intervention, although most silicone based products advise total wound closure before use.

Zinc Oxide Tape

Adhesive zinc oxide tape is sometimes used as an alternative to pressure garments or gels, in treating small hypertrophic scars. The rationale for its use is largely based on the work of Soderberg et al. (1982) who found it effective in reducing itching, redness and size. However, no control study was performed and no reports of similar studies have been published since. Clinically, some patients do report improvements in the appearance of their scars after wearing zinc oxide tape, and it is inexpensive and easy to use.

Splinting

Splints fabricated from low temperature thermoplastic materials are frequently used to prevent or correct the contractures that sometimes develop in association with hypertrophic scarring. The need to wear splints frequently continues beyond discharge from inpatient care, and splints are sometimes worn in conjunction with pressure garments for many months, as scar tissue matures.

In assessing the potential for hypertrophic scar development, the therapist must watch for restrictions of joint movement. Any burn that extends across a joint is liable to develop a deformity, commonly a flexion deformity, but certain areas are particularly at risk. These include the neck, axillary folds, elbow, knee, first web space and little finger. The scar tissue contracts insidiously, and deformities that may not have been apparent, or even anticipated, can develop surprisingly quickly when the patient is at home.

Contractures are most likely to occur in the first three months, and frequent outpatient appointments may be needed during this period in order to monitor the situation. Splinting is indicated at the earliest sign of contracture, as it is much easier to prevent a deformity than to correct an established one. At this stage, most splints are worn only at night or during periods of rest during the day. The exception to this is the conforming neck collar, which is commonly worn almost continually during the first three months, and removed only for washing, massage and exercise. A range of low-temperature thermoplastic materials is available, the therapist's choice depending on a number of factors, including conformability, strength of the material and patient preference.

Splint wearing is normally combined with a programme of exercise, and the occupational therapist will liaise closely with the physiotherapist in developing a programme of treatment that is closely tailored to individual patients' needs. Where there is an existing contracture, it is often best to fabricate the splint immediately after a session of physiotherapy, when the joint has been stretched to its maximum. Deep massage and the application of silicone gel over the contracture for thirty minutes prior to making the splint may also help to soften the skin and allow a few extra degrees of movement. At this stage, the contracture is only of the skin and underlying soft tissues and should respond well to treatment. As improvement is gained, the splint is altered (serial splinting), in order to maintain progress, and may continue to be worn even when full range of movement is achieved, since immature scar tissue is likely to re-assert its effect if unopposed.

Splints are commonly worn over pressure garments, or may be lined with silicone gel to afford a sustained softening of the tissue. Strapping is of particular importance as the straps themselves form an integral part of the splint. It is important to give patients, or their carers, clear explanations about the use of splints – their purpose, how and when to put them on, how long to wear them, and the need to check for skin damage. Since the patient will have been bombarded with information in this rehabilitative phase, it is helpful if splint instructions are written down as a ready reminder. Written instructions are never meant to replace frequent outpatient appointments however, and the patient needs to be reassured that help is available at the end of a telephone.

Medically Prescribed Treatment Methods

Scars occasionally remain resistant to pressure therapy, and the plastic surgeon may prescribe additional treatments to resolve particularly stubborn scars. Keloids respond less well to any type of treatment and if surgically excised have the tendency to recur. Additional treatments include the following:

- **Corticosteroids** have been proven to inhibit excessive collagen deposition (Cees et al., 1994). They may be applied topically as creams or adhesive tape, or by intralesional injection (sometimes multiple).
- **Surgical excision** is usually considered when the scar is mature, and if the conservative treatments described in the previous section have failed to give acceptable results. However, in some studies excision surgery alone has shown a 45–100% recurrence rate (Berman and Flores, 1998). Much depends on the surgical technique used, including the type of graft.
- **Radiotherapy** is sometimes used after excisional surgery to prevent recurrence of particularly unresponsive hypertrophic scars or keloids, but its use remains controversial for reasons of efficacy and safety (Berman and Flores, 1998).
- **Laser therapy** using the carbon dioxide, Nd:YAG and Argon lasers has been used with variable effect on hypertrophic and keloid scars. The pulsed dye laser has been shown to reduce erythema, increase pliability and reduce scar height (Berman and Flores, 1998).

Cosmetic Camouflage

Residual scarring can be the source of a great deal of emotional trauma, and a complete recovery, in terms of socializing, forming relationships and a return to employment, may not be achieved. This is particularly, but not exclusively, likely if the scars are highly visible and not normally covered by clothing. In these instances, cosmetic camouflage can be of great benefit. Often it is not started until pressure therapy is concluded, but patients should be made aware of it at an early stage so that they know they can consider its use when active treatment is no longer appropriate.

Camouflage is not simply a form of make-up; the art of choosing and applying the cover creams is taught by specially trained experts (Leveridge, 1991). Since 1975 the British Red Cross has trained volunteers in this field, and they offer a service in many hospitals, while in other Burns Units nurses, occupational therapists or physiotherapists have taken on the role. When patients have been shown how to apply the creams, they are able to obtain continuing supplies on prescription or by private purchase from several recognized suppliers. The creams are waterproof, which allows the wearer the freedom of swimming and bathing without fear of the scar becoming visible.

Unfortunately, not all scars can be completely disguised, particularly if there is altered skin texture or if the scar is raised. In these instances some improvement rather than resolution is usually possible, and further counselling may be needed if the patient remains unhappy with the final result. For some people, cosmetic camouflage is used as a temporary aid in rebuilding self-confidence, while for others it remains an essential and everyday part of their lives. Either way, it can produce remarkable results, not only visually, but also in terms of improved self-esteem.

Patient Education and Support

Prior to discharge, the patient is offered support and advice from the many members of the multidisciplinary Burns team. This situation may change after discharge from inpatient care, and it is not uncommon for the patient to feel unsure about aftercare during this period. Sensitive information giving by staff regarding the possibility of hypertrophic scar development can help to prepare patients for the rehabilitative phase of treatment. Showing 'before' and 'after' pictures, and visits from other patients wearing pressure garments can help, with therapists and nursing staff liaising closely to ensure that information is given in a consistent way and at times that are suited to the patient's needs.

Printed sheets and booklets designed to answer common questions can be a useful reference to the patient at home, together with telephone numbers for easy contact if help is required between outpatient appointments. Immediately after discharge, outpatient appointments will be frequent, perhaps daily, as the patient requires dressings, physiotherapy and occupational therapy. However, as the need for frequent attendances diminishes, new concerns may arise and there is a continuing need for information and support. After the first three to four months, apart from the plastic surgeon's outpatient clinic, it is often the pressure garment clinic that remains the patient's primary link with the Burns team. For this reason, it is the occupational therapist's role to provide continuing education and support and to act in liaison between other team members if late problems arise, for example, further skin breakdown, or the development of an unresponsive contracture.

Patients' questions regarding their burn scars are numerous; some of the commonly encountered topics are discussed below.

Itching

Itching is one of the most common and most distressing problems in the early months: it disturbs sleep and can lead to areas of skin breakdown in the grafts. A pilot study of functional outcomes in children with burn injuries found that itching was one of the prime causes of reduced function during the period of active scarring (Tyack et al., 1999). Patients need to know that itching is part of the normal healing process and will eventually resolve, but also that their general practitioner can prescribe medication to ease it.

Blisters and Spots

The formation of blisters and spots is quite common in the early months after healing and, while considered normal, can be a source of anxiety to patients. Good hygiene, careful massage and the wearing of correctly fitting pressure garments will usually prevent blister formation. The guidance for management of existing blisters is to cover with a light, non-stick dressing secured by the pressure garment, but if larger, open areas or infection develop, the advice of the general practitioner or Burns Unit staff should be sought. Small spots and blackheads frequently occur in grafted skin, and may be prevented or minimized by regular cleansing of the skin and the sparing use of cream.

Massage

Patients often ask how long regular massage is required to continue, on both donor and grafted areas. There are no hard and fast rules, but massage is generally recommended throughout the period of using pressure garments. Massage of donor sites is usually discontinued when the colour begins to fade and as long as the skin appears well hydrated.

Exposure to Heat, Cold and Sunlight

The body's ability to react to extremes of temperature is commonly affected by a burn injury, and patients frequently report that their scars feel more uncomfortable, itchy or painful during very hot or cold spells. In cold conditions, the advice is to wear extra layers of loose, warm clothing, to take particular care with extremities, and to limit time spent outdoors if at all possible. In hot weather, frequent tepid showers may be necessary in order to keep cool. Patients often express reluctance to wear pressure garments when the weather is very hot, and may need extra support to maintain motivation at these times.

It is of particular importance that patients are aware that active burn scars should be protected from exposure to sunshine, as they will be much more sensitive to the effects of the sun. In effect, this means avoiding direct sun for at least one year after the burn injury, and wearing extra protective clothing such as hats and tee-shirts. Unfortunately pressure garments alone do not protect against the sun as they are porous, but the use of a total sunblock, applied frequently, under garments should offer adequate protection. Patients often ask whether they should take foreign holidays in the first year after a burn, and much depends on whether they can tolerate higher temperatures and manage to avoid direct sun. If the area of burn scarring is extensive and actively hypertrophic, this might be quite difficult.

Swimming

Swimming is an excellent form of exercise post-burn and may be resumed as soon as all areas of skin are healed. Pressure garments may be removed or kept on while swimming, but if kept on must be rinsed well afterwards to eliminate chlorine or salt. Swimming should always be followed by thorough showering, drying and the application of cream.

Sport

Contact sports are best avoided in the first few weeks after healing, especially if grafts are in vulnerable areas such as the pretibial area. Gentler forms of exercise such as yoga or keep fit can be resumed when the skin is healed, and the stretching involved will be beneficial. For children in particular, being able to resume their usual sporting activities at school signifies a return to normality, and should be encouraged as far as possible.

Skin Colour

Patients frequently worry about the colour of their burn scars and the fact that the colour deepens when pressure garments are not worn, during bathing and when the body is cold. They need reassurance that this is quite normal and is due to changes in the blood's circulation. It can be limited by wearing the pressure garments as prescribed and where the burns are on the lower limbs, by avoiding standing still for long periods. Loss of pigment (hypopigmentation) is a different problem and may be extensive, especially in areas of partial thickness burn that were not grafted, as the melanocytes may still have been destroyed. Return of pigment is difficult to predict, but this is a concern that should not be underestimated. It can be particularly distressing for people with black skin. With time some improvement usually occurs, but if the return of pigment is incomplete cosmetic camouflage is often very effective.

Return to Work

Some patients are concerned about returning to work while their scars are still active, while others worry that they will lose their jobs if they are away for too long. For others, ongoing compensation claims complicate the situation and make planning for the future difficult. Each situation must be judged on its own merits, but the nature of some jobs, for example those that require a lot of standing or which involve working in extremes of temperature, may make them unsuitable for those who have suffered major burns. Patients may benefit from a work assessment in the occupational therapy department of a rehabilitation unit, or by being referred to the disablement employment advisor if retraining is indicated. Staff should not underestimate the importance of an early return to employment, not only for financial reasons, but also for the part it plays in restoring self-esteem.

Many factors have been identified that affect return to work after a burn injury. These include the availability of social support, size and severity of the burn, age of the patient and type of employment. One prospective study, carried out in America, found the pre-burn environment – particularly being employed at the time of injury – to be the strongest predictor of return to work after a severe burn (Wrigley et al., 1995).

Sometimes, a return to work is interrupted by the need for further surgical treatment, and patients may wish to discuss the timing of their surgery with the plastic surgeon so that work disruption is kept to a minimum.

Scar Resolution

Many patients ask what their scar will finally look like, a question that is difficult to answer in the early months. Some grafts settle so well that they eventually look like normal skin, although visual evidence of meshing may still be apparent. Other areas, commonly those that took longer to heal or became infected, do not completely lose their lumpy appearance. They resolve in that they become pale or even white, but with a texture that is obviously different from that of normal skin. Even with pressure therapy, some of the more aggressive scars do not flatten entirely. It is important to warn patients that they are likely to be left with some evidence of their injury, but the therapist must judge how much information to give at any one time.

Emotional Problems in Scar Management

Little has been mentioned so far regarding the patient's emotional response to onslaught treatments that extend far beyond the day of discharge from the Burns Unit. Jorgensen and Brophy (1975) have described three stages of psychological recovery from burns, and it is the third, recuperative, stage that mostly concerns scar management. If there is noticeable disfigurement or dysfunction, the patient may fear leaving the safety of the Burns Unit, where their condition is accepted and understood. They face the stares and questions of strangers, which may be dreaded, particularly if the injuries were self-inflicted or if the accident involved the death of another person.

The occupational therapist will be increasingly involved around the pre-discharge period, preparing the patient in practical ways, such as measuring for the first pressure garments, encouraging independence in activities of daily living and in discussion with the patient and family to emphasize the importance of regular follow-up. At this stage, the patient can be gently prepared for the possibility of scarring, and future treatments can be outlined.

Reluctance to leave the security of the Burns Unit is normal, but part of the patient's treatment prior to discharge will be to attend the occupational therapy department, perhaps for a kitchen assessment, and this may signal the first time that anyone other than the burns team and the patient's relatives have seen the burn wound. It is the first stage in a long process described by Malick and Carr (1982) as 'progressive desensitization' to the reactions of others to the patient's superficial deformity and disfigurement.

Once home, the patient is faced with the long process of rehabilitation, with its regime of exercise, splintage, massage and pressure garments. It does not help that the burn scars begin to look worse in the first few months. Withdrawal and even depression can follow, and this, in turn, leads to apathy and loss of motivation. During this stage, the patient is likely to need a great deal of support, information and encouragement. Meeting with other patients in an informal support network can be as valuable as staff support. Therapists should monitor closely the patient's levels of motivation and emotional status, offer counselling if this is within their expertise, or refer to another team member, such as the clinical psychologist. Appointments to check pressure garments may be used as informal counselling sessions, and gentle questioning can sometimes reveal hidden difficulties, such as sexual problems, persistent feeling of guilt or revulsion, sleep difficulties and alienation from other family members.

Finally, the sheer length of time of burn rehabilitation, sometimes many years, is something that depresses many patients at the outset. It is as if their lives will never return to normal. With support, advice and encouragement from the burns team, that need not be the case, and the close rapport that often develops between patients and staff is of benefit to both. Successful rehabilitation is marked by a gradual reduction of dependency on the staff as the patient gains confidence in resuming pre-burn interests and activities.

References

Ahn ST, Monafo WW, Mustoe TA (1989) Topical silicone gel: a new treatment for hyper-trophic scars. Surgery 106(4): 781–87.

Ahn ST, Monafo WW, Mustoe TA (1991) Topical silicone gel for the prevention and treat-ment of hypertrophic scar. Archives of Surgery 126(4): 499–504.

Baum TM, Busuito MJ (1998) Use of a glycerin based gel sheeting in scar management. Advances in Wound Care 11: 40–43.

Bieley HC, Berman B (1996) Effects of a water-impermeable, non-silicone-based occlusive dressing on keloids. Journal of the American Academy of Dermatology 35: 113–14.

Berman B, Flores F (1998) The treatment of hypertrophic scars and keloids. European Journal of Dermatology 8: 591–96.

Chang P, Laubenthal KN, Lewis RW et al. (1995) Prospective, randomised study of the effica-cy of pressure garment therapy in patients with burns. Journal of Burn Care and Rehabilitation 16(5): 473–75.

Cees JM, Van Den Helder MD, Hage JJ (1994) Sense and nonsense of scar creams and gels. Aesthetics of Plastic Surgery 18: 307–13.

Groce A, Meyers-Paal R, Herndon D et al. (1999) Are your thoughts of facial pressure trans-parent? Journal of Burn Care and Rehabilitation 20: 478–81.

Haq MA, Haq A (1990) Pressure therapy in treatment of hypertrophic scar, burn contractures and keloid: the Kenyan experience. East African Medical Journal 11: 785–93.

Jorgensen JA, Brophy JJ (1975) Psychiatric treatment modalities in burn patients. Current Psychiatric Therapies 15: 85–92.

Kischer CW, Linares HA, Dobrkovsky M et al. (1971) Electron microscopy of the hyper-trophic scar. In 29th Annual Proceedings of the Electron Microscopy Society of America.

Boston: Claitor's Publishing Division. p 302.

Larson DL, Abston S, Evans EB et al. (1971) Techniques for decreasing scar formation and contractures in the burned patient. Journal of Trauma 12: 807–23.

Lawrence JC (1987) The aetiology of scars. Burns 13: S3–S14.

Leung I, Ng M (1980) Pressure treatment for hypertrophic scars resulting from burns. Burns 6: 244–50.

Leveridge A (1991) Therapy for the Burn Patient. London: Chapman and Hall.

Linares HA, Larson DL, Willis-Galstaun BA (1993) Historical notes on the use of pressure in the treatment of hypertrophic scars or keloids. Burns Journal 19:17–21.

Malick MH, Carr JA (1982) Manual on Management of the Burn Patient. Pittsburg, PA: Harmaville Rehabilitation Center, Education Resource Division.

Patino O, Novick C, Merlo A (1998) Massage in hypertrophic scars. Journal of Burn Care and Rehabilitation 19: 268–71.

Perkins K, Davey RB, Wallis KA (1982) Silicone gel: a new treatment for burn scars and contractures. Burns 9: 201–4.

Quinn KJ (1987) Silicone gel in scar treatment. Burns 13: S33–S40.

Rivers E, Strate RG, Solem LD (1979) The transparent face mask. American Journal of Occupational Therapy 33: 100–13.

Sawada Y, Sone K (1990) Treatment of scars and keloids with a cream containing silicone oil. British Journal of Plastic Surgery 43: 683.

Sawada Y, Sone K (1992) Hydration and occlusion treatment for hypertrophic scars and keloids. British Journal of Plastic Surgery 45: 599.

Schons AR, Rivers E, Solem LD (1981) A rigid transplant face mask for control of scar hypertrophy. Annals of Plastic Surgery 6: 245–48.

Scott Ward R (1991) Pressure therapy for the control of hypertrophic scar formation after burn injury. A history and review. Journal of Burn Care and Rehabilitation 12(13): 257–61.

Tyack ZF, Ziviani J, Pegg S (1999) The functional outcome of children after a burn injury: a pilot study. Journal of Burn Care and Rehabilitation 16: 445–50.

Wrigley M, Trotman BK, Dimick A et al. (1995) Factors relating to work after burn injury. Journal of Burn Care and Rehabilitation 20: 367–73.

CHAPTER 14

Psychological Care following Burn Trauma

CHRISSIE BOUSFIELD

Burn injuries, a unique form of trauma, are in many respects one of the worst injuries that an individual can experience (Wachtel et al., 1983). According to the Department of Trade and Industry (1999), every 90 seconds someone in the United Kingdom receives burns or scalds as a result of an accident. Approximately 112 000 people visit Accident and Emergency departments per year and receive hospital treatment for burns and scalds, and at least a further 250 000 people visit GP surgeries. An estimated 7 765 individuals each year (21 per day) are admitted as inpatients suffering from severe burn injuries, and 211 (4 per week) die as a result.

The increasing survival rate of burns victims is the result of major advances in the critical care of burns (Feller et al., 1979; Curreri et al., 1980). However, a consequence of this reduced mortality is an increase in a new type of morbidity: the physical and psychological problems experienced by burn survivors (Ward et al., 1987).

The first detailed account of the psychological consequences experienced by victims of severe burns were described following the Cocoanut Grove fire disaster in Boston, Massachusetts (Adler, 1943). Since then, a succession of studies has been undertaken following the same theme, which have been reviewed by Malt (1980) and Tucker (1986). An unequivocal main finding in all of these studies is that burn injuries precipitate serious psychological distress. The distress may be minimal or remedial if well-timed and structured psychological care is integrated as part of burn management during the course of hospitalization. Psychological care means that expressed or anticipated needs are responded to, rather than being ignored, belittled, attacked or judged (Cresci, 1982).

232

The basic assumption of psychological care is the recognition and acceptance that all behaviour is determined by previous experience, by those factors of which the patient is aware, and by attitudes, conflicts and perceptions, of which the patient is totally unaware.

According to Cresci (1982), if consistent, appropriate psychological care on a Burns Unit is to be provided, then there are four basic requirements. First, all members of the multidisciplinary team should possess the ability to observe patient, family, and staff reactions in an objective, non-judgemental manner. Second, part of the patient's admission process should include an assessment of the family system, for example marital relationships, decision-making, previous coping mechanisms and response to injury. This will enable predictions of the patient's and family's adjustment to injury, surgery and hospitalization. The third factor is the ability of the staff to empathize. Avoiding emotional contact or becoming overly protective will demonstrate a lack of understanding by staff of patients' needs. Fourth, a working knowledge of factors predisposing to a burn injury, the psychological reactions and adaptations, the stages of recovery through which the patient and family will evolve, must be acquired. A combination of these four requirements seeks to provide members of the multidisciplinary team with a basic framework to guide the psychological care of patients following a burn injury during the course of hospitalization and beyond.

Throughout the course of this chapter, the author will focus on individuals prone to a burn injury, psychological reactions and the stages of recovery in more detail, concluding with a section on the importance of effective communication in psychological care and possible strategies and solutions for the future.

Factors Predisposing to a Burn Injury

Evidence in the literature suggests that some individuals are prone or predisposed to burn injuries (MacArthur and Moore, 1975).

A study undertaken by Noyes et al. (1979) focused on the relationship between stressful life events and burn injuries. The results indicated that over a 1-year period, 50% of adults admitted to a Burns Unit had a pre-existing history of physical and/or psychological conditions that had increased their susceptibility to the burn injury. Many of the individuals were also found to be unemployed, single and from poor socio-economic circumstances, and reported a significant increase in stressful life events in the year preceding the injury.

Steiner and Clark (1977) indicated that post-burn psychiatric conditions developed more frequently among patients who had a previous psychiatric history, and Bowden et al. (1980) pointed to a high incidence of burns among alcoholics. In 1983, Kolman also suggested that a large number of adults admitted to a Burns Unit came from disturbed family backgrounds, with unemployment, marital disharmony and poor housing conditions.

The results of these studies suggest, therefore, that in many cases burn injuries have their roots deep in the family setting, and imply that burn injuries may not always be purely incidental (Cresci, 1982). Individuals are often from dysfunctional depressed family settings, in which there may have been changes in the balance and structure of the family, such as a change in employment status, financial problems, a geographic move, divorce, remarriage, pregnancy or a physical or psychiatric illness prior to the burn injury.

Ward et al. (1987) suggested that it is more often the person rather than the injury that determines the emotional prognosis after burn trauma. It is worth bearing this fact in mind when dealing with individuals who present with poor coping strategies, inadequate psychological adjustment or major psychological dysfunctions during the course of hospitalization (Tobiasen and Hiebert, 1985; Buckhart, 1987; Roberts et al., 1987).

In comparison to adults, there is limited literature relating to the predisposing factors of a burn injury in children other than accident proneness. According to Burnside (1996) there are few published details on age, socio-economic status or prior school performance of children who have been burned. Langley et al. (1983) report a premorbid history of conduct disorders and the Child Accident Prevention Trust (1991) indicates a link between burn/scalding accidents and low economic status, poor housing, overcrowding and stress. Tarnowski et al. (1991) realistically note that as many of the child victims are toddlers they will not yet have been the subject of detailed public records.

Psychological Effects and Factors Predicting Adjustment Following a Burn Injury

There is clear evidence in the literature (Brown et al., 1985; Tucker, 1987) that problems relating to psychological adjustment in adults may be influenced by a variety of factors other than severity. Burnside (1996) suggests these factors include: the premorbid personality of the patient, the degree of disfigurement, visibility of burn scarring, employment status, effect on mobility, age and marital status of the patient, and the circumstances of the injury.

Cobb et al. (1990) and Malt and Ugland (1989) suggest the degree of psychological reaction is associated with the severity of the burn injury. Studies by Quested et al. (1988) and Wallace and Lees (1988), however, found no relationship between severity and psychological adjustment. In comparison, Brown et al. (1988) and Sheffield et al. (1988) found a link between adjustment and associated burn disability as opposed to severity of the injury. Brown et al. (1985) indicate that maladjustment is related to loss of occupational status, unemployment, avoidance in coping mechanisms and lack of involvement in recreational activities. Malt and Ugland (1989) note that the nature of the accident, prolonged hospitalization, deviant behaviour in hospital and the incidence of scarring all contributed to adjustment to the burn injury. Quested et al. (1988) indicated that the severity of the injury predicted the degree of disability but not the psychological adjustment. In addition, individuals displaying avoidance of coping strategies, poor problem solving skills, a lack of recreational activities and little social support tended to be less well adjusted.

The incidence of psychological effects in children following a burn injury is similar to those found in adults. There is no clear evidence to support the view that children with more severe burns show greater levels of disturbance (Burnside, 1996). While Chang and Herzog (1976) and Stoddard et al. (1989) reported such a relationship, six studies cited by Tarnowski et al. (1991) showed no clear links between severity and adjustment. In predicting outcome, Byrne et al. (1986) suggested maladjustment following a burn injury appears to improve over time. Age is also considered to be an important factor, with poorer outcomes in young children (Blackeney et al., 1988) and in adolescents, with boys showing more externalizing and girls more internalizing of problems (Bowden et al., 1980). There is also evidence of the negative effect of the injury to the child on the psychological functioning of the parent. Wright and Fulwiler (1974) found greater levels of emotional disturbance in the mothers than the children who had been burned.

Psychological Reactions Following a Burn Injury

For those readers who may be unfamiliar with the psychological effects of burn injuries, this section seeks to outline the psychological reactions of an adult following a severe burn injury during the course of hospitalization.

To be severely burned is both physically and emotionally a devastating experience (Noyes et al., 1971), and the individual concerned may experience extreme psychological reactions, which may compound the physical injury. It is an important part of psychological care that these reactions are understood and interpreted by members of the multidisciplinary team as part of the patient's normal defence and healing mechanisms (McGookin, 1991).

Because of the terrifying experience of the accident, the overwhelming events that follow, being rushed into hospital and the disorientation in an unfamiliar environment, it is not surprising that the patient is anxious and emotional on admission. However, it is worth noting that, at this stage, the patient may also be lucid, mentally clear and rational, even if he has sustained a major burn injury.

The physical appearance of the individual may be unpleasant, and members of the multidisciplinary team need to appreciate that relatives and other visitors who may come into contact with the patient will require considerable support and reassurance throughout.

The psychological reactions displayed by the patient are finite, temporary and often expected responses to the injury, and will resolve as the patient makes a physical recovery and becomes more independent. These reactions include withdrawal, denial, regression, anger or hostility, anxiety and depression.

Withdrawal is common in the acute phase of a burn injury, especially if it is severe or life-threatening, and the patient will show little interest in family, friends or external events.

Denial is a defence mechanism and may involve the individual denying the extent of the injury, loss of function, loss of life or injury to others. This protective defence mechanism relieves anxiety and external reality in the early stages (Blumenfield and Schoeps, 1993).

Regression is a normal adaptive mechanism, in which the individual may return to an earlier way of behaving or reacting in response to stress. According to Andreason et al. (1972b), the manifestations of regression are low tolerance to frustration, demanding infantile behaviour, hypochondriasis, poor emotional control, obstructiveness and exaggerated dependency needs, and members of the multidisciplinary team may be angered by the display of manipulative behaviour. Unsympathetic management, hostile reactions or joining in the patient's games will, however, only reinforce the behaviour. On the other hand, being overly concerned may promote regression to child-like behaviour.

Anger and hostility may continue from the time of the injury to full recovery, the basis of the anger being loss or threatened loss, and this is part of the grief response. The patient may not be aware of angry feelings and repress them, turning them inwards as depression, or he may project them or displace them onto another person.

Anxiety emerges because the individual experiences the injury as a dangerous situation that reawakens the basic fears and threats encountered during early childhood development (Blumenfield and Schoeps, 1993). Many of the feelings of anxiety come from the unconscious and relate to loss of body integrity, dependence, separation from family and friends, and loss of love and approval, or may be experienced as a punishment for previous transgressions (Blumenfield and Schoeps, 1993).

Depression is an expected response to any loss or threatened loss. Patients may verbalize sadness, are tearful, and show a poor appetite, weight loss, sleep disturbances and decreased self-esteem.

Differing personality styles can also be related to individual reactions to injury. Kahana and Bilbring (1968) described seven basic personality types in terms of psychological reactions: oral, compulsive, hysterical, masochistic, paranoid, schizoid and narcissistic. Recognizing individuals with a predominantly fixed style will allow members of the multidisciplinary team to understand patient/staff interactions that may occur during the stages of recovery.

In adults, the feelings of frustration, resentment, and guilt experienced during the period of hospitalization may produce an uncooperative and obstructive patient, leading to violent outbursts, abuse of staff and refusal of treatment. Responding with kindness and sympathy combined with firmness should be rewarded by successful management (Cason, 1981).

Adaptation and Stages of Recovery

Watkins et al. (1988) developed a seven stage method of assessing and assisting burn victims' psychological recovery. Each stage consisted of a dynamic reaction between cognitive (thinking) and affective (feeling) processes, resulting in the individual displaying adaptive behaviour, along with the most appropriate staff intervention.

Adaptive stages include survival, anxiety, pain, a search for meaning, recuperation, acceptance of loss, rehabilitation and reintegration of identity. Staff interventions include orientation, medication, validation, education, legitimization, commendation and termination.

Cresci (1982) and Price (1990) describe the course of recovery in three phases: the initial shock stage, an intermediate healing stage and rehabilitation.

The shock stage/acute phase coincides with the first 48–72 hours post-injury, when the patient is acutely ill and receiving treatment designed to support body organ function and fluid and electrolyte balance. At this stage, the patient is often disorientated or may be unconscious (Price, 1990). The effects of the burn injury, and the sensory and sleep deprivation associated with ongoing treatments, serve to prevent the patient from orientating himself to the environment (Paterson, 1987).

The individual may appear anxious, confused, frightened and frustrated, experiencing periods of agitation, hostility, denial and disorientation to time and place. Treating the underlying causes should alleviate these reactions (Cresci, 1982). Members of the multidisciplinary team should aim to provide simple information and orientation to the environment and treatment carried out, while anticipating hidden fears.

Relatives may also present acute grief reactions and guilt. Involvement in care will help to reduce helplessness, and encouraging ventilation of feelings and emotions will assist with communication and building up a therapeutic relationship.

The intermediate stage/healing phase comprises the following 2–6 weeks and coincides with intensive wound care management and the start of rehabilitation. At this stage, the patient focuses on pain and discomfort (Price, 1990) and, as time progresses, becomes more aware of the extent of the injury. Emotional outbursts, despair, hopelessness, grief and mourning over losses are evident. Relatives may feel unable to deal with these outbursts and are unsure how to respond. Members of the multidisciplinary team should seek to encourage and support relatives and friends in providing active involvement, reassurance and support.

The rehabilitation stage, which begins with the end of the initial surgical procedures and extends to discharge from hospital is the third stage. At this point, the patient re-establishes physical and psychological independence. In the short term, the individual may feel isolated or unloved, as people react to the injuries with fear, alarm or withdrawal. Discharge plans are formulated in accordance with individual patient needs and also those of family or carers. Whenever possible, social reintegration programmes should be arranged prior to discharge, to allow the opportunity and experience of meeting people outside the Burns Unit and be observed by others, to develop new skills in accepting a change in body image, and to enhance socialization skills for the future.

Noyes et al. (1971) comment that 'patients who have been exposed to the experience of a severe burn injury and recover without serious psychological sequelae' provide a 'moving testimony to the strength of the human adaptive potential'.

Understanding psychological processes in burn victims is still a relatively unexplored aspect of burn care and rehabilitation (Watkins et al., 1988). Reaction, adaptation, and the stages of recovery should be viewed as a continuous process throughout the course of hospitalization and discharge and, in some cases, for several years after the burn injury.

Effective Communication in Psychological Care

This final section focuses on the importance of effective communication in the psychological care of individuals following a burn injury. It seeks to identify the problems encountered by nursing staff on one Burns Unit, analyses them, and suggests possible strategies and solutions that could be realistically implemented in clinical practice to improve the quality of psychological care for the future.

The psychological aspects of burn patients' care are far-reaching (McGookin, 1991). The burns nurse requires a sound foundation in these matters, together with a variety of effective interpersonal and counselling skills, thus complementing the Burns Unit's multidisciplinary efforts to minimize psychological distress and facilitate the healing process. Therefore, communication is crucial for effective psychological care, because effective communication is the key to its achievement (Hyland and Donaldson, 1989).

A move towards primary nursing in one Burns Unit made nursing staff more aware of their roles and responsibilities in providing holistic care on an individual basis. Great emphasis was placed on maintaining high standards of physical care, but the psychological needs of patients were not met, for a variety of reasons: scant attention was paid by nurses when attempting to assess psychological vulnerability in patients early in the course of hospitalization; a nursing model and documentation that emphasised physical rather than psychological care was used; there were constraints within the clinical setting in terms of time priorities of care; perceived levels of good interpersonal skills were low; there was a lack of previous or adequate training in using therapeutic interventions; and patient interactions were identified as brief, ad hoc and superficial. On the basis of the problems identified, the situation was analysed further.

Evidence in the literature suggests that some individuals are more prone or predisposed to burn injuries than others (MacArthur and Moore, 1975). However, a review of the literature indicated the paucity of any appropriate assessment tools or strategies that could be used by nurses in the Burns Unit in order to highlight individuals at risk of psychological distress early in the course of hospitalization.

A review of adult admissions to the Burns Unit positively illustrated a variety of factors. Some patients appeared, more specifically than others, to have contributed to the occurrence of the burn injury, and not all the injuries appeared to be accidental. In several, a significant emotional crisis or major change in the pattern of living preceded the injury.

The nursing model and documentation in use was that of Roper et al. (1980), which is directed towards physical rather than psychological care. This appeared only to encourage a superficial level of questioning. There were no structured patient assessments, and little opportunity was given to allow patients to divulge either social or psychological concerns. The nature of the documentation also did not allow for the provision of written evidence of any nurse–patient interactions relating to the psychological care that had taken place, and of the resulting outcomes.

The clinical setting was the next target. Sathe (1983) suggests that the organizational culture might not encourage nurses to invite patients to talk about their problems or promote what Cassee (1975) called an open, two-way communication.

Reflecting on the clinical situation and the realities of managing the severely burned patient amid the typical pressures present in a busy specialist unit, the problems of lack of time, heavy workloads and perceived priority constraints were seen to influence the degree to which nurses were prepared to be facilitative in their interventions towards patients. A small number of nurses felt that psychological care was of paramount importance and that, in the long run, time thus invested was well spent. That view was neither universally held nor understood by others, and, in some cases, nurses felt that psychological care should be secondary to the more pressing needs of physical care.

In an attempt to assess the interpersonal skills of nurses within the unit, self perceptions of interpersonal skills were recorded. Using Heron's (1986) six category intervention analysis, nurses were asked to rank-order six intervention categories in terms of their perceived level of skills. The six categories are prescriptive (offering advice or making suggestions), informative (giving information or instruction), confronting (challenging the person's behaviour, attitudes or beliefs), cathartic (enabling the release of tension and strong emotions), catalytic (drawing out and encouraging further self-exploration) and supportive (validating or confirming the other person's self-worth).

The majority of nurses described themselves as being more skilled in informative, supportive and prescriptive roles and least skilled in being catalytic, cathartic and confronting. In general, these results reflect those of similar studies undertaken by Burnard and Morrison (1988) and Morrison and Burnard (1989), and supported Heron's (1975) statement that a wide range of practitioners in our society show a greater deficit in the skilful use of facilitative interventions (cathartic and catalytic) than they do in the skilful use of authoritative (prescriptive and informative) ones. According to Morrison and Burnard (1993), the reason for this may be that the facilitative approach takes time.

Catalytic, cathartic and confronting approaches involve an assessment of self that may be emotionally draining. The majority of nurses had also not received training either pre- or post-registration, in therapeutic interventions or in how to cope with the expression of personal problems and emotion. This view was reflected in studies undertaken by the Joint Board of Clinical Nursing Studies (1981), now the English National Board of Post Basic Studies, which found that, in most courses communication was not taught in any structured way. However, interpersonal skills training is an important aspect of nurse education today (Kagan, 1985; MacLeod Clark and Faulkner, 1987; Burnard, 1989).

In physically observing staff in their interactions with patients, it was possible to determine a lack of skills in maintaining effective interaction, for example, in using closed and leading questions, distancing themselves from patients, performing brief and superficial interactions, and blocking potentially difficult information as they appeared unsure how to deal with it, thereby preventing patients sharing concerns and absently ignoring patient cues. A general fear among nurses appeared to be that if they encouraged patients to disclose problems, strong emotions that they would be unable to deal with might be provoked. If effective communication is the tool of psychological care (Hyland and Donaldson, 1989), communication in the psychological care of individuals following burn trauma would be more effective by implementing the following strategies and solutions.

Owing to the paucity of any assessment tools, the first aim was to design an assessment tool in the form of a semi-structured questionnaire (Figure 14.1) that could be used by nurses in the Burns Unit as part of burn care management, as a measure to assess and predict patients who might be prone to psychological vulnerability (Bosworth and Regel, 1993). Factors influencing the design of this assessment tool were gleaned by a review of the literature, especially an article by Andreason et al. (1972a), which sought to examine the relationship of pre-morbid emotional and physical factors to the adjustment of burn patients following injury and hospitalization. The literature suggests that those patients who have adjusted poorly tended to have a greater frequency of changes or stresses in their life situation prior to the injury and implied that recent experience of major illness, accident or injury during life may be a contributing factor to adjustment during hospitalization. This information was not routinely gained from patients nor previously seen as being significant.

Questionnaire

Confidential - to be kept in the medical case notes

(To be completed by patient - with assistance from assessor)

Section I

A. Social History

1. Has anything happened recently in your life which has upset you or have there been any major changes in your life, e.g. job, house, etc?
2. What are your family circumstances?
   i.e. married/single/divorced/widowed.
3. Who is likely to visit?
4. Do you or your family have any contact with other agencies, i.e. social services, probation, etc?
5. Do you have a confidant - if yes, who is this?

B. Previous history of illness or injury

1. Have you experienced any major illness, accident or injury during your life (including childhood) YES /NO
   If yes, please give a brief description.
2. Did your life change in any way (however small) YES / NO If yes, how did you cope or adapt to the effects of this experience?
3. What additional factors (if any) do you feel would have helped you cope more efficiently?
4. During this time who did you feel gave you most help and support? i.e. family, partner, friend, other.
5. What form did this help and support take?

C. Psychiatric history

1. Have you or any member of your family ever suffered from nerves, e.g. anxiety/depression for which help was sought from your doctor?

YES/NO

If yes, please give a brief description.

2. Overview of mood.

- How are you in your mood (spirits)?
- How is your sleep pattern?
- How is your appetite at the moment?
- What is your concentration like at the moment?

D. Circumstances of burn injury

1. Could you give a brief account of how the injury occurred.

Assessor please tick

(a) Accidental

Deliberate – Self

– Others

(b) Work

Home

Leisure

Other - please comment

(c) Alone

Accompanied

2. How do you feel this accident has affected you?

3. Percentage of burn surface area?

Visible

Non-visible

Comments:

(contd)

Section II

Pain scale

1. During dressing changes and the pain you experience during this time, which category do you fit into? Tick appropriate box.

No pain	Slight discomfort	Moderate discomfort	Severe pain

2. At other times during the day which category do you fit into? Tick appropriate box.

No pain	Slight discomfort	Moderate discomfort	Severe pain

3. Is the amount of pain you are experiencing consistent, or does it fluctuate? If it fluctuates, please give a brief description.
4. Is the medication you are receiving adequately controlling your pain?

   YES / NO

Section III

Staff perspective (to be filled in after consultation and discussion with other disciplines)

1. How does the patient interact with staff and other patients?
2. How does the patient interact with relatives / friends?
3. Who visits, when and how often?
4. Other comments / relevant information.

Figure 14.1 The Psychological and Psychiatric Morbidity Questionnaire (Bosworth and Regel, 1993).

The questionnaire is wide ranging and open ended, in order that, during its use, nurses may follow up a question with probes or prompts to encourage patients to go into more depth with their answers.

Given the sensitivity of the information, reliability is of utmost importance. Patients often give answers that they think the nurses want to hear, or do not disclose information they feel may put them in an unfavourable light. Consideration should also be given as to whether other measures or assessment tools of a general nature, for example the Beck Depression Inventory (Beck et al., 1979) or the Hospital Anxiety and Depression Scale (Zigmond and Snaith, 1983) might be used in conjunction.

The second aim is to use the assessment tool as part of an assessment process for each adult patient, to elicit specific information not routinely gleaned from the previous documentation. This could highlight pre-existing physical or psychiatric conditions that might have increased the patient's susceptibility to the injury, making them more prone to complications that might affect the eventual outcome (Noyes et al., 1979). It may also be used to aid predictions of how the patient and family will adjust to injury, hospitalization and surgery. Another possible solution is to consider an alternative to the Roper nursing model that would focus on psychological care, for example that of Roy (1984).

Within the time constraints on the Burns Unit, and using the questionnaire as part of the assessment process, another solution would be to plan a series of structured interviews on each adult patient, undertaken by the patient's primary or associate nurse and lasting for approximately 30 minutes, once or (as the patient's condition dictates) twice a week from admission to discharge. Individualized care, and in particular primary nursing, leads to a better relationship between the nurse and the patient, as the patient is able to get to know and trust one nurse, who is therefore in a better position to provide psychological care (Hyland and Donaldson, 1989).

Providing psychological care means focusing on patients as people. Some nurses have a natural ability – they automatically listen, observe, empathize and communicate well – but most health care professionals need to develop these skills (Faulkner, 1992). In order to undertake the patient interviews, a series of training sessions would be required to outline the process and train staff in the appropriate skills required.

Preparation for the patient interviews is important, as ensuring privacy and maintaining a safe environment assists patients in disclosing problems and concerns, which would not otherwise be possible (Faulkner, 1992). Nursing staff need to be assertive about their need for time and privacy with the patient and avoid interruptions that may break the flow of the interview. The structure of the Burns Unit often allows the provision of single rooms, where confidential interviews may be carried out. The staff through training need to develop the verbal skills required for an effective interview as research suggests that most nurses do not exhibit the required skills (Faulkner, 1980; MacLeod Clark, 1982). What is encouraging is that, in experimental studies, nurses improved their skills dramatically after brief training (Maguire, 1982; Faulkner and Maguire, 1984).

These relevant skills include employing an appropriate questioning style, for example, open, closed or leading. An open question is one that does not restrict the respondent in any way and also allows expression of feelings. Closed questions give the patient a forced choice of answer but may be useful when facts are required. Leading questions are those which imply the preferred answer and, as such, are inappropriate in effective interactions (Faulkner, 1992). Other skills include encouraging precision and clarification, picking up cues, and at all times using a negotiating style that facilitates disclosure of current concerns. The nurse also needs to learn appropriate skilled opening and closing strategies, while maintaining effective control throughout the interview.

In the same way that verbal skills need to be developed to improve interaction between the nurse and the patient, the importance of non-verbal interaction has been well documented (Argyle, 1988). These skills include listening, the active use of silence, touch, the significance of gestures, eye contact and posture.

If the patient's problems are to be identified in a skilled way during an interaction, the encounter must be given structure and focus, together with a willingness on the part of the nurse to explore the patient's feelings, sometimes at a deep level, and to examine these without doing the patient any harm. On the part of the nurse, the need to negotiate, to assign some priority to assessing the patient's cues and to control diversions so that the focus is maintained until each sequence is closed, is required (Faulkner, 1992).

Helping patients to explore their feelings may help them to come to terms with these, but in doing so a number of emotions may be elicited that would normally be suppressed or contained. Nurses may require further training on the appropriate interventions. Talking does not solve problems, but interactions can be therapeutic.

It is intended that the interviews will highlight areas of psychological vulnerability and coping responses, and promote acceptance of injuries, improved understanding and more active involvement by the patient in treatment, pain relief and realistic preparation for the difficulties that may be encountered after discharge from hospital. Many emotional responses including anger, guilt, denial, fear, anxiety and sometimes depression and suicidal thoughts, may be encountered during the interviews. The nurse needs to build up a good therapeutic relationship with the patient in order to allow him to ventilate his feelings and to offer interventions.

Once the interview is complete, the information elicited should be recorded by the patient's primary or associate nurse on the appropriate documentation and stored in the patient's case notes, thereafter being reviewed by the supervising clinician at regular intervals and being updated after each interview.

Finally, in order to improve the low perceived levels of interpersonal skills highlighted in the early stages of treatment, a further training programme, together with active supervision and support for staff, could be set up. It is envisaged that training would include the following theoretical and practical elements: basic information gathering, counselling skills, establishing a therapeutic relationship, relationship enhancement methods and role play (and related experiential techniques). Because of the potential problem of developing facilitative skills, some nurses may find they become overinvolved in patients' problems, taking them home or feeling under stress because they, personally, cannot help. The provision of ongoing supervision and support is therefore essential.

Supervision is an important part of the learning process for anyone involved in counselling. The Burns Unit has access to a psychiatrist and an identified psychologist and psychotherapist, so one could be co-opted to the role of supervisor. Effective supervision provides support, monitoring of standards and personal opportunity to develop skills. People who work with other people's problems need care and support themselves. Supervision provides that support and helps to develop a more professional role, which increases the potential of using knowledge in practice. These ideas are reflected in the studies by Worthington and Roehike (1971), Urbano (1984) and Dryden and Thorne (1991).

The provision of regular staff support groups on the Burns Unit facilitated by a psychologist or psychotherapist should also be considered. The purpose of these would be to provide a forum for discussion, for raising controversial issues and to help staff express and clarify their feelings with attitudes towards work, each other, themselves, the patients and the patients' families. They could also be used to help staff develop new skills in communication.

Conclusion

The growing recognition of the importance of the burn patient's psychological needs means that all members of the multidisciplinary team must acquire a greater understanding of the processes involved in communicating with patients. Such an understanding may, in turn, facilitate an improvement in communication and provide holistic patient care.

Providing psychological care is an art, and the art of psychological care may be developed through experience (Hyland and Donaldson,

1989). If nurses emphasize psychological care in their management of burn care, they will develop their own psychological skills, skills that can be used in other situations and which involve the ability to understand people, to form warm caring relationships, and to help others achieve their goals.

Anyone who treats burn injuries has a professional and moral responsibility to investigate their cause. It is clear that there are no easy solutions to adjustment to a burn injury, but the patient's courage and confidence in his own abilities, and a well planned, comprehensive approach by staff using effective communication skills to meet the patient's psychological needs, can soften the impact of the injury and assist in developing trust and security between the patient, his relatives and staff on the Burns Unit.

References

Adler A (1943) Neuropsychiatric complications in victims of the Boston Cocoanut Grove disaster. Journal of the American Medical Association 123(17): 1098–1101.

Andreason NJC, Noyes R, Hartford CE (1972a) Factors influencing adjustment of burns victims during hospitalization. American Journal of Psychosomatic Medicine 34(6): 517–20.

Andreason NJC, Noyes R, Hartford CE (1972b) Management of emotional reactions in seriously burned adults. New England Journal of Medicine 286: 65–69.

Argyle M (1988) Bodily Communication. 2nd edn. London: Methuen.

Beck AT, Rush AJ, Shaw BF et al. (1979) Cognitive Therapy of Depression. A Treatment Manual. New York: Guildford Press.

Blackeney P, Herndon D, Desai M et al. (1988) Long term psychosocial adjustment following burn injury. Journal of Burn Care and Rehabilitation 61: 661–65.

Blumenfield M, Schoeps MM (1993) Psychological reactions to burns and trauma. In Blumenfield M, Schoeps MM (Eds) Psychological Care of the Burn and Trauma Patient. Boston: Williams and Wilkins. pp 94–121.

Bosworth C, Regel S (1993) The Psychological and Psychiatric Morbidity Questionnaire (PPMQ). A measure to assess and predict psychological and psychiatric morbidity in individuals following burn trauma. Journal of Clinical Nursing 2: 373–79.

Bowden ML, Feller I, Tholen D et al. (1980) Self esteem of severely burned patients. Archives of Physical Medicine and Rehabilitation 61: 449–52.

Brown G, Byrne B, Brown B (1985) Psychosocial adjustment of burn survivors. Burns Journal 12: 28–35.

Brown B, Roberts J, Brown G et al. (1988) Gender differences in variables associated with psychosocial adjustment to a burn injury. Research in Nursing and Health 11: 23–30.

Buckhart CS (1987) Coping strategies of the chronically ill. Journal of Nursing Clinics of North America 22: 543–50.

Burnard P (1989) Teaching Interpersonal Skills: a Handbook of Experiential Learning for Health Professionals. London: Chapman and Hall.

Burnard P, Morrison P (1988) Nurses' perceptions of their interpersonal skills: a descriptive study using six category intervention analysis. Nurse Education Today 8: 266–72.

Burnside I (1996) Psychological aspects of burn injuries. In Principles and Practices of Burns Management. Edinburgh: Churchill Livingstone. pp 443–51.

Byrne C, Love B, Browne G et al. (1986) The social competence of children following burn injury: a study of resilience. Journal of Burn Care 7: 247–52.

Cason JS (1981) Psychological and psychiatric problems. In Cason JS, (Ed) Treatment of Burns. London: Chapman and Hall. pp 266–72.

Cassee ET (1975) Cited in Cox C, Mead A (Eds) A Sociology of Medical Practice, Therapeutic Behaviour, Hospital Culture and Communication. London: Collier Macmillan.

Chang FC, Herzog B ((1976) Burns morbidity: a follow up study of physical and psychological disability. Annals of Surgery 183: 34–37.

Child Accident Prevention Trust (1991) Burns and Scalds. Milton Keynes: CAPT.

Cobb N, Maxwell G, Silverstein P (1990) Patient perception of quality of life after burn injury: results of an eleven years survey. Journal of Burn Care and Rehabilitation 11: 330–33.

Cresci JV (1982) Emotional care of the hospitalised thermally injured. Cited in Hummel R (1982) Clinical Burn Therapy. Bristol: John Wright. pp 475–507.

Curreri PW, Braun DW, Shires GT (1980) Burn injury: analysis of survival and hospitalisation time for 937 patients. Annals of Surgery 192: 472.

Department of Trade and Industry (1999) Government Consumer Safety Research – Burns and Scalds Accidents in the Home. London: DTI.

Dryden W, Thorne B (1991) Training and Supervision for Counselling in Action. London: Sage.

Faulkner A (1980) The student nurse's role in giving information to parents. Unpublished MLitt thesis, University of Aberdeen. Cited in Faulkner A (1992) Effective Interaction with Patients. London: Churchill Livingstone: Edinburgh. pp 1–8.

Faulkner A (1992) Effective Interaction with Patients. London: Churchill Livingstone: Edinburgh. pp 1–8.

Faulkner A, Maguire P (1984) Teaching Assessment Skills. Cited in Faulkner A (Ed) (1984) Recent Advances in Nursing Communication. Edinburgh: Churchill Livingstone. pp 61–67.

Feller I, Crane K, Flanders S (1979) Baseline data on the mortality of burn patients. Quality Review Bulletin 7(4): 4.

Heron J (1975) Six Category Intervention Analysis. Human Potential Research Project. Guildford: University of Surrey.

Heron J (1986) Six Category Intervention Analysis. 2nd edn. Human Potential Research Project. Guildford: University of Surrey.

Hyland ME, Donaldson ML (1989) Psychological Care in Nursing Practice. London: Scutari Press. p 2.

Joint Board of Clinical Nursing Studies (1981) General Nursing Council for England and Wales: A Report. London: General Nursing Council.

Kagan C (1985) Interpersonal Skills in Nursing Research and Applications. London: Croom Helm.

Kahana RJ, Bilbring GL (1968) Lectures in Medical Psychology. New York: International Universities Press. p 246.

Kolman P (1983) The incidence of psychopathology in burned adult patients – a critical review. Journal of Burn Care and Rehabilitation 416: 430–36.

Langley J, McGee R, Silva P et al. (1983) Child behaviour and accidents. Journal of Paediatric Psychology 8: 181–89.

MacArthur J, Moore F (1975) Epidemiology of burns: the burn prone patient. Journal of the American Medical Association 231: 259–63.

McGookin C (1991) Psychological problems of the burned adult. Cited in Leveridge A (1991) Therapy for the Burn Injured Patient. London: Chapman and Hall. pp 69–85.

MacLeod Clark J (1982) Nurse–patient verbal interaction. Unpublished PhD thesis, University of London. Cited in Faulkner A (1992) Effective Interaction with Patients. London: Churchill Livingstone: Edinburgh. pp 1–8.

MacLeod Clark J, Faulkner A (1987) Cited in Davis B (Ed) Teaching in Nurse Education. Nurse Education Research and Developments Communication Skills. London: Croom Helm.

Maguire P (1982) Doctor–Patient Skills in Social Skills and Health. London: Methuen.

Malt U (1980) Long term psychological follow-up studies by burned adults: a review of the literature. Burns Journal 6: 190–97.

Malt U, Ugland OM (1989) A long term follow up study of burned adults. Acta Psychiatrica Scandinavica Supplement 80: 94–102.

Morrison P, Burnard P (1989) Students and trained nurses' perceptions of their own interpersonal skills: a report and comparison. Journal of Advanced Nursing 14: 321–29.

Morrison P, Burnard P (1993) Caring and Communication. 3rd edn. London: Macmillan.

Noyes R, Andreason NJC, Hartford CE (1971) The psychological reaction to severe burns. American Journal of Psychosomatic Medicine 11: 416–22.

Noyes R, Frye SJ, Slymen DI et al. (1979) Stressful life events and burn injuries. Journal of Trauma 19(3): 141–44.

Paterson R (1987) Psychological management of the burn patient. Topics in Acute Care and Trauma Rehabilitation 1(3): 25–39.

Price B (1990) The burn patient. In Price B (Ed) Body Image Concepts and Care. Hertfordshire: Prentice Hall. pp 183–99.

Quested KA, Patterson DR, Boltwood MD (1988) Relating mental health and physical function to rehabilitation status at three months post burn. Journal of Burn Care and Rehabilitation 9: 87–89.

Roberts JG, Browne G, Steiner D et al. (1987) Analysis of coping responses and adjustment: stability of conclusions. Nursing Research 36(2): 94–97.

Roper N, Logan W, Tierney AJ (1980) Nursing and the activities of living. In Roper N, (Ed) The Elements of Nursing. Edinburgh: Churchill Livingstone. pp 73–280.

Roy C (1984) Introduction to nursing – an adaptation model. Cited in Aggleton P, Chambers H (1992) Nursing Models and the Nursing Process. London: Macmillan. pp 83–99.

Sathe V (1983) Implications of corporate culture – a manager's guide to action. Organisational Dynamics 12: 5–23.

Sheffield CG, Irons GB, Mucha P et al. (1988) Physical and psychological outcome after burns. Journal of Burn Care and Rehabilitation 9: 172–77.

Steiner H, Clark WR (1977) Psychiatric complications of burned adults – a classification. Journal of Trauma 17: 134–43.

Stoddard F, Norman D, Murphy M (1989) A diagnostic outcome study of children and adolescents with severe burns. Journal of Trauma 29: 471–77.

Tarnowski KJ, Rasnake LK, Gavaghan-Jones MP et al. (1991) Psychosocial sequelae of paediatric burn injuries: a review. Clinical Psychology Review 11: 371–98.

Tobiasen JM, Hiebert JM (1985) Burns and adjustment to injury. Do psychological coping strategies help? Journal of Trauma 25: 1151–55.

Tucker P (1986) The burn victim – a review of psychosocial issues. Australian and New Zealand Journal of Psychiatry 20: 413–20.

Tucker P (1987) Psychosocial problems among adult burn victims. Burns Journal 13: 7–14.

Urbano JM (1984) Supervision of counsellors, ingredients for effectiveness. Counselling 50: 7–16.

Wachtel TL, Kahn V, Frank HA (1983) Rehabilitation of the burn injured patient. Current Topics in Burn Care. Rockville, MD: Aspen Systems Corporation. pp 217–20.

Wallace LM, Lees J (1988) A psychological follow up study of adult patients discharged from a British Burns Unit. Burns Journal 14: 39–45.

Ward HW, Moss RL, Darko DF et al. (1987) Prevalence of post burn depression following burn injury. Journal of Burn Care and Rehabilitation 8(4): 294–97.

Watkins PN, Cook EL, May SR et al. (1988) Psychological stages in adaptation following a burn injury: a method for facilitating psychological recovery of burn victims. Journal of Burn Care and Rehabilitation 9(4): 376–84.

Worthington EL, Roehike HJ (1971) Effective supervision as perceived by beginning counsellors in training. Journal of Counselling Psychology 26: 64–73.

Wright L, Fulwiler R (1974) Long range emotional sequelae of burns: effects of children and their mothers. Paediatric Research 8: 931–34.

Zigmond AS, Snaith RP (1983) The hospital anxiety and depression scale. Acta Psychiatrica Scandinavica 67: 361–70.

CHAPTER 15

Burn Trauma and Post-Traumatic Stress Disorder

STEPHEN REGEL

> I did within these six days see smoke still remaining of the late fire in the City; and
> it is strange to think how this very day I cannot sleep at night without great
> terrors of fire, and this very night could not sleep until almost 2 in the morning
> through thoughts of fire.

So recorded Samuel Pepys in his diary on 18 February 1667, six months
after the Great Fire of London in 1666 (Latham and Matthews,
1970–83). Pepys' account is perhaps one of the earliest thoroughly documented descriptions of a major disaster and its aftermath. His accounts of
the fire and its psychological sequelae provide a detailed and fascinating
account of his own and others' reactions to the effects of the fire. There is
also ample evidence to suggest from his accounts that he experienced
symptoms of Post-Traumatic Stress Disorder (PTSD) (Daly, 1983).
Despite this, and many other earlier accounts (Trimble, 1985), the
concept of PTSD was not officially recognized as a serious mental health
problem until 1980, when it was included in the psychiatric diagnostic
handbooks (American Psychiatric Association, 1980).

The diagnostic criteria were revised in 1987 and underwent a further
revision in 1994 (APA, 1994). The current edition of the *Diagnostic and
Statistical Manual of Mental Disorders* (DSM-IV) states that in order to meet
the diagnostic criteria for PTSD, the requirements are:

> The development of characteristic symptoms following exposure to an extreme
> traumatic stressor involving direct personal experience of an event that involves
> actual or threatened death or physical injury, or other threat to one's physical
> integrity; or witnessing an event that involves death, injury or a threat to the
> physical integrity of another person; or learning about unexpected or violent
> death, serious harm, or threat of death or injury experienced by a family member
> or other close associate.

In addition, the person has been exposed to a traumatic event in which both the following were present – Criterion A: (1) the person experienced, witnessed, or was confronted with an event or events that involved actual or threatened death or serious injury, or a threat to the physical integrity of others and (2) the person's response involved intense fear, helplessness, or horror. Furthermore, three distinct groups of symptoms are known to arise following a traumatic event:

Criterion B: Re-experiencing intrusive phenomena
Criterion C: Avoidance and numbing
Criterion D: Hyperarousal symptoms

In order to fulfil the diagnostic criteria of PTSD, the individual must experience at least one (or more) symptoms from B, at least three (or more) from C and at least two (or more) from D (see Figure 15.1). The implications for individuals suffering from burn trauma are twofold:

- The size or extent of the injury will not necessarily be an indication of whether the individual will develop symptoms of PTSD.
- There is an indication that the development of PTSD is often related to the way an individual interprets and makes sense of his experience, rather than to the experience per se.

The Epidemiological Evidence – a Brief Review

While there are numerous references in the psychiatric and psychological literature to what we now know to be PTSD, it was research in the USA with Vietnam War veterans which highlighted the syndrome and supplied much of the data on which the earlier diagnostic criteria were based (Blanchard et al., 1982).

Since then, there has been considerable research into PTSD with rape victims (Burgess and Holmstrom, 1974; Foa et al., 1992; Rothbaum et al., 1992) and victims of disaster, most notably in the UK with the Bradford City Football Club fire (Duckworth and Charlesworth, 1988), the sinking of the *Herald of Free Enterprise* (Hodgkinson, 1990) and the King's Cross underground station fire (Sturgeon et al., 1991). In the USA, one of the worst fire disasters occurred in 1942 at Boston's Cocoanut Grove nightclub, where a celebration turned to tragedy when a reveller accidentally set fire to an artificial palm tree. The fire, which spread suddenly, resulted in the deaths of almost 500 people. This disaster provided researchers

B. Re-experiencing symptoms (need 1)
1. Recurrent, intrusive, distressing recollections of the event, e.g. images, thoughts or perceptions
2. Recurrent distressing dreams of the event
3. Acting or feeling as if the traumatic event were recurring (flashbacks)
4. Intense psychological distress at exposure to internal or external cues
5. Reactive psychological arousal to internal or external cues that symbolise or resemble an aspect of the trauma

C. Avoidance and numbing (need 3)
1. Avoidance of thoughts, feelings or conversations associated with the trauma
2. Avoidance of activities and situations
3. Inability to recall an important aspect of the trauma
4. Diminished interest and participation in significant activities
5. Feelings of detachment and estrangement from others
6. Restricted range of affect (e.g. unable to have loving feelings)
7. Sense of foreshortened future

D. Heightened arousal (need 2)
1. Sleep disturbance
2. Irritability and anger
3. Concentration difficulties
4. Hypervigilance
5. Exaggerated startle response

Figure 15.1 PTSD DSM-IV Criteria.

with a valuable insight into both bereavement processes and reactions (Lindemann, 1944). There was also evidence to suggest that many survivors suffered from post-traumatic stress, exhibiting symptoms such as flashbacks, panic attacks, extreme tension, breathlessness and an inability to concentrate (Cobb and Lindemann, 1943). Another major fire disaster, again in the USA, which has been extensively studied for the effects of post-traumatic stress, was the Beverly Hills Supper Club fire of 1977, which resulted in 165 people losing their lives (Green et al., 1983).

Epidemiological evidence suggests that PTSD can constitute a major health problem. There are few studies that have attempted to estimate the extent of PTSD after traumatic incidents in the general population. Such studies have put the rate at between 1 and 3% of the population (Helzer et al., 1987; Davidson et al., 1991). These studies, however, have been conducted in the USA, and at present there are no figures for the UK. In disasters, estimates of PTSD tend to be much higher, for example between 22 and 50% (Raphael, 1986; Curran et al., 1990). One of the most recent epidemiological surveys (The National Comorbidity Survey), designed to study the distribution, correlates and consequences of psychiatric disorders in the United States, estimated lifetime prevalence of PTSD at 7.8%. Survival analysis showed that more than one third of people with an index episode of PTSD fail to recover even after many years (Kessler et al., 1995).

Burn Trauma and PTSD

Within the last decade, there has been an emerging interest in the multifaceted nature of post-traumatic psychopathology (Roca et al., 1992; Sturgeon et al., 1991; Taal and Faber, 1997) and PTSD following burn injury (Perry et al., 1992; Bryant, 1996). Almost all the published research attempting to assess PTSD following burn trauma, with few exceptions (Taal and Faber, 1997; Ehde, Patterson et al., 1999) have used the DSM-IIIR diagnostic criteria (APA, 1987). Whilst the above studies have indicated that post-traumatic psychopathology is not uncommon in burn survivors, long-term prospective outcome studies which aim to assess the prevalence of PTSD, using standardized measures and clinical interviews, based on the current DSM-IV diagnostic criteria for PTSD are lacking. In addition, many of the studies are retrospective with an absence of standardized assessment of psychopathology and PTSD post trauma.

The current diagnostic criteria for PTSD also include the diagnosis of acute stress disorder (ASD), comprised of dissociative intrusive, avoidant and arousal symptoms. The diagnosis can be made as early as three days following the traumatic event. Given that there is some evidence that a diagnosis of ASD within one month post trauma is predictive of PTSD at six months (Harvey and Bryant, 2000), this has important clinical implications for the early identification and intervention for those at risk of chronic PTSD. It also suggests that in some cases acute PTSD may not be a 'normal' response to trauma. In addition, few studies have examined the impact of psychological interventions. Those that exist have to be viewed with some caution (Bisson et al., 1997). There have nevertheless, been a few detailed descriptions of treatment in PTSD of burn survivors (Sturgeon et al., 1991; Regel, 1997).

It would be hardly surprising if burn injury, which is a painful, frightening and extraordinary traumatic event, precipitated post-traumatic symptoms in some burns survivors. Andreason and Norris (1972) described transient 'phobic' and 'traumatic' neuroses in many burns survivors in a study that predates DSM-III by at least 8 years. Attempts to predict the development of PTSD in burn trauma have, by and large, been inconclusive. White (1981) found that over one-third of 86 patients admitted for 7 days or more to a Burns Unit, who were followed up one year after their accident, had marked psychological sequelae. While this study indicated that premorbid vulnerability, i.e. previous history of psychological disorder, could be an important predictor of PTSD, the overwhelming majority of victims who developed post-traumatic stress did not have a past psychiatric history. Other factors found to be important were age, social class and whether patients lived on their own or with a large family. There is also no clear relationship between area of injury and the frequency and severity of psychological side-effects. Perry et al. (1992) acknowledged limitations in their study of predictors of PTSD after burn injury because of the absence of standardized assessment of psychopathology prior to the trauma. However, despite this shortcoming, high rates of PTSD were found in their sample, even at a 1-year follow-up.

Notable exceptions to the paucity of literature on burn trauma and PTSD are two papers by Courtemanche and Robinow (1989) and Sturgeon et al. (1991), which concentrate on specific case examples and treatment strategies used. Sturgeon et al. (1991) provide a comprehensive and graphic account of the psychological sequelae and treatment of some of the most severely physically damaged survivors of the King's Cross fire in 1987. Many were troubled by nightmares (invariably involving flames); all described a heightened sense of vigilance in everyday situations, for example crossing the road. They also experienced an intense sense of the frailty of human life and an expectation of further disasters. Many reported flashbacks, disturbed sleep, avoidance of common activities and emotional difficulties on the anniversary of the disaster, all symptoms characteristic of PTSD. The lesson to be learned here is, as Sturgeon et al. (1991) conclude, 'that early psychological contact is vital for the emotional and physical well being of the patient in the early stages of recovery'.

The development of PTSD in children post-burn has been studied, but again the literature is sparse. Stoddard et al. (1989) found that when compared with other clinical samples of children, the burn sample had especially high levels of psychiatric disturbance, including PTSD. Some believe that the burn treatment itself becomes a traumatic event and that, for some children, the longer hospitalization is extended, with its daily cycle of dressing changes and physiotherapy, the more regressed and withdrawn they become (Sieck, 1990).

While the presence of PTSD does not, in many cases, seem to correlate with the size of the burn, nurses working in this area of critical care should be aware of PTSD as a common and treatable cause of psychological disturbance in the burn patient, especially as the burn injury is often more than an adequate stressor.

Assessment and Treatment of PTSD

Assessment of a patient suffering from PTSD can be conducted in a number of ways, but the prime function of the assessment process is to gather enough information to arrive at a decision on what would be the most appropriate form of intervention or treatment. It is quite usual for many people, post trauma, to experience a number of psychological difficulties, and burn trauma is no exception. It would be erroneous to assume, however, that every burn trauma patient will suffer psychological distress. The prime function of the assessment process is to gather enough information in order to arrive at a decision as to the most appropriate form of clinical intervention. Knowledge and awareness of the course of recovery, signs and symptoms of post-traumatic psychopathology, ASD and PTSD are crucial in identifying the early beginnings of long-term chronic distress. Therefore, a knowledge and awareness of the symptomology of PTSD would enable nurses and other professionals to be vigilant for symptoms that persist for at least one month post-burn.

Conducting a full assessment may often be beyond the skill and time constraints of many nurses in busy Burns Units, but a recognition that there may be problems and a referral for specialist assessment would be an appropriate course of action. The identification of the symptoms indicative of PTSD can, however, be picked up at primary nurse/keyworker level by:

- A knowledge and awareness of the diagnostic criteria for PTSD
- A good relationship and rapport with the patient
- Possession of basic interviewing or counselling skills

Once this has been done, a decision can then be made on whether a referral for specialist assessment and treatment is indicated, or whether the patient would benefit more from some support at ward level. If there is a doubt, a consultation with a psychiatrist, nurse specialist in liaison psychiatry or clinical psychologist would help to clarify the situation and indicate further intervention, if necessary.

Formal assessment can be carried out using structured clinical interviews, for example the Clinician Administered PTSD Scale DSM-IV (CAPS: Blake et al., 1992). The CAPS is a diagnostic tool and is more appropriate as a research instrument, but it is nevertheless well validated and was developed to measure cardinal and hypothesized signs and symptoms of PTSD. It also provides a method to evaluate the frequency and intensity of individual symptoms as well as the impact of the symptoms on social and occupational functioning, the overall intensity of the symptoms and the validity of the ratings obtained. It uses a time frame of one month, in keeping with the diagnostic criteria for the presence of PTSD symptoms.

The aforementioned assessment tool is often more in use for research purposes, and therefore a more likely and equally effective framework of assessment would be a three-systems analysis, which takes the view that anxiety (a significant component of PTSD) is not a unitary concept but is made up of three components:

- *Autonomic* – the physiological manifestations of anxiety
- *Behavioural* – the effects of anxiety on the individual's behaviour
- *Cognitive* – the thoughts an individual experiences when anxious

PTSD is often complex in its presentation and also rarely found on its own. It has been suggested that a major focus for ongoing trauma research should be on the evaluation of prevention and treatment methods. In addition, it has been postulated that inadequate assessment prior to intervention often leads to poor outcomes (Alexander, 1996). There is a need to identify:

- trauma-specific normal and pathological reactions in the absence of pre-existent psychopathology;
- pre-existent psychopathology which has been triggered by the burn trauma;
- co-morbidity – the presence of another major psychiatric disorder, e.g. depression, anxiety, substance abuse, in response to the trauma (Alexander, personal correspondence).

Therefore a multi-modal approach to assessment is advocated and needs to include these four main areas:

- A structured interview
- A formal mental state examination
- 3-systems cognitive behavioural assessment (the patient's cognitive, behavioural and physiological responses to the trauma)
- The use of appropriate psychometric tests

The use of psychometric questionnaires and rating scales is a useful adjunct to the assessment process. However, they must be interpreted and integrated into the patient's self-report of symptomology. While there are many such measures in use to assess the wide range of post-traumatic reactions, the most reliable and well validated instruments for use with this population are described in Figure 15.2. Rating scales are also useful for providing a guide to the individual's progress and highlighting specific areas that may need closer attention.

Each individual will experience different levels of intensity and severity of each of the three systems, and careful assessment can therefore provide valuable information on where to target an intervention as far as PTSD is concerned. Of course, anxiety is not the only presentation; PTSD is often seen in conjunction with other disorders, most commonly depression and substance abuse. Therefore, a wide-ranging assessment focusing down to examine the specific components of PTSD is indicated (for a useful guide see Scott and Stradling, 1992: 10–13).

If a patient is thought to be suffering from PTSD and this is confirmed by formal assessment, the next step is to choose the most appropriate intervention. Almost all treatment for PTSD is psychologically orientated and is aimed at dealing with the range of emotional and behavioural problems outlined earlier. There is evidence that supportive counselling is only of general, rather than specific, use in PTSD sufferers (Duckworth and Charlesworth, 1988), and that the manifestation of PTSD as a specific disorder requires specialized treatment.

Cognitive Behavioural Therapies for Burn Trauma

Cognitive behavioural therapies (CBT) have, over the past few years, been used successfully in the treatment of PTSD (Frank et al., 1988; Richards and Rose, 1991; Foa et al., 1992; Richards et al., 1994). For example, Blake and Sonnenberg (1998) recently reviewed 29 studies on CBT for PTSD and found compelling evidence that PTSD symptoms can be ameliorated using cognitive behavioural therapies. The two most common therapeutic strategies are:

- Those that help the survivors to 'emotionally process' the memories of the trauma and overcome their avoidances.
- Those that teach survivors additional coping skills and anxiety management techniques.

The Hospital Anxiety and Depression Scale (HADS): Zigmond and Snaith (1983)
This is a brief 14-item self-report questionnaire used for detecting states of depression and anxiety. A cut-off score of 11 in each subscale indicates a 'definite' case of anxiety or depression. In an inpatient setting, this would be more sensitive then the GHQ-28.

General Health Questionnaire - GHQ-28: Goldberg (1981)
This is a self-rating scale for screening for psychiatric morbidity in the general population. The threshold/cut-off point for identifying 'psychiatric caseness', i.e. the likelihood that the individual could be classified as a psychiatric case, is 7. However, if used with a physically injured population it would be more appropriate to raise the threshold/cut-off point to 13 or above. A note of caution is advised with the GHQ-28. If given in the early stages post injury it is often inevitable that the patient will score a false positive as the questionnaire asks about the individual's general health and well-being 'over the past few weeks', and therefore it is highly likely they will return a high score.

Impact of Events Scale (IES): Horowitz (1979)
This self-rating scale is also widely used in research and clinical practice and measures the degree of psychological distress caused by exposure to traumatic events. The time frame for the frequency of symptoms is over the 'past seven days'. It has two subscales; Intrusion corresponds to the first axis of PTSD, Reexperiencing Phenomena and Avoidance corresponds to the second axis, the Avoidance/Numbing criteria. Whilst there are various published cut-off points, a useful guide is 30.

The Clinician Administered PTSD Scale DMS-IV (CAPS): Blake et al. (1992)
The CAPS is a diagnostic tool and is more appropriate as a research instrument, but it is nevertheless well validated and was developed to measure cardinal and hypothezised signs and symptoms of PTSD. It also provides a method to evaluate the frequency and intensity of individual symptoms as well as the impact of the symptoms on social and occupational functioning, the overall intensity of the symptoms and the validity of the ratings obtained. It uses a time frame of one month in keeping with the diagnostic criteria for the presence of PTSD symptoms.

PTSD symptom checklists (even if adhering to the DSM-IV criteria) are not a satisfactory method of assessing the absence or presence of PTSD as there is a danger of over- or under-diagnosis without careful corroboration of the patient's self-report of frequency and intensity of symptoms.

Figure 15.2 Measures for Trauma and PTSD.

Specific interventions include:

- *Graded exposure in real life* – This involves the individual confronting previously avoided anxiety-provoking situations, until the anxiety subsides.
- *Imaginal exposure* – This is a technique that involves direct exposure to memories of the trauma and involves the use of audiotaped material.

As with real life exposure, this can also be graded and, with repeated practice, will eventually result in a reduction in anxiety and other related symptoms.

- *Cognitive therapy* – This often integrates both of the above and is also shown to be effective.
- *Eye Movement Desensitization and Reprocessing* (EMDR) is a relatively new technique (which sits comfortably in the cognitive behavioural repertoire) in the treatment of PTSD (Shapiro, 1995; Wilson et al., 1995).

EMDR is a relatively new and effective treatment for PTSD. Despite the ongoing debate surrounding its use, there is now a growing body of scientific literature on the technique and a number of studies are confirming its effectiveness in the treatment of PTSD (Spector and Read, 1999). The author has successfully used the technique on numerous occasions for PTSD following burn trauma.

In essence, EMDR involves pairing memories/disturbing thoughts and the resultant emotions with repeated saccadic (rapid and rhythmic) eye movements, resulting in the desensitization of the memories. A similar pairing of memory and a chosen positive cognition, with further eye movements, constitutes the reprocessing component. The precise mechanism for clinically reported change is as yet unclear and is still the subject of considerable ongoing research. The available evidence is that the treatment effects of EMDR are maintained at follow-up. There is also clear evidence that exposure, both to avoidance situations and traumatic memories, provides clinically significant areas for treatment interventions in PTSD. A cognitive behavioural approach which also utilizes EMDR (if appropriate) therefore offers a cost-effective, integrative, pragmatic and flexible framework for treatment for PTSD.

Cognitive therapy is a form of psychotherapy based on a theory of emotional disorders (Beck, 1967). It is a structured form of psychotherapy designed to alleviate symptoms and help patients learn more effective ways of coping with their psychological difficulties. The therapeutic mode of cognitive therapy is problem-orientated and semistructured. It is aimed at correcting the combination of psychological and situational problems that may be contributing to the patient's distress. The label 'cognitive therapy' is used because the techniques employed are directed at changing distortions in patients' cognitions. This includes the way in which situations and stressors are appraised, assumptions about themselves, the world and the future, and the beliefs and attitudes that are presumed to increase their vulnerability to emotional problems.

This is a treatment approach based on historical, theoretical and empirical grounds (Blackburn and Davidson, 1990). Many individuals often find that their beliefs and assumptions about themselves, others and their world have been 'shattered' as a result of their experience of trauma (Janoff-Bulman, 1985). The PTSD sufferer's belief in personal invulnerability, their perceptions of the world as meaningful and comprehensible, in their assumptions that other people can be trusted, and in their views of themselves as being a competent and worthwhile person, can be severely challenged. Self-questioning, feelings of insecurity, unworthiness and weakness, and perceptions of threat and danger might be evident. The world might be viewed as threatening, and the likelihood of future recurrence might be seen as high. While this particular feature of PTSD is often experienced by individuals who have been victimized, for example by violent crime, it is also a common feature experienced by anyone who has suffered any form of physical trauma. Therapy aims to address this and helps the sufferer to come to terms with the experience.

All the techniques and strategies described above should always be carried out as individually tailored treatment packages, after thorough assessment and only with the cooperation and collaboration of the patient. The duration of treatment will vary in individual cases; however, average treatment programmes may take place over 12 sessions.

Post-traumatic Stress Disorder – a Case Study

Jane was a 29-year-old mother of two who was referred by the consultant psychiatrist for treatment following a serious accidental explosion at her home 18 months previously. The accident occurred a few days before Christmas. Jane was sitting in her living room by the window wrapping Christmas presents, and her 2-year-old son Robert was playing on the living room carpet. Her husband was momentarily out of the room. Without warning, the back boiler exploded, virtually demolishing the living room and causing severe damage estimated at £12000.

Robert was seriously injured, suffering a depressed fracture of the frontal lobe of the brain and 12% burns, which required grafting, the areas of most concern being his right forehead (the eyebrow being missing) and the right side of his torso. Jane sustained burns to both legs, mostly superficial, with scattered areas of full thickness. She also received a head injury requiring stitches, sustained when she was hit by flying debris. The accident was serious and dramatic enough to receive headline coverage in the local newspaper, and the senior fire officer attending was quoted as saying, 'If the Lord was on anyone's side, he was on theirs.'

Both mother and son were taken to the local Accident and Emergency department and then admitted to the Burns Unit, where they received treatment. By the time Jane was referred for assessment, she had given birth to a baby girl who was 7 months old, and Robert was making a significant recovery, although he was still being followed up.

Shortly after the explosion, Jane went through a period of clinical depression, which was characterized by appetite and weight loss, diurnal mood variation and bouts of tearfulness. Her irritable bowel syndrome symptoms were exacerbated, and she experienced an increase of migraineous headaches. By the time she was seen by the consultant psychiatrist, she was felt no longer to be suffering from a clinical depression but was nevertheless suffering from marked anxiety reactions, characterized by a variety of symptoms needing specialist psychological intervention.

In the period since the accident, following her initial bout of depression, Jane continued to experience a variety of symptoms which met the diagnostic criteria for PTSD. She was unable to discuss her son's injuries (which were severe) or her own. She would engage in a variety of avoidance behaviours, characterized by an inability to watch television programmes and read magazines or newspaper articles containing material that served as a reminder of her own experiences. If confronted with any of the above situations, she would experience marked symptoms of panic, for example palpitations, tremors, headaches and sweating. This would then have a significant effect on her mood, leading to irritability and tearfulness. Jane also exhibited a significant degree of obsessional behaviour, which resulted in a preoccupation with and frequent checking of appliances such as the gas fire and the cooker. This would often cause her enough anxiety to lead her back to the house more than once after she had left, to make numerous physical checks.

Her relationship with her husband was also put under considerable strain, and she found that she was becoming overprotective and overconcerned with her son's welfare, the latter inevitably having implications for his future psychological development and well-being. Jane also found that she was unable to discuss the accident with anybody she might meet on a casual or social basis, the reason being that, as she had never adequately 'emotionally processed' her experience, she would inevitably become extremely distressed and consequently withdrawn from the situation.

Jane was also experiencing bouts of anxiety and depression, which were triggered by the continuing treatment Robert required because of his injuries. Both she and her husband (not unnaturally) found his continuing care a constant source of worry and a strain. Jane also had marked concern about Robert's ability to integrate with other children, owing to the cosmetic nature of his injuries, and she worried that this might cause some problems at school and then in later life; to some extent, these concerns were not without substance. Jane also experienced feelings of guilt and anger about the incident and her part in Robert's aftercare. She felt that she could have done more at the time of the accident to help to remove him from the scene of the explosion. She recalled that at the time of the accident, she made every attempt to try to reach her son, but was so bewildered, shocked and frightened that she could not locate him in the room, being in darkness and also handicapped by her own injuries. Consequently, she made for the nearest chink of light and stumbled free to get help. She began to see this as an act of selfishness rather than the only course of action open to her at the time.

At the assessment, she was given a rationale for treatment and a fairly detailed explanation of what a cognitive behavioural approach to her difficulties would entail. While she was not unnaturally apprehensive, she was nevertheless extremely motivated to engage in treatment, as she felt she was considerably debilitated by her symptoms. She was also extremely concerned that her behaviour would begin to affect Robert adversely. Before treatment commenced, her husband was seen and his aid enlisted as co-therapist. Her health visitor was also contacted and informed of the treatment planned.

Jane's treatment consisted of the following components:

- *Cognitive anxiety management training* – This consisted of a variety of strategies that were aimed at enhancing her coping skills, including the use of relaxation therapy, teaching Jane diaphragmatic breathing exercises and educating her about PTSD and all the contributing factors that led to the development and maintenance of her emotional and behavioural problems. She was also taught the principles of exposure therapy and how to measure her anxiety.
- *Exposure in vivo (real life)* – This involved Jane facing up to a number of situations that she had previously avoided. As there were a variety of situations, the programme was graded, and Jane devised her own hierarchy of feared situations. As mentioned earlier, exposure is a tech-

nique whereby individuals have to confront feared situations until their anxiety reduces to a manageable level. This process is known as habituation and is used commonly with many phobic problems. Jane inevitably found this technique quite difficult; sessions would sometimes last up to four hours and involve a significant degree of discomfort and hard work on her part.

- *Exposure in imagination* – This component was very similar to that outlined above, but concerned exposing Jane to a variety of distressing thoughts and traumatic imagery concerning the accident. She was asked to describe it in the first person, and present tense, as though it were actually occurring. This was then audiotaped, and she would then listen to this for as much as five or six times a week, replaying the tape on each occasion until she noticed a reduction in her anxiety. By the seventh session, habituation had taken place and she found that she was getting 'bored' and that her mind was 'wandering', evidence, therefore, that the traumatic imagery and memories were no longer as potent.

- *Cognitive restructuring* – This involved Jane keeping a detailed diary of her thoughts and emotions throughout therapy, and was specifically aimed at getting her to emotionally 'reprocess' her traumatic experience. She was eventually able to challenge and modify her beliefs about not having acted more appropriately at the time of the incident, and was able to accept that she did everything humanly possible at the time and in the circumstances.

Jane had received 14 sessions, totalling approximately 24 hours of therapy time when she was discharged. At discharge, Jane had improved by approximately 80% in all areas, as indicated by all rating scales and measures used. She was able to discuss the accident without undue anxiety and also discuss the injuries that Robert had received. She was also able to read newspaper reports about her accident and watch television documentaries or read previously disturbing newspaper and magazine articles. Jane also reported that she was far less irritable at home, experienced fewer significant fluctuations in mood and felt that she had, by and large, come to terms with her experience. She worked extremely hard in treatment and was highly motivated throughout, which was an undoubted contributing factor to the significant progress she had made. Jane was seen up to the year after the end of treatment for follow-up, and she had continued to maintain her progress. Robert had continued to improve, and while it was felt that he might have some difficulties with language and concentration after the accident, he was making excellent progress at school, was socializing well and had many friends. It was clear that despite his injuries, which were far more serious, he was psychologically unaffected by the accident.

Summary

As highlighted earlier, many, but not all, burn victims develop PTSD. Good physical and psychological nursing, remedial and medical care will often be enough to allow the majority of individuals to come to terms with their trauma and deal with it appropriately. In the light of the evidence, however, PTSD may manifest itself in many individuals who suffer a burn injury. Other factors, for example the part that significant others may have played in the trauma and the impact this will have had on all concerned, also need to be taken into account.

Assessment, perhaps at an informal level at first, followed by a more thorough formal assessment process, is essential. Sensitivity on the part of nursing, remedial and medical staff is of paramount importance in terms of gaining the patient's confidence and trust, thus allowing him to disclose traumatic and painful memories. Many individuals suffering from PTSD can feel set apart from others because of their symptoms and their experience. They may be hesitant to discuss events surrounding their trauma, and may even report fears that they may be going 'mad'. Therefore, a sound knowledge base is extremely important in order that their thoughts, feelings and behaviours can be acknowledged and 'normalized' in the context of their experience.

A number of effective treatment strategies have been developed for individuals suffering PTSD, and access to treatment should be sought and made available at an early stage of the disorder. Treatment will not only diminish the effects of this particularly disabling disorder, but also encourage and allow for the most complete rehabilitation possible. Nurses and remedial staff are often best placed to identify the disorder in its infancy and seek consultation and supervision as to further intervention strategies.

Artz (1979) once suggested that 'the need for psychiatric assistance (in the care of burn patients) should be rare'. There is now a wealth of literature to confirm psychological disturbance following burn injury (Wallace and Lees, 1988; Watkins et al., 1988; Ehde, Patterson et al., 1999; Tedstone and Tarrier, 1997). Knowledge of PTSD as a specific psychological sequela of burn trauma is becoming increasingly common, mainly

through greater awareness and reporting of the disorder in the psychological and psychiatric literature. It is also clear that, in the arena of
psychological care, it is an area that warrants continued empirical
scrutiny, especially as psychological assessment, treatment and evaluation
are essential components of the overall care and rehabilitation of the
burn victim.

References

Alexander DA (1996) Trauma research: a new era. Journal of Psychosomatic Research 41(1):
    1–5.
APA (1980) Diagnostic and Statistical Manual of Mental Disorders. Washington: American
    Psychiatric Association.
APA (1987) Diagnostic and Statistical Manual of Mental Disorders. 3rd edn (revised).
    Washington: American Psychiatric Association.
APA (1994) Diagnostic and Statistical Manual of Mental Disorders. 4th edn. Washington:
    American Psychiatric Association.
Andreason NJC, Norris AS (1972) Long term adjustment and adaptation mechanisms in
    severely burned adults. Journal of Nervous and Mental Disease 154: 352–62.
Artz CP (1979) Psychological considerations. In Artz CP, Moncrief JA, Pruitt BA, (Eds) Burns:
    A Team Approach. Philadelphia: WB Saunders. pp 35–37.
Beck AT (1967) Depression: Clinical, Experimental and Theoretical Aspects. New York:
    Hoeber.
Beck AT, Ward DH, Mendelson M et al. (1961) An inventory for measuring depression.
    Archives of General Psychiatry 4: 561–71.
Bisson JI, Jenkins PL, Alexander J (1997) Randomised controlled trial of psychological debrief-
    ing for victims of acute burn trauma. British Journal of Psychiatry 171: 78–81.
Blackburn I, Davidson K (1990) Cognitive Therapy for Depression and Anxiety. Oxford:
    Blackwell.
Blake D, Weathers F et al. (1992) Clinician Administered PTSD Scale. National Centre for
    Post Traumatic Stress Disorder, Boston
Blake DD, Sonnenberg RT (1998) Outcome research on behavioural and cognitive treat-
    ments for trauma survivors. In Follette VM, Ruzek JI, Abueg FR, (Eds) Cognitive
    Behavioural Therapies for Trauma. New York: Guilford. pp 15–47.
Blanchard EB, Kolb LC, Pallmeyer TP et al. (1982) A psychological study of Post Traumatic
    Stress Disorder in Vietnam veterans. Psychiatric Quarterly 54: 220–29.
Bryant RA (1996) Predictors of post–traumatic stress disorder following burns injury. Burns
    22(2): 89–92.
Burgess WW, Holmstrom LL (1974) Rape trauma syndrome. American Journal of Psychiatry
    131(9): 981–86.
Cobb S, Lindermann E (1943) Neuropsychiatric observations on the Cocoanut Grove fire.
    Annals of Surgery 117: 814–24.
Courtemanche DJ, Robinow O (1989) The recognition and treatment of the Post Traumatic
    Stress Disorder in the burn victim. Journal of Burn Care and Rehabilitation 10(3): 247–50.
Curran PS, Bell P, Murray G et al. (1990) Psychological consequences of the Enniskillen
    bombing. British Journal of Psychiatry 156: 479–82.
Daly RJ (1983) Samuel Pepys and Post Traumatic Stress Disorder. British Journal of
    Psychiatry 143: 64–68.

Davidson JRT, Hughes D, Blazer DG et al. (1991) Post Traumatic Stress Disorder in the community: an epidemiological study. Psychological Medicine 21: 713–21.

Duckworth DH, Charlesworth A (1988) The human side of disaster. Policing 4: 194–210.

Ehde DM, Patterson DR et al. (1999) Post traumatic stress symptoms and distress following acute burn injury. Burns 25: 587–92.

Foa EB, Rothbaum BO, Riggs DS et al. (1992) Treatment of Post Traumatic Stress Disorder in rape victims: a comparison between cognitive behavioural procedures and counselling. Journal of Counselling and Clinical Psychology 59: 715–23.

Frank E, Anderson B, Stewart BD et al. (1988) Efficacy of cognitive behaviour therapy and systematic de-sensitisation in the treatment of rape trauma. Behaviour Therapy 19: 403–20.

Goldberg D (1981) The General Health Questionnaire 28. NFER-Nelson.

Green BL, Grace MC, Lindy JD et al. (1983) Levels of functional impairment following a civilian disaster: the Beverly Hills Supper Club fire. Journal of Consulting and Clinical Psychology 51: 573–80.

Hammarberg M (1992) PENN Inventory for Post Traumatic Stress Disorder: psychometric properties. Psychological Assessment: A Journal of Consulting and Clinical Psychology 4: 67–76.

Harvey AG, Bryant RA (2000) Two-year prospective evaluation of the relationship between Acute Stress Disorder and Post-traumatic Stress Disorder. American Journal of Psychiatry 157(4): 626–31.

Helzer JE, Robbins LN, McEvoy L (1987) Post Traumatic Stress Disorder in the general population: findings from the epidemiological catchment area survey. New England Journal of Medicine 317: 1630–34.

Hodgkinson PE (1990) The Zeebrugge disaster. III. Psychological care in the UK. Disaster Management 2: 131–34.

Home Office (1983) Fire Statistics. London: HMSO.

Home Office (1991) Disasters: Planning for a Caring Response. London: HMSO.

Horowitz MJ, Wilner N, Alvarez MA (1979) Impact of event scale: A measure of subjective stress. Psychosomatic Medicine 41(3).

Janoff-Bulman R (1985) The aftermath of victimization: rebuilding shattered assumptions. In Figley CR (Ed) Trauma and its Wake: the Study and Treatment of Post Traumatic Stress Disorder. New York: Bruner Mazel. pp 15–35.

Kessler RC, Sonnega A, Bromet E (1995) Post-traumatic stress disorder in the national comorbidity survey. Archives of General Psychiatry 42: 1048–60.

Latham R, Matthews W (1970–83) The Diary of Samuel Pepys, 11 vols. London: Bell and Hyman.

Lindemann E (1944) Symptomatology and management of acute grief. American Journal of Psychiatry 101: 141–48.

Ochitill H (1984) Psychiatric consultation to the Burns Unit: the psychiatrist's perspective. American Journal of Psychosomatic Medicine 25: 697–702.

Perry S, Difede J, Musngi G et al. (1992) Predictors of Post Traumatic Stress Disorder after burn injury. American Journal of Psychiatry 149(7): 931–35.

Raphael B (1986) When Disaster Strikes: A Handbook for the Caring Professions. London: Hutchinson.

Regel S (1997) Staff support on the Burns Unit. In Bosworth C (Ed) Burn Trauma – Nursing Management and Care. London: Baillière Tindall. pp 201–10.

Richards DA, Rose JS (1991) Exposure therapy for post traumatic stress disorder: four case studies. British Journal of Psychiatry 158: 836–40.

Richards DA, Lovell K, Marks IM (1994) Post-traumatic stress disorder: evaluation of a behavioural treatment program. Journal of Traumatic Stress 7(4): 669–80.

Roca RP, Spence RJ, Munster AM (1992) Post traumatic adaptation and distress among adult burn survivors. American Journal of Psychiatry 149(9): 1234–38.

Rothbaum BO, Foa EB, Riggs DS et al. (1992) A prospective examination of post traumatic stress disorder in rape victims. Journal of Traumatic Stress 5: 455–75.

Scott MJ, Stradling SG (1992) Counselling for Post Traumatic Stress Disorder. London: Sage.

Shapiro F (1995) Eye Movement Desensitization and Reprocessing: Basic Principles, Protocols and Procedures. New York: Guilford Press.

Sieck HS (1990) Post traumatic stress disorder. Journal of Burn and Rehabilitation 11(1): 96 (letter; comment).

Spector J, Read J (1999) The current status of eye movement desensitization and reprocessing (EMDR). Clinical Psychology and Psychotherapy 6: 165–74.

Spitzer RL, Williams JBW (1985). Structured Clinical Interview for DSM-II-R: Patient Version. New York: Biometrics Research Department, New York State Psychiatric Institute.

Stoddard TJ, Norman DK, Murphy JM (1989) A diagnostic outcome study of children and adolescents with severe burns. Journal of Trauma 29(4): 471–77.

Sturgeon D, Rosser R, Shoenberg P (1991) The Kings Cross fire. Part 2: The psychological injuries. Burns 17(1): 10–13.

Taal LA, Faber AW (1997) Dissociation as a predictor of psychopathology following burns injury. Burns 23(5): 400–3.

Tedstone J, Tarrier N (1997) The investigation of the prevalence of psychological morbidity in burn-injured patients. Burns 23(7/8): 550–54.

Trimble MR (1985) Post traumatic stress disorder: history of a concept. In Figley CR, (Ed) Trauma and its Wake: the Study and Treatment of Post Traumatic Stress Disorder. New York: Brunner Mazel.

Wallace LM, Lees J (1988) A psychological follow-up study of adult patients discharged from a Burns Unit. Burns Journal 14: 39–45.

Watkins PN, Cook EL, May SR et al. (1988) Psychological stages in adaptation following burn injury: a method for facilitation of psychological recovery of burn victims. Journal of Burn Care and Rehabilitation 9: 376–84.

Weiss D, Horowitz MJ, Wilner N (1984) The stress response rating scale: a clinician's measure for rating the response to various life events. British Journal of Clinical Psychology 23: 205–15.

White AC (1981) Psychiatric study of severely injured burn victims. MD thesis, University of Birmingham.

Wilson SA, Becker LA, Tinker RH (1995) Eye movement desensitisation and reprocessing (EMDR) treatment for psychologically traumatised Individuals. Journal of Consulting and Clinical Psychology 63(6): 928–37.

Wing JK, Babor T, Brugha et al. (1990) SCAN: schedules for clinical assessment in neuro-psychiatry. Archives of General Psychiatry 47: 589–93.

Zigmond AS, Snaith RP (1983) The hospital anxiety and depression scale. Acta Psychiatrica Scandinavica 67: 361–70.

CHAPTER 16

Staff Support on the Burns Unit

STEPHEN REGEL

At present, there are constant and often significant changes in the modern NHS, and the notions of stress and crisis will be familiar, if uncomfortable, themes for many nurses and allied professions. Thus, many nurses have not only to live with the uncertainty of change on an organizational basis, but also to cope with demanding environmental and professional situations. While no health-care professional is immune to these pressures, there is evidence that suggests that many areas of nursing, particularly those areas we think of as critical care environments, for example Accident and Emergency departments, Intensive Care Units and Burns Units, are often the most vulnerable to stress, and in need of much support (Huckaby and Jagla, 1979; Bishop, 1983; Jacobsen, 1983; von Baeyer and Krause, 1983).

The questions that invariably spring to mind are: are staff in these areas supported and, if so, what is the nature of that support and who provides it? This chapter is primarily concerned with the development and maintenance of staff support on a Burns Unit. There are, however, a number of other issues that are of relevance when discussing the nature and provision of staff support in this and other areas of critical care nursing. Therefore, the main issues under discussion will be:

- The nature of stress, the importance of the role of cognitions (thoughts) and their influence on emotions and behaviour
- The case for staff support
- A comprehensive and flexible model for staff support on a Burns Unit

The Nature of Stress

Many explanations of stress tend to be somewhat simplistic, in that they do not allow for variations in individual circumstances or events. Since the early 1980s, much more sophisticated models of stress have evolved, thus giving us a greater understanding not only of the nature of stress, but also of how to deal with it more effectively. Lazarus (1981) noted that individuals are not mere victims of stress, but that two factors in particular determine the nature of stress. These are:

- How they appraise stressful events (primary appraisal)
- How they appraise their coping resources and options (secondary appraisal)

The individual's appraisal processes influence the relationship of transaction between the individual and the social environment, which is constantly changing. Meichenbaum (1985) also proposes the notion that stress and coping are transactional in nature. The concept of stress has been defined in a variety of ways. Some researchers have defined stress as a condition of the environment, for example work stressors, raising children or the stress of competition. According to this view, stress represents a set of external forces impinging upon the individual or the group. Another common view of stress relates to the individual's response when placed in a challenging or threatening environment.

At this point, it would be appropriate to examine the influential role played by an individual's cognitions (thoughts and images) and feelings, experienced before, during and after an event. Given that cognitions influence stress, it is worth considering this concept in more detail. The concept of cognitions can be divided into three different areas, namely:

- Cognitive events
- Cognitive processes
- Cognitive structures

Cognitive Events

Cognitive events are conscious, identifiable thoughts and images. Beck (1976) describes these as automatic thoughts; they invariably appear in shorthand form, are almost always unquestioned and believed, are often expressed as '*shoulds*', '*oughts*' or '*musts*', are relatively idiosyncratic, and are difficult to turn off. They also appear plausible and valid. Meichenbaum (1977) has described such cognitive events as a form of internal dialogue, the sort of 'little conversations' one has with oneself, either prior to, during or after an event. This dialogue incorporates, among other things, attributions, expectations, self-evaluation and related or irrelevant thoughts and images.

The nature and content of such cognitive events can significantly influence how one feels and behaves. Therefore, individuals under stress tend to become self-focused and often display a variety of self-defeating thoughts and feelings, which will further increase emotional disturbances. Thus, individuals prone to stress are loaded to make one-sided, extreme, absolute and global judgements, often tending to personalize events and engage in cognitive distortions, such as polarization (black and white dichotomous reasoning), magnification and exaggeration (overemphasis on the most negative possibilities in a given situation), and overgeneralization. These distortions often occur in an automatic, unconscious fashion (Beck, 1984).

Cognitive Processes

The term 'cognitive processes' refers to the ways in which we automatically or unconsciously process information, including how we store, retrieve and search for information. These processes shape our schemata, i.e. our beliefs and assumptions about ourselves, others and our world. Most of the time, we do not think about the way we think or how we appraise situations, how we selectively attend and recall events or how we selectively seek information consistent with our beliefs. For example, individuals who feel strongly that the world *should* be fair are likely to be hypervigilant for signs of potential injustice and misread events as personal slights. This would, in turn, affect their mood and behaviour.

Cognitive Structures

'Cognitive structures' encompass the tacit assumptions, beliefs and meanings that influence habitual ways of construing oneself and the world. Cognitive structures can be thought of as schemata, which are mental organizations of experience. These are the ways in which an individual interprets his world and makes sense of experiences. Therefore, the way in which we interpret, perceive, appraise and evaluate events significantly influences our emotions and behaviour. The work of Beck (1984) indicates that stressful life events can trigger such schemata, and views such schemata as specific sensitive areas or specific emotional vulnerabilities that result in individuals' predilections to overreact. Such hypersensitivities or cognitive structures act as templates that influence the way in which situations are appraised and that guide cognitive processes, emotions and behaviours.

The work of Lazarus, Beck, Meichenbaum and others has made a significant contribution to our understanding of anxiety and the nature of stress. Most importantly, their work has given substance to the notion that high levels of stress are largely brought about by an individual's interpretation of an event, rather than the event per se.

Another important factor in our understanding of the nature of stress is the role played by life events. A considerable amount of evidence, stemming from the work of Holmes and Rahe (1967), indicates that certain life events that cause change increase an individual's vulnerability to stress-related illness. These life events involve change of some kind, for example in health, family relationships, economic and living conditions, education, religion and social affairs. They range in seriousness from major life crises, such as the death of a partner, to relatively minor events, such as going on holiday or receiving a parking ticket.

The only difficulty with this early attempt to classify and describe life events (even though it holds much relevance today) is that it is unidimensional and deals only with stress. As mentioned previously, cognitive appraisal is important, as perceptions of a stressful event may vary from one individual to another. An important point that needs to be made here is that one individual's life event becomes another's. This is especially relevant in areas of critical care nursing, for example the Burns Unit, where nurses have to contend not only with high levels of stress caused by distressing procedures, but also with a variety of psychosocial factors. A significant proportion of burn injuries occur in the context of stressful life events. Adults with a burn injury often have psychiatric conditions that increase their susceptibility to injury. Many victims are also single, unemployed and from disadvantaged backgrounds, which increases their vulnerability (Noyes et al., 1979). A number come from disturbed family backgrounds, in which unemployment, poor housing and relationship problems may complicate the situation (Kolman, 1983).

In view of the above, many nurses can be and very often are touched by the lives of the individuals they nurse. A high level of emotional and personal involvement, rather than being viewed in negative terms, should be supported, and a framework provided whereby that support can be accessed on a personal and professional level. The nature of support needs to be tangible and flexible in order to respond to the demands that staff face in such a challenging environment.

The Case for Staff Support

Many studies have provided evidence that nurses in specialized areas are vulnerable to stress (Shubin, 1978; Maslach, 1981; Jacobsen, 1983; Beaver et al., 1986). Bailey (1985) suggests that nurses and medical staff are often more at risk than are those they care for. Melia (1987) notes the main concern for many nurses as being issues of control or power regarding decisions pertinent to care. Individuals who feel they have no control over what is happening to them or what they do have been found to experience high levels of stress (Weiss, 1972; Cohen, 1980). There is further evidence that individuals who think they have no control over events can learn to become helpless. This 'learned helplessness' in turn leads to stress (Seligman, 1975).

Nurses may often be faced with making decisions of enormous responsibility without the immediate support of a team and without immediate access to supervision. Another area of stress in nursing is in the professional arena, in which nurses may feel undervalued or taken for granted. In the present climate, competition for employment is intense, which is inevitably a source of tension and dissatisfaction. Inadequate and poor communication can lead to misunderstandings and misinterpretation of intentions and behaviour, thus creating an environment in which the stress is constantly perpetuated because opportunities are never taken to resolve outstanding organizational and interpersonal issues (Cassee, 1975). Stress in the area of critical care nursing is an acknowledged concern, and there is recent evidence in the literature to highlight this (Llewelyn, 1989; Wright, 1991). It would be pertinent at this point to move on to examine a specific example of staff support and discuss a number of issues of relevance, in an attempt to answer the questions posed in the introduction to this chapter.

Staff Support on the Burns Unit – a Working Model

It is not the intention here to discuss at any length the mechanisms of setting up a support group. That is comprehensively covered by a number of authors (Burnard, 1991; Nichols and Jenkinson, 1991; Wright, 1991) whose works are worthy of scrutiny for those readers considering either setting up or leading a support group. Llewelyn (1989) makes a good point in advising caution in applying some of the techniques advocated, as they can be beneficial if chosen as individual coping strategies, but can be counterproductive if imposed on people without consideration or regard for individual circumstances.

Antebi (1993) described the work of the psychiatrist on a Burns Unit and the setting up of a consultation-liaison service. The model for staff meetings and support was multidisciplinary (excluding medical staff – no reasons are given other than to say that they approached the psychiatrist separately for discussions). The meetings were held weekly; the content was decided by staff and was usually based around teaching on a specific psychological or psychiatric problem, followed by discussion of 'problem' patients. No pressure was exerted for staff to attend, although there appeared to be a core group of regular attenders. However, psychiatrists at registrar and senior registrar levels rotate, so consistency and continuity may be a problem, as may their availability in any given circumstances.

The literature on providing support for staff in critical care settings is sparse and often tends to be of a psychodynamic orientation (Parish et al., 1997). The authors describe a reflective practice group in an ICU. There was no planned agenda and indicate that the nature of the sessions were very non-directive, with the facilitators often acting as a 'mirror'. Typical questions for example, might be 'What is the atmosphere like in here at the moment?' It is clear that the authors adopted a fairly psychodynamic perspective, indicating influences from Yalom (1985). Interestingly, they also describe that the hospital chaplain had facilitated previous support work and whilst there had never been any criticism of the chaplain's abilities and qualities, some individuals experienced difficulties with the religious connotations of his role. There was little objective measure of the group's success other than that the group continued to meet and was operating for over two years (Parish et al., 1997). A number of other authors (Burnard, 1991; Nichols and Jenkinson, 1991; Wright, 1991) have described supportive interventions and these are worthy of scrutiny for those readers considering either setting up or leading a support group. However, Llewelyn (1989) quite rightly advises caution in applying some of the techniques advocated, as they can be beneficial if chosen as individual coping strategies, but can be counterproductive if imposed on people without consideration or regard for individual circumstances.

Before setting up or facilitating a support group it is essential to make an assessment of need within the context of the environment. Liaison mental health nurses may be called upon to facilitate support groups in areas with which they have regular contact. However, as yet there has been little in the consultation liaison literature that describes such involvement (Regel and Davies, 1995). There is potential for a significant demand for mental health skills in critical care areas. Our clinical experience of staff support in critical environments such as Intensive Care and Burn Trauma over the past decade has indicated that knowledge and skills in the assessment and management of the mechanisms and processes of problems that manifest in these areas has been invaluable. These include:

- Knowledge of normal and pathological responses to trauma and bereavement
- Knowledge and skills in management of acute anxiety responses
- Crisis intervention, defusing and debriefing skills

Assessment should involve detailed discussions of perceived need with Unit staff of all grades and disciplines and the support groups should ideally be multidisciplinary in nature, though this may not always be possible for a variety of reasons (Antebi, 1993). A working knowledge of the environment and the stressors experienced will provide an invaluable insight into the stressors encountered within that environment, not to mention a 'feel' and sensitivity for the dynamics and personalities within the Burns Unit. Parish et al. (1997) also highlighted the importance of management support for such ventures, e.g. in the form of funding for the facilitators and most importantly, 'permission' to leave the workplace. Without this type of support for such ventures, they are doomed to failure. The next section describes some practical strategies for implementing staff support groups.

This input, which by its nature is a consultation-liaison psychiatry service, has five main features:

- *Consultation* – which could encompass a wide range of activities, for example training or advice and guidance on specific or general issues.
- *Supervision* – for assessment or intervention.
- *Staff support* – either individual or group. This could include case discussion and emerging themes.
- *Teaching* – on specific psychological problems and their management.
- *Clinical input* – as and where appropriate, to patients who require therapy or counselling. This could also be purely for assessment, to establish or clarify a psychological care plan.

Certain practical problems have to be acknowledged and worked around, given the intrinsic nature of the environment. Therefore the basic format or ground rules of the group setting are as follows:

- Confidentiality is paramount, especially if the group at any point deals with the personal issues of those present at the time.
- Interruptions are, within reason, acceptable (given the demands of the Burns Unit).
- Staff members will not be discussed in their absence.
- Managerial and organizational aspects will be discussed only if all those concerned are present.
- The format of the group is flexible, but the main focus is the presentation of a case history and the discussion of any emergent themes (Figure 16.1).
- Specific teaching requests can be made and planned in advance.

In addition to the above, other features, for example problem-solving (Sobel and Worden, 1981) and psychological debriefing (Dyregrov, 1989), can be built into or form an essential part of staff support.

Common to many problem-solving programmes is a formula that involves the following steps and is useful for case management:

- Define the stress or stress reaction to be problem-solved
- Establish realistic goals
- Generate a wide range of alternative solutions
- Imagine or consider others' reactions to similar stressors
- Evaluate the pros and cons of each proposed solution, and rank solutions in order, from the least to the most practical and desirable
- Possibly rehearse chosen strategies
- Try out the most acceptable and feasible solution
- Reconsider the original problem in the light of the attempt at problem-solving
- Expect some failures, but reward oneself for effort

Another important aspect of staff support is 'Critical Incident Stress Debriefing' (CISD). This is essentially based on a crisis intervention model, developed by Mitchell (1983). The technique was further articulated and refined by Dyregrov (1989), who coined the term 'Psychological Debriefing' (PD). These two terms are often used interchangeably to describe the same process. (For the purposes of clarity in this chapter, PD

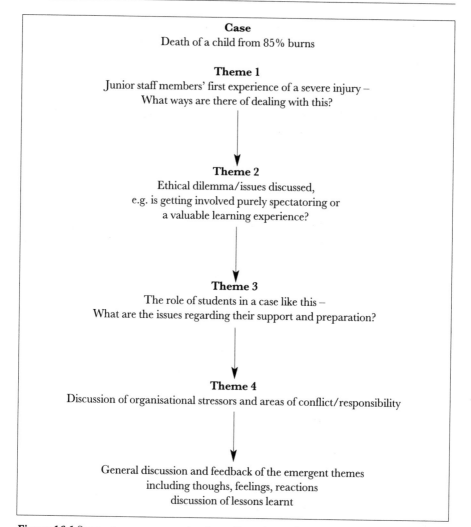

Figure 16.1 Support group – example of case discussion and emergent themes.

will be used throughout this section.) PD or a variant of the model is now widely used with emergency service personnel (Mitchell and Dyregrov, 1993), the armed forces (Jones and Roberts, 1998) and in a variety of other situations where individuals or groups have been exposed to a traumatic event (Tehrani, 1994; Flannery and Penk, 1996).

Dyregrov defined Psychological Debriefing (PD) as:

> . . . a group meeting arranged for the purpose of integrating profound personal experiences both on the cognitive, emotional and group level, and thus preventing the development of adverse reactions.

> (Dyregrov, 1989: 25)

Thus, it is a process which when used appropriately could be an invaluable tool in the repertoire of a support group facilitator. The aim of a debriefing is to minimize the occurrence of unnecessary psychological suffering after a traumatic incident, by allowing the ventilation of emotions, reactions and experiences. Although designed for groups, it can also be extremely helpful for individuals who have been involved in any way in a serious trauma, for example staff involved in a major incident or dealing with seriously injured adults and children (as in the examples used earlier). However, there has been considerable controversy of late as to the efficacy of PD, prompting calls for the use of the technique to be stopped (Wessley et al., 1998). The debate surrounding the efficacy and utility of PD with survivors and professional groups following exposure to traumatic events has become muddled and confused, primarily because of the methodology of the recent research. This is an important issue and an attempt will be made here to disentangle some of the issues for the sake of clarity and in view of the implications for practice in the context of staff support.

Psychological Debriefing in Context

Mitchell (1983), writing about 'Critical Incident Stress Debriefing', described it as a structured intervention utilizing six phases (not seven, as is so often referenced), which were:

- the Introductory phase
- the Fact phase
- the Feeling phase
- the Symptom phase
- the Teaching phase
- the Re-entry phase

Mitchell did not describe a seven-stage model till five years later (1988a, 1998b). It was to be used as an organized approach to the management of stress responses in the emergency services. He stated that it 'entails either an individual or group meeting between the rescue worker and facilitator who is able to help the person talk about his feelings and reactions to the critical incident' (1983: 37). He went on to state that 'follow-up CISD may be performed with the entire group, a portion of it, or with an individual' (1983:39). Note the use of the word 'individual', since this is important for the debate and we shall return to this later. All through the 1980s PD was widely used with the emergency services and a number of other survivor and professional groups in the US, Australia, New Zealand, Scandinavia and throughout Europe, including the UK. In Mitchell's defence, he never claimed that it would prevent PTSD, but that it might merely help ameliorate long-term consequences.

The Debate on the Evidence

In 1994, the first questions were raised about its efficacy, with calls for more research into its application, using randomized controlled trials (Raphael et al., 1995; Bisson and Deahl, 1994). Finally two randomized controlled trials (RCTs) were published. The studies were carried out with injured burn trauma (Bisson et al., 1997) and road traffic accident survivors (Hobbs et al., 1996). Both studies demonstrated negative effects among the intervention groups. The influential Cochrane Review, a systematic review of the published literature in this area, concluded:

> There is no current evidence that psychological debriefing is a useful treatment for prevention of post traumatic stress disorder after traumatic incidents. Compulsory psychological debriefing for victims of trauma should cease.
> (Wessley et al., 1998)

Advocates of PD argued that these studies were an unfair test of PD/CISD as it applied a technique meant for groups to individuals and that 'debriefing conducted individually is essentially single shot exposure and has considerable potential to harm the individual by sensitising them to their memories' (Richards, 1997). Moreover, these were injured individuals and therefore there were a number of other variables to consider. For example, it was suggested that early interventions following serious illness or injury should be discouraged as physical healing needs to take place before psychological healing can begin (Dyregrov, 1998). However, there is ample evidence that early interventions following serious injury or illness can be effective, especially the psycho-educative components (Bordow and Porritt, 1979; Bennett and Carroll, 1993; Clare and Singh, 1994; Raphael, 1977; Bunn and Clarke, 1979). The educational aspect of PD is one of the most important elements of the process as it provides a framework for understanding normal and pathological responses to the illness or traumatic event.

Detractors of PD argued that here at last was evidence that PD as an early intervention was ineffective and therefore should cease, especially in this age of clinical governance and evidence-based practice. However, this has only served to blur the issues surrounding the nature and process of PD. The recent RCTs with burn trauma and RTA victims are not without their limitations. In the Bisson et al. (1997) study on burn trauma, the authors admitted that the vagaries of randomization meant that all the subjects with the highest levels of subjective life threat, previous psychological morbidity and previous psychological treatment ended up in the intervention group. In addition, the authors viewed PD as a treatment and described it as 'intense imaginal exposure to a traumatic incident' (Bisson et al., 1997: 80). Intense imaginal exposure is a therapeutic technique, which is often used in the treatment of trauma survivors (Richards and Lovell, 1999). Anyone familiar with PD, trained and experienced in the process knows full well that it involves *discussion about the event*, rather than an intense imaginal reliving of the experience. Clearly, this is a significant issue, particularly as PD was never intended as a treatment or counselling strategy; nevertheless, the notion of counselling has become synonymous with PD. Again, this only serves to cloud the issue further. It begs the question – what *did* the intervention involve? PD is not counselling and the differences are clear (Dyregrov, 1998).

Finally, it would be wholly fitting to conclude this chapter on staff support by discussing the extremely important role of the facilitator. It is the author's view that facilitators should be trained and experienced in psychological models of care and involved in clinical practice. They should possess counselling or psychotherapy skills in both group and individual settings. They should also have a knowledge, in general terms, of the clinical environment in which support is to be provided, for example the client group, the types of psychosocial and psychological problems experienced, and an awareness of relevant literature and research. A technical knowledge is not always essential, especially if the facilitator is only providing staff support; however, if he is to fulfil a number of other functions, as mentioned earlier, some knowledge is desirable. This can be gained by attendance at ward reviews and spending time with staff in clinical situations.

The choice of facilitator for a support group can be difficult. Given the variety of counselling and psychotherapeutic models available, one way to arrive at the decision would be to arrange meetings with possible facilitators and members of the ward or unit. Staff could then have the opportunity to discuss their needs and learn about the counselling and psychotherapeutic orientation of the prospective facilitator. The choice will inevitably be determined by the style, orientation and personality of the individual and whether the staff feel he or she would meet their needs. Some models of staff support and methods such as those suggested by

Burnard (1991) may be acceptable to some but not others. A framework of support and supervision is also essential (albeit even at peer level) for anyone engaged in consultation-liaison work, especially as this is a growing area of need and is still in a relatively embryonic stage of development in nursing (Tunmore, 1994; Regel and Davies, 1995; Regel, 1995).

The notion of staff support is therefore starting to be recognized as an important area of need in many challenging critical care environments. A further acknowledgement is that the demands of today's rapidly changing NHS and the pressures created by those changes give the case for providing a framework for staff support of even greater urgency. In the caring professions, we are often notorious for not looking after those who provide the care. In a recent report published by the Health and Safety Executive, Cox (1993) argues that at least part of the effects of any stress management programme (whatever its nature) are due to the way they alter workers' perceptions of and attitudes to their organizations and hence organizational culture. He also argues that poor organizational culture might be associated with an experience of stress, while a good organizational culture might weaken the effects of stress on health. Therefore senior managers and clinicians should take a leaf out of the book of successful corporate organizations (especially in the new 'corporate culture' of the NHS) and adopt a relatively simple rule: Look after your staff and they become more productive and cost-effective, not to mention a more contented workforce.

References

Antebi D (1993) The psychiatrist on the Burns Unit. Burns 19(1): 43–46.

Armstrong K, O'Callaghan W, Marmer CR (1991) Debriefing Red Cross disaster personnel: the multiple stressor debriefing model. Journal of Traumatic Stress 4: 581–93.

Bailey RD (1985) Coping with Stress in Caring. Oxford: Blackwell Scientific.

Beaver RC, Sharp ES, Cotonis GA (1986) Burnout experienced by nurse-midwives. Journal of Nurse Midwifery 31: 3–15.

Beck A (1976) Cognitive Therapy and the Emotional Disorders. New York: International Universities Press.

Beck A (1984) Cognitive approaches to stress. In Woolfolk R, Lehrer P, (Eds) Principles and Practice of Stress Management. New York: Guilford Press.

Bennett P, Carroll D (1993) Intervening with cardiac patients. Health Psychology Update 14: 3–6.

Bishop V (1983) Stress in the intensive care unit. Occupational Health 35(12): 537–43.

Bisson JI, Deahl MP (1994) Psychological debriefing and prevention of post traumatic stress – more research is needed. British Journal of Psychiatry 165: 717–20.

Bisson JI, Jenkins PL, Alexander J (1997) Randomised controlled trial of psychological debriefing for victims of acute burn trauma. British Journal of Psychiatry 171: 78–81.

Bordow S, Porritt D (1979) An Experimental Evaluation of Crisis Intervention. Social Science and Medicine 13A: 251–56.

Bunn TA, Clarke AM (1979) Crisis intervention: an experimental study of the effects of a brief period of counselling on the anxiety of relatives of seriously injured or ill hospital patients. British Journal of Medical Psychology 52: 191–95.

Burnard P (1991) Coping with Stress in the Health Professions – a Practical Guide. London: Chapman and Hall.

Cassee E (1975) Therapeutic behaviour, hospital culture and communication. In Cox C, Mead A, (Eds) A Sociology of Medical Practice. London: Collier Macmillan.

Clare L, Singh K (1994) Preventing relapse in psychotic illness: a psychological approach to early intervention. Journal of Mental Health 3: 541–50.

Cohen S (1980) After effects of stress on human performance and social behaviour: a review of research and theory. Psychological Bulletin 87: 578–604.

Cox T (1993) Stress research and stress management: putting theory to work. Health and Safety Executive Contract Research Report No. 61/1993. London: HMSO.

Dyregrov A (1989) Caring for workers in disaster situations: psychological debriefing. Disaster Management 2: 25–30.

Dyregrov A (1998) Psychological debriefing – an effective method? Traumatology – The International Electronic Journal of Innovations in the Study of the Traumatization Process and Methods for Reducing or Eliminating Related Human Suffering.

Flannery RB, Penk WE (1996) Program evaluation of an intervention approach for staff assaulted by patients: preliminary inquiry. Journal of Traumatic Stress 9(2): 317–24.

Hobbs M, Mayou R, Harrison B (1996) A randomised controlled trial of psychological debriefing for victims of road traffic accidents. British Medical Journal 313: 1438–39.

Holmes TH, Rahe RH (1967) The social readjustment rating scale. Journal of Psychosomatic Research 11: 213–18.

Huckaby LMD, Jagla B (1979) Nurses' stress factors in the intensive care unit. Journal of Nursing Administration 9(2): 21.

Jacobsen SF (1983) Nurses' stress in intensive and nonintensive care units. In Jacobsen SF, McGrath HM, (Eds) Nurses under Stress. Chichester: John Wiley and Sons.

Jones N, Roberts P (1998) Risk Management Following Psychological Trauma: A Guide for Royal Marine Corps Combat Stress Trauma Practitioners (4th Edition). Headquarters Royal Marines, Whale Island, Portsmouth, UK.

Kolman P (1983) The incidence of psychopathology in burned adult patients – a critical review. Journal of Burn Care and Rehabilitation 416: 430–36.

Lazarus R (1981) The stress and coping paradigm. In Eisdorfer C, (Ed) Models for Clinical Psychopathology. Englewood Cliffs, NJ: Prentice Hall.

Llewelyn S (1989) Caring: the cost to nurses and relatives. In Broome A, (Ed) Health Psychology – Processes and Applications. London: Chapman and Hall

Maslach C (1981) Burnout: The Cost of Caring. New York: Prentice Hall.

Meichenbaum D (1977) Cognitive Behaviour Modification: An Integrative Approach. New York: Plenum/Press.

Meichenbaum D (1985) Stress Inoculation Training. New York: Pergamon Press.

Melia K (1987) Everyday ethics for nurses. Nursing Times 83(3): 28–32.

Mitchell JT (1983) When disaster strikes . . . the critical incident debriefing. Journal of the Emergency Services 8: 36–39.

Mitchell JT (1988a) Development and Functions of a Critical Incident Stress Debriefing Team. Journal of the Emergency Services: 43–6.

Mitchell JT (1988b) The History, Status and Future of Critical Incident Stress Debriefings. Journal of the Emergency Services: 47–51.

Mitchell JT, Dyregrov A (1993) Traumatic stress in disaster workers and emergency personnel. In JP Wilson, B Raphael, (Eds) International Handbook of Traumatic Stress Syndromes. New York: Plenum Press. pp 905–14.

Nichols K, Jenkinson J (1991) Leading a Support Group. London: Chapman and Hall.

Noyes R, Rye SJ, Slymen DJ, Canter A (1979) Stressful life events and burn injuries. Journal of Trauma 19(3): 141–44.

Parish C, Bradley L, Franks V (1997) Managing the stress of caring in ITU: a reflective practice group. British Journal of Nursing 6(20): 1192–96.

Parkinson F (1993) Post Traumatic Stress. London: Insight Press.

Raphael B (1977) Preventive intervention with the recently bereaved. Archive General Psychiatry 34: 1450–54.

Raphael B, Meldrum L, McFarlane AC (1995) Does debriefing after psychological trauma work? British Medical Journal 310: 1479–80.

Regel S, Davies J (1995) The future of mental health nurses in liaison psychiatry. British Journal of Nursing 4: 1052–56.

Regel S (1995) The role and contribution of mental health nurses in liaison psychiatry. Proceedings of 21st International Conference on Mental Health Nursing: 'Celebrating a New Era'. Canberra, Australia.

Richards D (1997) The current status of psychological debriefing and PTSD. Keynote address to the South Yorkshire Trauma and Debriefing Network, Doncaster Royal Infirmary.

Richards D, Lovell K (1999) Behavioural and cognitive behavioural interventions in the treatment of PTSD. In Yule W, (Ed) Post Traumatic Stress Disorders – Concepts and Therapy. Chichester: Wiley.

Seligman MEP (1975) Helplessness. San Francisco: Freeman.

Shubin S (1978) Burnout: the professional hazard you face in nursing. Nursing 8: 22–27.

Sobel H, Worden J (1981) Helping Cancer Patients Cope: A Problem Solving Intervention for Health Care Professionals. New York: MBA/Guilford Press.

Tehrani N (1994) Debriefing individuals affected by violence. Counselling Psychology Quarterly 7(3): 251–59.

Tunmore R (1994) Encouraging collaboration. Nursing Times 20: 66–67.

Von Baeyer C, Krause L (1983) Effectiveness of stress management training for nurses working in a burn treatment unit. International Journal of Psychiatry in Medicine 13: 13–125.

Weiss JM (1972) Influence of psychological variables on stress induced pathology. In Porter R, Knight J, (Eds) Physiology, Emotion and Psychosomatic Illness. New York: American Elsevier. pp 253–65.

Wessley S, Rose S, Bisson J (1998) A systematic review of brief psychological interventions ('debriefing') for the treatment of immediate trauma related symptoms and the prevention of post traumatic stress disorder. The Cochrane Library – 1998 Issue 4.

Wright B (1991) Sudden Death – Intervention Skills for the Caring Professions. Edinburgh: Churchill Livingstone.

Yalom ID (1985) The Theory and Practice of Group Psychotherapy. New York: Basic Books.

Index